Contributors

Lynette A. Ament, RN, CNM, MSN, PhD(c)
University of Wisconsin Medical School
and Marquette University College of Nursing
Milwaukee, Wisconsin

Mary A. Bowden, RN, MSN, WHNP
Naval Medical Center
San Diego, California

Margaret M. Burns, RN, PhD
Bay State Medical Center
Springfield, Massachusetts

Peggy L. Chinn, RN, FAAN, PhD
University of Colorado School of Nursing
Denver, Colorado

Ellen Dore, RN, MS
Lakewood, Colorado

Elizabeth A. Ely, RN, PhD
University of New Hampshire
Durham, New Hampshire

Georgia L. Gardner, RN, BSN, MS
Pueblo Community College
Pueblo, Colorado

Marcia Garman Laux, RN, MSN
Lake Shore Technical College
Sheboygan, Wisconsin

Mary M. Lepley, RNC, MS, CNS, WHCNP
University of Colorado School of Nursing
Denver, Colorado

Susanna Meissner-Cutler, RN, BSN, JD
Parker, Colorado

Patricia Moores, RN, PhD
Beth-El College of Nursing
Colorado Springs, Colorado

Christine Sullivan, RN, MSN, CNM, CNAA, PhD
Bixby Medical Center
Adrian, Michigan

Toni M. Vezeau, RNC, PhD
Seattle University
Seattle, Washington

Preface

Nationwide, there is a trend for increased nursing liability. This is due in part to tort reform, the increased litigiousness of society, and increased professional accountability for nursing practice. Maternal-child nursing (obstetrical, neonatal, and pediatrics) is a particularly high-risk practice area. Improper treatments related to birth are among the primary allegations in malpractice suits against nurses. According to the National Nurses Claims Data Base (ANA, 1991), 70% of all claims against nurses occur in the hospital setting and 35% of all hospital claims occur in obstetrics. Claims for neurologically impaired infants are among the highest injury awards, and out-of-court settlements are also large ($250,000 to $900,000). Should an adverse outcome develop, the unique nature of obstetric/newborn care (e.g., care of two patients; lifelong ramifications of injury), increased public expectations in limited childbearing (e.g., fewer pregnancies with increased psychological investment; belief that hospital birth is "safe") and technologic advances in maternal-child care, including nurse specialization, all increase the risk for nursing legal liability.

When solutions for the "malpractice crisis" are offered, rarely does prevention enter the discussion. Rather, tort reform (limiting damages), defensive medicine (ordering unnecessary costly tests), and ceasing high-risk practice are seen as viable solutions. However, tort reform laws have been overturned on appeal (e.g., in Texas, Kansas); defensive medicine is costly to all Americans; and ceasing obstetrical/newborn and pediatric practice is not an option for hospitals. Thus, we are left with the challenge of preventing situations that may lead to litigation.

This book is written from a feminist perspective. Because the majority of nurses are women—only 4% of all nurses are male, and in the maternal-child setting fewer than 0.01% of nurses are male (US Department of Health and Human Services, 1994)—we have chosen to use the feminine pronoun when referring to nurses. We believe the evolution of nursing strongly parallels the evolution of women (Grissum & Spengler, 1976).

This book is divided into four parts. Section I presents a conceptual overview: accountability, empowerment, legal and professional aspects, risk management/continuous quality improvement, and a proactive, professional practice model. Sections II through IV explore actual cases in each specialty area, the relevant standard of care, and utilization of the model to solve the case proactively. To maintain confidentiality, the names of patients, families, professional care providers, and institutions have been changed. If the case has resulted in a jury verdict by trial, and thus is in the public domain, the case is legally referenced (i.e., plaintiff's vs. defendant's names) to facilitate the reader's further research of the case.

Combined, the coeditors have more than 30 years of experience reviewing nursing malpractice, both defendant and plaintiff cases. It is the philosophy of the coeditors and contributing authors that the *practicing clinical nurse* is the main line of defense against patient injury and subsequent legal liability. We are struck with the fact that parents, babies, and children do not need thousands of dollars worth of equipment (many already have such equipment) to prevent damage. Rather, a nurse, thinking and practicing within the standard for professional nurses and advocating for the patient, is able to prevent injury using herself as the tool. Preventing legal liability, and more importantly, impairment or death to women, babies, and children, will in turn prevent economic and social catastrophes for the community and society.

This book is the first in a series about legal aspects of clinical practice. Subsequent books planned will deal with medical-surgical and psychiatric nursing practice as well as advanced nursing practice. These books will utilize the professional practice model presented here as well as address the concepts of interdependent practice, responsibility, and accountability. All books will utilize a similar case-presentation format exploring true cases from inpatient and outpatient settings.

For information about seminars/workshops on risk management and legal aspects of maternal-child nursing practice, an accredited home study/risk management program (completion of this program reduces by 10% the professional liability insurance premium through McGinnis and Associates), institutional/organizational risk management consultations, or legal consultations (defense and plaintiff), contact Sandra L. Gardner, RN, MS, CNS, PNP, 12095 East Kentucky Avenue, Aurora, Colorado 80012, telephone (303) 367-1072, fax (303) 367-1072.

Acknowledgments

We wish to acknowledge the knowledge and expertise of the following people: Sally Olds, RN, MS, for her thoughtful dialogue and editorial assistance; Mary Fran Hazinski, RN, MS, for her pioneering work in critical care pediatrics and to whose work we referred for criteria in assessing pediatric intensive care nursing; Dr. Dennis Mahoney, Susanna Meissner-Cutler, and Brian Lampert for their vast knowledge of the medical/legal system; Jeanne K. Bruner, BSN, MS, PhD, Texas Woman's University, for her review of the manuscript; and our clinical colleagues—practicing nurses who spurred us on in writing about this important topic. Lastly, we would like to thank Patricia Cleary, our editor extraordinaire, for her confidence in us and her recognition of the urgency of publishing this work, and Marla Nowick, Sondra Glider, Antonio Padial, and Laura Bonazzoli for their expert editorial assistance.

References

American Nurses Association. (1991). *Prevention and you*. Washington, D.C.: Author.

Grissum, M. & Spengler, C. (1976). *Woman power and healthcare*. Boston: Little, Brown.

US Department of Health and Human Services. (1994). *Registered nurse population of 1992*. Washington, D.C.: Author.

Contents

Section III Model Application in Neonatal Care

Section IV Model Application in Pediatric Care

1

Accountability for Professional Nursing Practice

Mary I. Enzman Hagedorn, RN, PhD, CNS, CPNP
Sandra L. Gardner, RN, MS, CNS, PNP

In today's changing health care system, the responsibilities of and the accountability for professional practice has not changed. Regardless of the health care setting, professional nurses are morally, ethically, and legally accountable for their nursing judgments and actions. The editors will present the concepts of personal and professional empowerment as the basic criteria for approaching patient care. In addition, they provide a proactive model for professional practice that illuminates the importance of patterns of knowing, critical thinking, nursing therapeutics/skills, and communication in advocating and providing care in both highly technical and community-based settings. This model provides nursing with the tools not only to advocate for patients, but to practice professionally rather than technically. The cases presented in this book are actual malpractice cases either under litigation or settled with monetary awards. In each instance, the nurse failed to provide basic nursing care, monitor the situation, and advocate for the patient. Similar cases occur commonly in the chaotic environment where nurses practice.

While most nurses assume that they will never be named in a lawsuit—and it is true that few are—their professional actions may still be the focus of a suit. In addition, the employing agency is liable for employee negligence if named as the defendant in a lawsuit. This book proposes several ways to limit nursing liability.

First, nurses must develop *caring relationships* with patients and families. Poor relationships between health care providers and the patient can prompt patients and families to file malpractice suits (Hickson, et al., 1992). Those patients and families who sue for malpractice are not necessarily the ones who are harmed the most. Often the patients and families who are angry and believe that they have been treated in a curt, uncaring way will file claims. Quality nursing care, effective communication skills, and a caring, respectful attitude, will assist the nurse in developing a positive rapport with patients and families, thereby reducing the risk of being named as a defendant in a malpractice suit. In addition, the nurse should educate all patients and families about the care being provided and address complaints in a caring, nondefensive, attentive, and timely manner (Ladebauche, 1995).

Nurses must *maintain clinical competence.* Nurses today practice in a highly technical and complex clinical milieu. Acuity is high and many areas of clinical practice, including home care, are creating new challenges for professional nurses. Nurses must maintain competence through professional reading, continuing-education offerings, and participation in institutional inservice programs. Records must be maintained of the attendance and participation in such programs. Lack of knowledge does not excuse the nurse from accountability and responsibility for patient safety and welfare. This book challenges each professional nurse to identify her own gaps in knowledge, practice, and the law. Nursing, as a profession, requires lifelong learning and updating to provide competent, current practice.

Know your legal responsibilities as a nurse. State nurse practice acts legally define nursing practice and mandate skills and responsibilities of the professional nurse. Nurses must know these laws and adhere to them. In addition, nursing practice is defined by institutional policies and procedures that are designed to support the standard of practice, particularly in the event of a malpractice suit. If clinical practice is found to be inconsistent with institutional policies and procedures, nurses are obligated to inform the appropriate resource people, including quality-assurance managers and risk-management personnel (Ladebauche, 1995).

Define appropriate assignments. In response to the rising health care costs, many agencies, attempting to restructure and "down size" services provided, use unlicensed assistive personnel (UAPs) in a variety of settings. These individuals are trained to assist professional nurses in providing patient care activities as delegated by and under the supervision of the registered professional nurse (ANA, 1994). To limit their own liability, nurses must review role expectations and the preparation of UAPs under their supervision. Nurses must remember that state nurse practice acts grant the legal authority to perform nursing acts *only* to professional nurses. Work assignments must be consistent with job descriptions and expertise.

Nurses must *take action* when a patient's condition deteriorates. The standards of clinical practice mandate that the nurse take immediate action to safeguard the patient (ANA, 1983, 1991). A major area of potential litigation results from failure to properly assess patients and communicate all untoward changes in their condition immediately. Specific information communicated to the physician, as well as the physician's orders and instructions, must be documented. In addition, if medical support is inadequate, the nurse must immediately report the problem by following the agency's chain of command. She must document the time and date of the notification, who was notified, the information communicated to that person, and response/orders, specific interventions implemented, and patient response (Lilley & Guanci, 1994). In addition, nurses must be alert to other common situations in clinical practice that signal potential harm and take timely and appropriate action. The accompanying box lists the most common causes of nursing liability.

Common Causes of Nursing Liability

- Medication and treatment errors
- Failure to supervise patient safety
- Burns from equipment
- Failure to monitor and report changes
- Failure to report incompetent care

From Fishbach, F. (1991). *Documenting care: Communication, the nursing process, and documentation standards.* Philadelphia: F.A. Davis. Adapted with permission.

Defensively document all patient care, treatments, and interventions. Accurate medical records that document legally relevant information related to patient status, medical care, and nursing care, and reflect adherence to standards of practice and policies and procedures are critical for limiting nursing liability (Ladebauche, 1995). All nursing documentation must clearly indicate all of the individualized, goal-directed nursing care—based on the nursing process—that was provided for the patient. State nurse practice acts and regulating agencies (e.g., JCAHO) identify the nursing process as the acceptable method of planning and implementing nursing care. Nursing assessments at admission, ongoing assessments, interventions, patient monitoring, patient response to care, and action taken must be documented. In the event of litigation, time gaps, information squeezed between lines, crossed out entries, omission of key facts and other "red flags" may be damaging to the nurse's defense. The most common "red flags" in documentation are listed in the box below.

Changes in reimbursement procedures and decreased average length of stay have increased the importance of *discharge planning* (Ladebauche, 1995). JCAHO documentation criteria require evidence of discharge instructions and the patient's/family's understanding of discharge instructions. Teaching must be specific, and individualized, and consider the literacy and comprehension of the patient/family. Instructions for patients/families on how to assess for signs of problems must be given in both verbal and written form.

Red Flags in Documentation

- Time gaps
- Improbable events
- Omission of key facts
- Limited nursing assessments
- Altered records
- Omission of safety interventions
- Unsigned chart entries

From Fishbach, F. (1991). *Documenting care: Communication, the nursing process, and documentation standards.* Philadelphia: F.A. Davis. Adapted with permission.

In addition, complete verbal and written instructions should accompany any teaching regarding treatments and discharge medications.

The practice of nursing is becoming more complex and nurses are being placed in situations that, if mismanaged, can result in litigation. The need to prevent liability through proactive, preventive strategies and accurate documentation is essential.

References

American Nurses Association. (1983). *Standards of maternal-child health nursing practice.* Washington, D.C.: Author.

American Nurses Association. (1991). *Standards of clinical practice.* Washington, D.C.: Author.

American Nurses Association. (1994). *Registered nurses and unlicensed assistive personnel.* Washington, D.C.: Author.

Fishbach, F. (1991). *Documenting care: Communication, the nursing process, and documentation standards.* Philadelphia: F.A. Davis.

Hickson, G., Wright, E., Githens, P., and Sloan, F. (1992). Factors that prompted families to file medical malpractice claims following perinatal injuries. *Journal of the American Medical Association, 267,* 1359–1363.

Ladebauche, P. (1995). Limiting liability to avoid malpractice litigation. *The American Journal of Maternal/Child Nursing, 20*(5), 243–248.

Lilley, L., and Guanci, R. (1994). Getting back to basics. *American Journal of Nursing, 94,* 15–16.

2

Empowering Women: A Theoretical Perspective

Peggy L. Chinn, RN, PhD, FAAN

Feminism is the radical notion that women are people.
Anonymous

For over two decades of my life working to empower women, including myself, I have not yet been able to shake the paradoxical emotions that this work arouses in me. I feel immense rage that we are even in a situation where the work is necessary. I feel despair that we never quite get the job done. I feel great joy as time and again I experience, for myself and in solidarity with other women, a sense of accomplishment in small and big ways. I feel wonderment at the immense resourcefulness that women bring to our work. I feel tremendous respect for the insight and the dignity that women demonstrate in the face of incredible odds. I feel pain about and disappointment in the limitations that we face day in and day out, limitations that defy our explanation and often even our comprehension.

The idea of empowering women has at least three levels that are not yet completely accounted for in any single theoretical framework: the individual, the small but significant group, and the sociopolitical context. The first level—that of the individual—is the level most frequently addressed by people who use the word *empowerment.* On the individual level, empowerment is a process that women must undertake for themselves; others cannot do so on their behalf. It is a personal accomplishment, struggle, process, that happens within and that leads to action on one's own behalf. In my view, while personal empowerment is an important aspect of personal growth, the individualistic view of empowerment also connotes an untenable sense of personal responsibility, even blame, for whether or not empowerment happens.

Empowerment as a concept implies that there is more than one actor in a situation—that a person is in a situation in which greater power is called for in relation to other people or circumstances. Thus, the second level of consideration—that of the small but significant group—is more significant in moving toward a meaningful model of empowering women. Individual approaches to personal growth can lead to such desired outcomes as personal inner peace, strength, resolution of hurts of the past, clarity of purpose, or resolve to make and carry through with a decision. Empowerment, which is grounded in relationships with others, develops in a context of interaction with others. Empowerment defined as "the ability to enact one's own will and love for self in the context of love and respect for others" (Wheeler & Chinn, 1991, p. 2) requires a group context. In the context of the group, women are able to move beyond a sense of individual responsibility (and guilt) when efforts to empower fall short. Instead, the power of the group comes forth to ground experience in larger social realities, the politics, the constraints, and the collective strength of women working together.

This grounding of experience in the larger social reality leads to consideration of the third level—that of the sociopolitical context. This context can be as immediate as the dynamics of an organization or a family system, or as large as the sociopolitical culture or legal system. Seen from an individual perspective, this context is largely out of the individual's scope of control or influence. However, in many ways the empowerment of women can be approached only at the sociopolitical level through united action. In fact, many of the gains of this century that have led to the empowerment of women can be attributed to this level of focus. For example, without the ability to hold bank accounts, nurses who established the early schools of nursing in this country were severely limited in their ability to exercise their values and will in shaping nursing education. As laws and cultural practices changed to make it possible for women to have bank accounts, to own property, and eventually to secure credit in their own name and in their own right, the range of possible exercise of will expanded significantly. Still today, I experience time and again the utter despair of women in the face of social and political realities that no amount of individual will can change. If we hold only to the individual view of empowerment, women are defeated before we begin. Instead, empowerment can come from recognizing the realities of the social and political situation, and turning our rage, and finally our collective action, in a direction that can lead to real social and political change.

The question remains: Where to begin? In my experience, the starting point has always been the small but significant group. I emphasize the concept *small* but *significant:* small because there are limits to the context in which individuals can work effectively, and significant because important interactions in small groups can have far-reaching effects. From this center grows both the individual, personal sense of strength and power within the context of love and respect for others, and a sense of political possibility to change the larger social and political situation.

The key dynamic that leads to empowerment within a small but significant group is that of empowering dialogue. In her theory of liberation, Freire (1970) sets forth conditions for empowering dialogue that inform my own empowering group-process approaches.

The first condition for empowering dialogue is love for the world and for the individuals in the small group. Dialogue begins with a process of naming the world, of identifying the experiences within the world, and moving toward deep understanding of the personal and political meanings within what is named and described. Freire (1970) states, "The naming of the world, which is an act of creation and re-creation, is not possible if it is not infused with love" (p. 77). The act of love is a commitment to the cause of liberation—to the project of empowerment.

The second condition for empowering dialogue is humility, or the disciplined and determined sense that I learn and grow in my ability to act in the world to the extent that I respectfully join with others in this project. Arrogance is projecting ignorance onto others, making dialogue impossible. At the point of dialogue, there are only individuals "who are attempting, together, to learn more than they now know" (Freire, 1970, p. 79).

The third condition for empowering dialogue is faith, or the conviction that the power to create and transform, even when thwarted in concrete situations of oppression, tends to be reborn (Freire, 1970, p. 79). This condition of faith is what sustains a vision of possibility even in the face of seemingly insurmountable odds.

These three conditions create a horizontal relationship of mutual trust in which true dialogue is possible. Failures that lead to the common refrain "we need to learn to trust each other" reflect in actuality the need to step back and take a long look at what it means to come to a group with the intention of empowerment. Trust is not the starting point. Rather, love, humility, and faith lead to and create mutual trust.

There are identifiable characteristics of true empowering dialogue. When these characteristics flourish, you know that empowering dialogue is happening.

Hope is the abiding expectation that something will come of our efforts. Even when the group or individuals experience real despair in the face of great odds, there emerges a larger sense that there is a possibility that our efforts will lead, eventually, to what we desire.

The other characteristic of empowering dialogue is critical thinking. Critical thinking in empowering dialogue is far more than problem solving. It is seeing beyond the layers of mystification and, in the process of seeing, constructing a vital link between what is known, what each individual experiences, and the sociopolitical realities of the situation. Freire distinguishes critical thinking characteristics of empowering dialogue as follows:

- Thinking that discerns an indivisible solidarity between the work and individuals, admitting of no dichotomy between them
- Thinking that perceives reality as process, as transformation, rather than as a static entity
- Thinking that does not separate itself from action, but constantly immerses itself in temporality without fear of the risks involved (Freire, 1970, pp. 80–81)

Nurses who are committed to working with women in ways that can lead to empowerment have a key opportunity to influence individuals, groups, and the large sociopolitical contexts all at once. The ways in which nurses can and do work toward empowerment are various and rich. Our challenge is to begin at home—with the women and nurses with whom we work.

References

Freire, P. (1970). *Pedagogy of the oppressed.* New York: Seabury Press.

Wheeler, C., & Chinn, P. (1991). *Peace and power: A handbook of feminist process.* (3rd ed.). New York: National League for Nursing Press.

3

Empowering Women in the Practice Setting

Patricia Moores, RN, PhD

Empowerment is the ability to enact one's own will and love for self in the context of love and respect for others.
Wheeler & Chinn, 1991, p. 2

Proactive risk management does not begin in the administrative offices or behind the door marked Risk Manager. Proactive risk management begins at the bedside with staff nurses (Napiewocki, 1985). Empowered nurses practice according to the standards of professional practice and standards of care (ANA, 1991). The empowered nurse, viewing herself in a collaborative, collegial role, advocates for the patient to prevent injury or harm, thus avoiding cause for litigation. However, all too often the institution or organization does little to empower nurses and may reward, either overtly or covertly, powerlessness. Organizations proactively seeking to prevent litigation will provide the atmosphere to empower nursing staff and reward empowered professional nursing practice. This chapter discusses individual and organizational aspects in the development of empowerment.

Issues Associated with a Lack of Empowerment

Several authors have advanced the empowerment of nurses as a means of resolving identified nursing problems (Joel, 1989; Martin, 1990; Porter, Porter, & Lower, 1989; Sovie, 1990). These historical problems include the demonstration of oppressed group behaviors, difficulties with image and gender issues, cycles of national nursing shortages, and feelings of vulnerability (Cox, 1991; Dykema, 1985; Flynn & Heffron, 1989; Marriner-Tomey, 1990; Martin, 1990; Moores, 1993; Muff, 1982). Each of these problems can potentially be linked to a lack of empowerment for nurses, particularly staff nurses, and may thus impact risk management (Joel, 1989; Martin, 1990).

The negative image of nursing has been explored and described by Kalish and Kalish (1982a, 1982b) as well as other authors (Meleis, 1985; Muff, 1982). Gender-specific issues are key to nursing's negative image. The nursing workforce has always been predominantly female. Gender-related issues in nursing historically parallel the status of women.

Women are often perceived as less intelligent and skilled than men. Muff (1982) cites one nursing stereotype held by the general public: that of the ignorant nurse who needs the direction and protection of the physician to provide safe nursing care. Three images of nurses from the past still haunt the development of nursing for the present and the future. First, the image of the nurse as servant stems from the Protestant work ethic of the sixteenth to the nineteenth centuries (Bridges, 1990; Marriner-Tomey, 1990; Muff, 1982). When perceived as subservient, nurses will not be effective as patient advocates.

The second image of nursing still impacting on its development is the identification of nursing as an oppressed group with a resultant loss or lack of power (Cox, 1991; Dykema, 1985; Hedin, 1986). The literature in nursing on powerlessness includes studies of the behavior of oppressed groups (Roberts, 1983), verbal abuse (Cox, 1991), and sexual harassment (Libbus & Bowman, 1994). Characteristic behaviors of oppressed groups include lack of autonomy, exhibited self-hatred, fear of success, and dependency on and submissiveness to a dominant group (Gaventa, 1980). Freire characterizes the oppressed as having an existential duality in which they find that they cannot exist authentically without freedom and yet are afraid of that freedom. The oppressed are both the oppressed and "the oppressor whose consciousness they have internalized" (Freire, 1970, p. 32).

The third image, self-deprecation and passivity, results when the oppressed group internalizes the derogatory opinion. Any struggle for freedom and self-affirmation results in a tendency to react passively and with alienation. Nurses and women in a paternalistic society have been socialized and conditioned to accept the powerless role (Dykema, 1985). Feelings of powerlessness and passivity lead to poor decision making and/or fear of making a decision and thus potentially put patients at risk.

This nation has experienced recurrent nursing shortages for the past 40 years (Abdellah, 1990; McKibbin, 1990). However, the nursing shortage of the 1990s resulted from the increased demand for nursing care services. Nursing shortages have been cyclic, and trends suggest that in the twenty-first century critical shortages of registered nurses will again occur (Moses, 1992). The ending of the most recent shortage reflected a reduction in the demand for nurses rather than the resolution of underlying nursing problems (e.g., poor image of nursing, salary compression, and control of practice external to the profession). The reduced demand for registered nurses has resulted from a sharply increased use of unlicensed assistive personnel (UAPs), increasing the risk for hospitalized patients (ANA, 1994; Bergman, 1991). Also, any shortage of nurses endangers patient safety (Flood & Diers, 1988; Nyberg, 1991; Prescott, 1991a, 1991b).

As a result of the context in which nurses practice, staff nurses feel vulnerable (Moores, 1993). Contextual conditions of staff nursing include control over nursing practice by others (i.e., physicians and managers), the responsibility for patient care without authority to change it, and the institutional hierarchy of the hospital. Nurses contend with being demeaned during professional interactions with physicians and others as well as having their professional competence devalued. Staff nurses also feel vulnerable because of their perceptions about power and its use, if not against them, then certainly not in their favor. Staff nurses also repeatedly deal with situations where patient status is either potentially or severely compromised. The individual nurse may also feel vulnerable because she questions her clinical ability to handle a crisis situation. Feelings of vulnerability may place the nurse in a precarious risk-management situation.

Empowerment

Empowerment has been advanced as a means to resolve or at least ameliorate the problems of the nursing shortage, oppressed group behavior, negative nursing image, and vulnerability (Joel, 1989; Kramer, 1990; Sovie, 1990). Empowerment can be conceptualized as either a process or as an outcome (Gibson, 1991). Empowerment may be an internal process of either personal competence (Zimmerman & Rappaport, 1988), control, or mastery over one's own life (Kreisberg, 1992). Empowerment may also be an external process during which a portion of someone else's power is appropriated, that is, either granted, gained, or usurped (Brown, 1987; Joel, 1989; Strasen, 1989a; Wilson and Laschinger, 1994).

Becoming Empowered

Stuart (1986) describes using strategic contingency theory to attain organizational power. She regards empowerment as the effective utilization of four principles: increasing connections, becoming irreplaceable, demonstrating nursing assets, and participating in high-level decision making. Carlson-Catalano (1992, 1993) identifies four empowering strategies for student nurses and clinical nurse specialists including: (a) extending the problem-solving skills used in the nursing process to other problems or analytic nursing, (b) implementing planned change projects or change activity, (c) developing skills to value and access experienced colleagues or collegiality, and (d) learning how to obtain mentoring or sponsorship. Moores (1993) regards empowerment as a maturational process during which the nurse evolves through at least three phases including: (a) reacting to threats, (b) confronting challenges, and (c) collaborating to resolve problems.

Five processes—confidence, comfort, competence, credibility, and control (the five Cs)—underlie the development of an empowered self (Figure 3-1). The environment in which the staff nurse functions is an intervening variable in this growth process. Systems either facilitate or impede the development of empowerment.

Self-Empowerment

Central to the model of the five Cs is the development of an empowered self. An empowered staff nurse embodies control, confidence, credibility, competence, and confidence (Moores, 1993). Each of these attributes develops and evolves as the staff nurse matures in nursing.

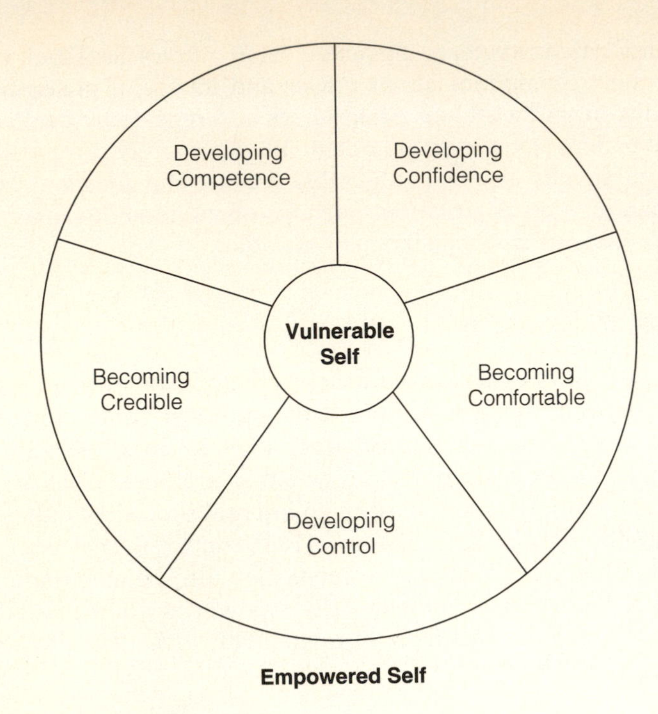

Figure 3-1 The five Cs of empowerment.

Reprinted with permission, Moores, 1993.

Developing Control Moores (1993) defines control as personal and situational. Personal control involves learning emotional self-control. Situational control involves participating in the control of a situation: making and acting on patient care decisions. Control of a nursing situation develops through three stages: being given control, assuming control, and sharing control.

In the first stage of developing control, the staff nurse makes decisions and carries out changes only after perceiving that permission has been given. The nurse who describes being given control is somewhat similar to the advanced beginner in the study by Benner, Tanner, and Chelsa (1992). These authors found that the advanced beginner feels responsible to complete nursing tasks that are either implied or ordered in the medical or nursing care plans.

Assuming control in a nursing situation involves being able to make decisions without permission, but potentially having someone retrospectively determine that those decisions were incorrect (Moores, 1993). The third stage of control in the nursing situation encompasses mutual decision making and being able to share control or give up control of the situation to someone else.

Recognition of these stages enables colleagues and managers to tailor their directions to and expectations of nurses, especially those new to nursing.

Advanced beginners (Benner, 1984) are often uncomfortable with control issues and need the guidance of an expert nurse to verify decisions and assist with control issues.

Becoming Competent For the staff nurse, competence means feeling capable to do the job of nursing by providing good nursing care to patients (Moores, 1993). Feelings of competence emerge as the staff nurse develops a nursing knowledge base and successfully resolves nursing conflicts. The process of becoming competent is an evolution from feeling inept to feeling competent. Assessing perceived and actual competence is an important component to minimize patient risk. The nursing manager needs to structure a safe environment for the staff nurse to obtain competence. The individual nurse needs to seek out opportunities to gain competence.

Becoming Credible For staff nurses, becoming credible involves developing trust in their own judgment (Moores, 1993). This developmental process incorporates both gaining credibility with others and becoming credible with self. The external aspect of gaining credibility with others develops first through the process of interacting with other nurses, health team members, patients, and families. Although she relies on others to establish credibility in the beginning, the nurse eventually determines her credibility through self-evaluation rather than by relying on the judgment and feedback of others. Credibility results, in part, because other people believe in, trust, and respect the staff nurse. The nurse develops credibility with her peers and herself through the interactions that occur in shared clinical situations.

Becoming credible with self develops as the staff nurse learns to trust her own judgments rather than relying on the judgment and feedback of others and becomes self-reliant. Self-reliant nurses trust their own self-evaluation rather than depending on others. Nurses who have not yet achieved this stage of self-credibility need more support and feedback to manage patient problems.

Developing Confidence Confidence denotes the ability of the nurse to take action in a nursing situation (Moores, 1993). Confidence is crucial to feeling empowered. Although her self-confidence develops in response to resolving nursing situations, the staff nurse must possess an underlying sense of self-esteem or self-worth. Therefore, increasing confidence includes having self-esteem and developing self-confidence. Mentors are key in the process of increasing confidence.

An initial lack of belief in self-ability, or lack of self-esteem, means that the nurse will not take risks if she feels little or no capability to resolve the event. Self-valuing is important if the nurse is to believe in her abilities. Litigious events sometimes occur because a nurse does not value herself or her judgments and therefore does not advocate for the patient. Mentors help the staff nurse develop self-valuing.

Mentors are important in the development of self-confidence. Mentorship correlates with one of Bandura's (1977) psychological procedures of self-efficacy. In his theory, Bandura proposes that certain psychological procedures create and strengthen self-efficacy. Efficacy involves the expectation that one can successfully perform the behavior needed to obtain the desired outcome. One of Bandura's procedures involves verbal persuasion or leading people to believe, through the use of positive suggestion, that they can cope successfully. Mentors can increase confidence in other nurses by offering encouraging suggestions and predicting success. Boyd, Collins, Pipitone, Balk, and Kapustay (1990), in their discussion of the opening of a new unit, show how mentors or resource nurses provided support for less experienced nurses. By reminding the less experienced nurses that they "were empowered to act," the resource nurses coached and supported these nurses (p. 1228).

Becoming Comfortable A sense of comfort develops as the staff nurse acquires the ability to predict outcomes of nursing problems or situations (Moores, 1993). This three-part process evolves as follows: (a) being comfortable in the environment, (b) feeling comfortable with familiar patients, and (c) feeling comfortable predicting probable responses. When the staff nurse feels comfortable or able to predict a possible outcome, she feels more empowered.

Nurses first develop comfort within a predictable environment. When the new nurse begins practicing, she feels comfortable in a familiar environment where she can locate items, can find resources, and knows the personnel. Nurses at this level of comfort should not be placed in an unfamiliar situation (i.e., "floated"), especially in areas with potentially unstable patients.

In the second stage of becoming comfortable, nurses learn to anticipate possible problems, identify treatments commensurate with diagnoses, and become comfortable with a variety of patients. The staff nurse no longer depends on familiar surroundings to engender feelings of comfort and knows how to manage seriously ill patients (in her specialty). Feelings of comfort extend to interactions with other staff. When a nurse predicts the probable response of either colleagues or physicians, she is comfortable presenting new ideas or recommending alternative therapies to improve patient care and reduce risk.

Phases of Empowerment

A new staff nurse moves from feeling vulnerable to feeling empowered through the development of the underlying processes of control, credibility, comfort, confidence, and competence (Moores, 1993). The staff nurse moves through three phases in the development of an empowered self. The process evolves from: (a) reacting to threatening situations, (b) confronting nursing challenges, and (c) collaborating to resolve problems. Each of these maturational phases of threat, challenge, and collaboration follows similar sequences in relationship to interactions. The sequences include assessing risks, taking action, and determining success.

Reacting to a Threat The first phase of becoming empowered is that of reacting to a threat. Threats are situations in which the nurse perceives that she is lacking, to some degree, one or more of the five Cs (Moores, 1993). Because of her perceived lack of ability, the staff nurse experiences fear or anxiety when faced with the situation. The nurse, in the reactive phase, recognizes the situation as threatening, assesses the risk of taking action, selects and implements strategies, and then determines the success of her actions. If she selects and uses passive strategies, she remains at the level of threat for similar situations. If she selects active strategies and feels successful, she progresses in her feelings of empowerment (Figure 3-2).

Once she recognizes a situation as a threat, the nurse makes an unconscious risk assessment before deciding which strategies to use. Assessment results in the selection of either active interpersonal strategies to deflect the threat or passive intra/interpersonal strategies to salvage the ego or avoid the situation. At the conclusion, the staff nurse evaluates her effectiveness in managing the situation. Successful resolution of a threat depends on the staff nurse feeling good about her participation in the outcome. A feeling of empowerment emerges from resolution of the threat.

Unsuccessful resolution of a threat may keep the nurse at the reactive level. The nurse may use self-empowering strategies to move to the challenge phase with this situation. A staff nurse may emotionally withdraw after either the use of passive strategies or the unsuccessful use of active strategies (Figure 3-3). Emotional withdrawal results in self-talk and the development of self-empowering or active intrapersonal strategies (e.g., rehearsing to be assertive, giving self permission to try, and emulating a mentor's behavior). Following development and employment of self-empowering strategies, the nurse moves into the phase of confronting challenges. Rehearsing to be assertive includes mentally identifying the problem, planning what can be done, and then talking to oneself about the threat.

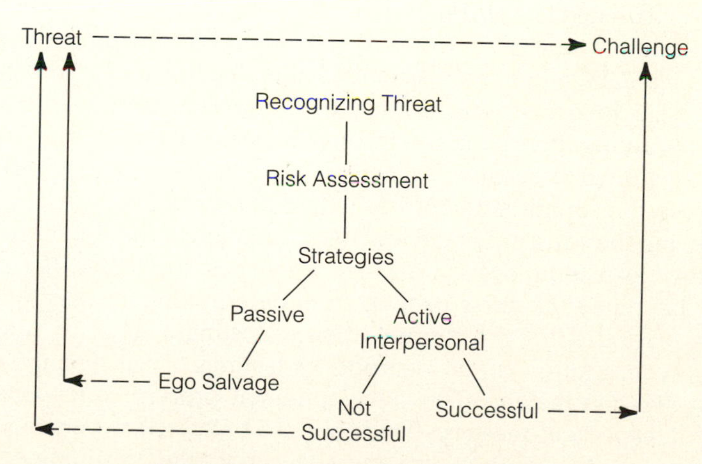

Figure 3-2 Model of reactive phase.

Reprinted with permission, Moores, 1993.

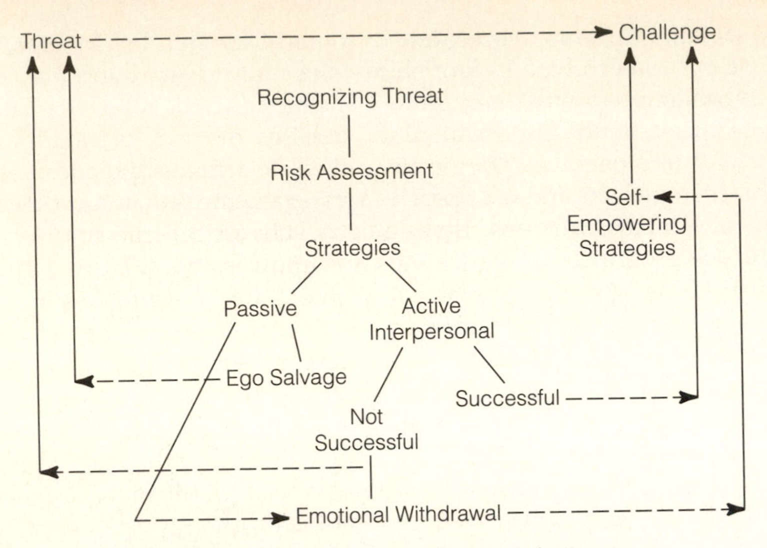

Figure 3-3 Transition from threat to challenge.

Reprinted with permission, Moores, 1993.

Emulating a mentor's behavior is similar to one of Bandura's (1977) psychological procedures of self-efficacy. The psychological process of relying on vicarious experience assists others to derive self-expectations of potential success. Managers and colleagues facilitate self-empowering strategies in nurses who are in a phase of reacting to threat. The strategy of rehearsing, especially, can be very productive for new or threatened nurses.

Confronting a Challenge During the second phase of becoming empowered, confronting challenges, nursing practice issues are perceived as challenges. A challenge is a situation that was threatening in the past but that the nurse is now able to confront, thereby changing the outcome (Moores, 1993). Threatening situations become challenges for nurses in three ways. Each of these three mechanisms affect the degree of ascertained risk: (a) situations becoming more common through repeated experiences, (b) making conscious choices to perceive a situation as a challenge, and (c) identifying a change in the situation that reduces the degree of risk.

Following the risk assessment and determination of the situation as a challenge, the nurse employs confrontive strategies to resolve the situation. During this phase the nurse evolves from determining success by virtue of winning or controlling the confrontation to feeling a sense of autonomous mastery. Feeling autonomous incorporates feelings of self-reliance and independent decision making. This developmental process corresponds to the theoretical aspects of mastery. Bandura (1977) states that personal mastery arises from effective performance and affects both the beginning of and persistence in a behavior. Pearlin and Schooler (1978) define mastery as the belief that one's life changes are under one's own control. According to

Younger (1991), the important elements of mastery include certainty, change, acceptance, and growth. All four elements are important to the staff nurse as she begins to feel autonomous.

Continuing to feel successful in confronting challenges and developing autonomy, the nurse becomes more empowered and begins to collaborate rather than confront. Some situations remain threatening, while others challenge her. The mature nurse views much of her practice as empowered collaboration.

Collaborating to Resolve a Problem The third phase of becoming empowered is empowered collaboration. This phase involves a sense of continuing development without a finite ending point or completion. The nurse competently manages the situation. Responses become natural, and the feeling of empowerment is internalized. This response corresponds to Benner's (1984) "intuitive grasp" of nursing situations by expert nurses.

In this phase, the nurse feels capable of interacting as an equal with other health care providers and collaborates to accomplish goals and resolve problems. In the collaborative phase, empowered nurses communicate their feelings about working cooperatively. The collaborative phase is simultaneous yet sequential. This process is instantaneous and interactive in each situation. The nurse appraises consequences, implements strategies, and determines success. In the collaborative phase, the nurse appraises the potential consequences of her actions. Appraisal continues as the situation progresses. Crucial to this process are interaction and collaboration with others. Collaborative strategies focus on a sense of partnership.

Now the nurse feels confident regarding nursing knowledge, competent to resolve nursing problems, and comfortable anticipating or predicting the outcomes of situations. She defines a sense of credibility mainly through self-evaluation and shares control of the situation with colleagues, physicians, and patients.

Empowered Nursing Practice

Empowered nursing practice includes several components: (a) supportive systems that facilitate empowerment, (b) motivated nursing management, and (c) involved, interested staff. Empowerment is a growth process that goes beyond management sharing power with staff (Moores, 1993; Vogt & Murrell, 1990).

Individual nurses can help empower newer, less experienced nurses by assisting in the development of credibility and control (Moores, 1993). Mentorship by experienced nurses develops both confidence and competence. Nurses sharing stories and having active discussions of clinical situations are examples of self-empowering strategies. Other self-empowering strategies include: (a) supportive interactions, (b) moving toward self-actualization, (c) valuing and creating change, (d) seeking increased responsibility, (e) being patient with self, and (f) appreciating new ideas (Vogt & Murrell, 1990).

Nursing administrators must anticipate incidents that make nurses feel vulnerable. Once incidents are identified, nursing administrators need to provide nurses the resources to develop and refine skills or implement small group problem solving (Moores, 1993). Nursing administrators can make certain that other departments and physicians are aware of the values and contributions of the nursing role. Additionally, administrators must promote an environment for collaborative practice and interactions among the health care team.

Prescott and Bowen (1985) report that not all of the disagreements between nurses and physicians had a negative impact on patient care. Seventy percent of physicians and 69% of nurses described the relationships as positive. However, most of the interactions were described as competitive, with only 14% of physicians and 7% of nurses describing any type of collaborative activity. If the final phase of empowerment involves collaboration, and nurses feel that they are collaborating with physicians only 7% of the time, nursing administrators need to encourage and support the development of strategies that enable collaboration.

Fagin (1992) remains optimistic that changes in nursing education, collaborative practice models, and the pressure for health care reform will enhance the development of collaboration between nurses and physicians. Improving the interactional process between nurses and physicians would improve patient outcomes. Knaus, Draper, Wagner, and Zimmerman (1986) found that the interaction and communication among nurses and physicians had a direct impact on improving the prospective outcome for patients in the critical care unit. Enhanced communication improves survival rates.

Nursing administrators are responsible for developing an environment where professional interactions create feelings of value (Moores, 1993). Nursing managers must commit time and energy to aid staff in developing positive self-concepts (Strasen, 1989b). Characteristics of empowering leaders include: (a) providing challenges for staff nurses, (b) setting nurses up for success, and (c) letting go of control (Keller, 1991).

Interventions for empowering staff include: (a) recognizing and valuing individual differences, (b) delegating responsibility and power, (c) being direct and encouraging others to be direct, (d) identifying and clarifying common goals, (e) verbalizing support for others, (f) using conflict-resolution skills, and (g) establishing participative management systems (Vogt & Murrell, 1990). Administrators must use positive feedback to reinforce feelings of success. Provision of positive feedback is not forthcoming from many nursing managers (Moores, 1993). Providing new nurses with rehearsal sessions, whether for responding to a cardiac arrest or intervening with an irate physician, helps nurses develop empowerment. Recognition and provision for peer mentorship influences the development of empowered nurses (Moores, 1993).

A Supportive System

A supportive system can either provide the foundation for an individual nurse to become empowered or create a milieu or environment that makes the nurse feel unempowered (Moores, 1993). Certain management strategies can assist the nurse in her maturational process of becoming empowered. Blanket policies designed to "empower" staff nurses may not be effective because each nurse is at a different phase of empowerment. The properties of a supportive system include: (a) risk taking, (b) risk reduction, (c) self-valuing, and (d) recognition of the nurse as a team member.

Vogt and Murrell (1990) recommend several interventions to move the system toward empowerment: (a) trust people, (b) create a shared vision, (c) plan for change, (d) maintain an orientation toward excellence, (e) make information readily and widely available, (f) value autonomy, (g) sustain a clear ethical framework, (h) flatten the hierarchy, (i) open communication channels, and (j) have staffing patterns that reflect empowerment. Dveirin and Adams (1993) promote aspects of empowerment that include: (a) participation in creating the organization's mission and vision, (b) control over resources, (c) meaningful incentives, (d) an environment of trust and respect, (e) clear boundaries, and (f) access to education, training, and information.

By providing a supportive system, managers facilitate and encourage the development of an empowered nursing staff. Staff nurses can choose to use active strategies to create change rather than passive strategies (e.g., inaction, withdrawal, and complaining) (Moores, 1993).

Promoting Self-Valuing Systems where nurses feel demeaned or not valued do not promote empowerment (Moores, 1993). A supportive system has an orientation of respect for the person and for the freedom to question. Nurses want the difficult job of nursing recognized.

Supporting Risk Taking A system that promotes empowerment provides structure without rigidity (Moores, 1993). This type of structure encourages taking on new roles and expressing creative ideas. Nurses want the freedom to take on new roles with some direction from the manager. Gunden and Chrissman (1992) identify teaching, modeling, and coaching as some of the methods to empower staff nurses through leadership behavior. Thyen, Theis, and Tebbitt (1993) describe a self-governed team approach where mistakes were analyzed and plans developed for corrective action.

For creativity to exist, systems must be flexible and open to change. Kramer (1990) reports that magnet hospitals fostered experimentation, recognition of individual competence, and autonomy. These hospitals have designed open flexible systems that encourage the development of empowerment.

Recognizing the Nurse as Team Contributor Nurses perceive themselves as important team members (i.e., of the health care and nursing teams) in the provision of health care. A supportive system recognizes and strengthens this belief. The health care team includes all of the participants in patient care: nurses, physicians, patient, family, and others. Nurses want to be regarded as equal participants in the patient care process, in a collegial relationship with all members (Moores, 1993). The nurse has unique, valuable knowledge regarding patient care unavailable from any other source.

All nurses providing care to patients constitute a nursing team. Nursing team interactions have several dimensions. Members of the team assist individual nurses. Nursing team members interact with each other to provide good care but maintain separate individual responsibility. Team members evaluate care provided by all members to maintain good patient care and team functioning. Team members also provide support and cohesiveness during crisis or conflict (Moores, 1993).

The development of self-managed teams has been identified as a means of empowering the nursing work force (Kerfoot & Uecker, 1992; Thyen et al., 1993). Self-managed teams have evolved from aspects of self-governance and total quality management (Sovie, 1992). Team membership is important to nurses regardless of their phase of empowerment. A supportive system augments and develops these relationships and enhances the developmental process of becoming empowered.

Reducing Risk of Error Reducing risk of error or failure through a supportive system enhances the staff nurse's development of empowerment. Risk reduction includes provision of a system that supports knowledgeable patient care and reduces risk of error or failure. Staff nurses want a system that supports continuity and knowledgeable patient care. Staffing and "floating" repeatedly surface as issues that negate feelings of empowerment. When most staff nurses float, they feel (and therefore are) inadequate to care for their assigned patients (Moores, 1993). Nurses are also concerned about staffing levels affecting safe patient care (Moores, 1993).

Systems must provide resource people when nurses are in unusual situations. When feeling threatened, nurses need peer support and have also identified a need for someone to validate and advise (Moores, 1993). Systems that provide peer support and encourage mentorship reduce the risk of error, especially for new nurses (Moores, 1993).

References

Abdellah, F. (1990). Reflections on a recurring theme. *Nursing Clinics of North America, 25*(3), 509–516.

American Nurses Association. (1991). *Standards of clinical nursing practice.* Washington, D.C.: Author.

American Nurses Association. (1994). *Registered professional nurses and unlicensed assistive personnel.* Washington, D.C.: Author.

Bandura, A. (1977). Self-efficacy: Toward a unifying theory of behavioral change. *Psychological Review, 84*(2), 191–215.

Benner, P. (1984). *From novice to expert.* Menlo Park, CA: Addison-Wesley Nursing.

Benner, P., Tanner, C., & Chelsa, C. (1992). From beginner to expert: Gaining a differentiated clinical world in critical care nursing. *Advances in Nursing Science, 14*(3), 13–28.

Bergman, E. (1991). Nurse extenders now found in 97% of hospitals. *American Journal of Nursing, 91*(9), 88–90.

Boyd, M., Collins, L., Pipitone, J., Balk, E., & Kapustay, P. (1990). Theory Z as a framework for the application of a professional practice model in increasing nursing staff retention on oncology units. *Journal of Advanced Nursing, 15,* 1226–1229.

Bridges, J. (1990). Literature review on the images of the nurse and nursing in the media. *Journal of Advanced Nursing, 15*(7), 850–854.

Brown, C. (1987). Power and images of nursing in the lived world of nurse administrators. Unpublished doctoral dissertation, University of Colorado.

Carlson-Catalano, J. (1992). Empowering nurses for professional practice. *Nursing Outlook, 40*(3), 139–142.

Carlson-Catalano, J. (1993). Application of empowerment theory for CNS practice. *Clinical Nurse Specialist, 7*(6), 321–325.

Cox, H. (1991). Verbal abuse nationwide, part 1: Oppressed group behavior. *Nursing Management, 22*(2), 32–35.

Dveirin, G., & Adams, K. (1993). Empowering health care improvement: An operational model. *The Joint Commission Journal, 19*(7), 222–232.

Dykema, L. (1985, Sept). Gaventa's theory of power and powerlessness: Application to nursing. *Occupational Health Nursing,* 443–446.

Fagin, C. (1992). Collaboration between nurses and physicians: No longer a choice. *Academic Medicine, 67*(5), 295–303.

Flood, S., & Diers, D. (1988). Nurse staffing, patient outcome and cost. *Nursing Management, 19*(5), 34–39, 42–43.

Flynn, J., & Heffron, P. (1989). *Nursing: From concept to practice* (2nd ed.). Norwalk, CT: Appleton & Lange.

Freire, P. (1970). *Pedagogy of the oppressed.* New York: Continuum Publishing Corporation.

Gaventa, J. (1980). *Power and powerlessness.* Urbana: University of Illinois Press.

Gibson, C. (1991). A concept analysis of empowerment. *Journal of Advanced Nursing, 16,* 354–361.

Gunden, E., & Chrissman, S. (1992). Leadership skills for empowerment. *Nursing Administration Quarterly, 16*(3), 6–10.

Hedin, B. (1986). A case study of oppressed group behavior. *Image, 18*(2), 53–57.

Joel, L. (1989). Empowerment of the staff nurse: A means to an end and an end in itself. *The Kentucky Nurse, 37*(1), 12–15.

Kalish, P., & Kalish, B. (1982a). The image of nurses in novels. *American Journal of Nursing,* 82(8), 1220–1224.

Kalish, P., & Kalish, B. (1982b). Nurses on prime-time television. *American Journal of Nursing,* 82(2), 264–270.

Keller, B. (1991). A study of empowering nurses within the context of a health-care organization. Unpublished doctoral dissertation, University of Colorado.

Kerfoot, K., & Uecker, S. (1992). The techniques of developing self-managed teams: The nurse manager's role. *Nursing Economics, 10*(1), 70–71, 78.

Knaus, W., Draper, E., Wagner, D., & Zimmerman, J. (1986). An evaluation of outcome from intensive care in major medical centers. *Annals of Internal Medicine, 104*, 410–418.

Kramer, M. (1990). The magnet hospitals: Excellence revisited. *Journal of Nursing Administration, 20*(9), 35–44.

Kreisberg, S. (1992). *Transforming power: Domination, empowerment, and education.* New York: State University of New York Press.

Libbus, K., & Bowman, K. (1994). Sexual harassment of female registered nurses in hospitals. *Journal of Nursing Administration, 24*(6), 26–31.

Marriner-Tomey, A. (1990). Addressing the nursing shortage. In C. Little (Ed.), *Nursing and health care: The supplement.* New York: National League for Nursing.

Martin, C. (1990). A response from an educational perspective. *Nursing Clinics of North America, 25*(3), 561–568.

McKibbin, R. (1990). *The nursing shortage and the 1990's: Realities and remedies.* Kansas City, MO: American Nurses Association.

Meleis, A. (1985). *Theoretical nursing: Development and progress.* Philadelphia: J.B. Lippincott.

Moores, P. (1993). *Becoming empowered: A grounded theory study of staff nurse empowerment.* Ann Arbor: UMI Dissertation Services. Order number 9401789.

Moses, E. (1992). RN shortage seen for 21st century: As I see it. *American Nurse, 24*(7), 5.

Muff, J. (1982). *Socialization, sexism and stereotyping.* St. Louis: Mosby.

Napiewocki, J. (1985). Want to cut liability claims? Look to your staff nurse. *Hospitals*, 75.

Nyberg, J. (1991). The nurse as professnocrat. *Nursing Economics, 9*(4), 244–247, 280.

Pearlin, L., & Schooler, C. (1978). The structure of coping. *Journal of Health and Social Behavior, 19*(3), 2–21.

Porter, R., Porter, M., & Lower, M. (1989). Enhancing the image of nursing. *Journal of Nursing Administration, 19*(2), 36–40.

Prescott, P. (1991a). Forecasting requirements for health care personnel. *Nursing Economics, 9*(1), 18–24.

Prescott, P. (1991b). Nursing intensity: Needed today for more than staffing. *Nursing Economics, 9*(6), 409–414.

Prescott, P., & Bowen, S. (1985). Physician-nurse relationships. *Annals of Internal Medicine, 103*, 127–138.

Roberts, S. (1983, July). Oppressed group behavior: Implications for nursing. *Advances in Nursing Science*, 21–30.

Sovie, M. (1990). Redesigning our future: Whose responsibility is it? *Nursing Economics, 8*(1), 21–26.

Sovie, M. (1992). Care and service teams: A new imperative. *Nursing Economics, 10*(2), 94–100.

Strasen, L. (1989a). Redesigning patient care to empower nurses and increase productivity. *Nursing Economics, 7,*(1), 32–35.

Strasen, L. (1989b). Self-concept: Improving the image of nursing. *Journal of Nursing Administration, 19*(1), 4–5.

Stuart, G. (1986). An organizational strategy for empowering nursing. *Nursing Economics,* 4(2), 69–73.

Thyen, M., Theis, R., & Tebbitt, B. (1993). Organizational empowerment through self-governed teams. *Journal of Nursing Administration, 23*(1), 24–26.

Vogt, J., & Murrell, K. (1990). *Empowerment in organizations.* San Diego: Pfeiffer & Company.

Wheeler, C., & Chinn, P. (1991). *Peace and power: A handbook of feminist process.* (3rd ed.). New York: National League of Nursing Press.

Wilson, B., & Laschinger, H. (1994). Staff nurse perceptions of job empowerment and organization commitment. *Journal of Nursing Administration.* 24(45), 39–47.

Younger, J. (1991). A theory of mastery. *Advances in Nursing Science, 14*(1), 76–89.

Zimmerman, M., & Rappaport, J. (1988). Citizen participation, perceived control, and psychological empowerment. *American Journal of Community Psychology, 16*(5), 725–750.

4

Maternal-Child Nursing and the Law

Susanna Meissner-Cutler, RN, BSN, JD
Sandra L. Gardner, RN, MS, CNS, PNP

The maternal-child nurse is a professional with special training, skill, and knowledge in the care of the pregnant woman, newborn, and infant/child (ANA, 1983; NAACOG, 1990, 1991). In her practice, the maternal-child nurse undertakes multiple legal, moral, and ethical obligations for which she is held accountable and responsible. The maternal-child nurse is accountable to her patient, profession, and employer (ANA, 1985). Failure of the maternal-child nurse to meet her obligations can result in liability in her profession, liability in her employment, a civil suit, or a criminal conviction.

The practice of nursing is distinct from the practice of medicine because nursing professionals have their own independent responsibility to patients. Members of society served by nursing expect the professional nurse to be competent and accountable. In turn, to a large degree, the public permits the profession to set standards of conduct for its members (see Chapter 6). To assist in preserving the public's health, safety, and welfare, all states regulate the practice of nursing. Only those individuals meeting the licensing criteria (i.e., education and testing) may practice as professional nurses. Criteria for practice include appropriate education and licensing. The maternal-child nurse is considered a specialist in professional nursing. In *Planned Parenthood v. Vines* (1989) the court held that a labor and delivery nurse was considered a specialist (i.e., an expert with superior knowledge and skill). As such, the practice of maternal-child nursing generally requires additional education, training, and experience. However, the scope of practice for a maternal-child nurse is also determined by regulation, education, training, and experience. This scope of acceptable practice determines where professional liability may attach for the maternal-child nurse. To provide the best possible quality of care to the patient and to defend the care rendered, the maternal-child nurse must "understand the law and standards by which nursing care is measured" (McRae, 1993, p. 411).

Protracted Liability of Maternal-Child Nursing Specialist

Statute of Limitations

All states have passed legislation setting forth a specific time limit during which a person, having a cause of action for damages due to professional negligence, is required to file a lawsuit. This time limit for filing suit is termed the statute of limitations. After the term of the statute of limitations has expired, a lawsuit may not be filed. A lawsuit will be dismissed if it is determined that the term of statute of limitations expired prior to the date of filing.

The time limit for filing suit varies from state to state but generally ranges from 1 to 6 years from the date of the negligence resulting in injury. However, in the case of a minor (most often defined as a child under the age of 18 years) the term of the statute of limitations may not begin to run until that child reaches the age of majority (greater than 18 or 21 years of age, depending on state law). If there is not a specific statutory provision describing the time limits for filing professional negligence claims, the professional negligence action is generally governed by the statute of limitations for actions for personal injuries (most other claims for damages to the person). All nurses should know the terms of the statute of limitations for professional negligence in the state in which they practice. For the maternal-child nurse, this knowledge is of particular importance in light of the varying nature of patients and care provided, and the potential for a prolonged period of liability. For instance, a surgical nurse caring for an adult patient having a cholecystectomy has a significantly shorter period of exposure for liability than the maternal-child nurse, who may be called upon to defend her care of a minor many years into the future.

Not only the term of the statute of limitations but also its application differs among the states. The time period may begin to run from (a) the date of the act causing the injury (*Olsen v. St. Croix Valley Memorial Hospital*, 1972), (b) the date of last treatment by the particular nurse, or (c) the "date of the discovery" of the injury (*Teeters v. Currey*, 1974). The date of discovery is the date that the patient knew or should have known of the injury (*Renslow v. Mennonite Hospital*, 1977). For example, a maternal-child nurse might fail to administer an ordered RhoGAM (Rh_o immune globulin) injection to an Rh-negative patient who has just delivered an Rh-positive child. Several years later, this same patient becomes pregnant and develops antibodies to the Rh-positive fetus, causing injury to the child's brain, nervous system, and other organs. Even though more than 2 years have passed since the failure to administer RhoGAM, the patient did not and reasonably would not have learned of the omission until she again became pregnant and delivered a sensitized Rh-positive child. In this instance, the 2-year discovery rule stipulates that the term of the statute of limitations commences at the time the patient knew or should have known of the failure to receive the RhoGAM (i.e., when she delivered the second child).

Discovery

In some states, the date of "discovery" may be defined not only as the time that the patient knew or should have known of the injury but also as the time that the patient learned its cause (i.e., that the injury was caused by professional negligence). For instance, suppose an infant is diagnosed with cerebral palsy as a result of fetal distress at the time of delivery. However, not until the child is 1 year of age do the parents learn that the fetal distress could and should have been recognized and remedied so that the child would not have sustained injury. Here, the term of the statute of limitations may begin at the time that the parents first learned that professional negligence, causing their child to sustain injury, had occurred. "Discovery" often occurs after parents have consulted a specialist about the child's special needs. Many states recognize the discovery rule and place a limit on the time of discovery through a statute of repose (i.e., providing an outside limit or maximum time to invoke the discovery rule). For example, if the term of the statute of limitations is 2 years from the date of discovery a suit might have to be filed no more than 3 years from the date of the injury (date of the act that caused the injury) despite the date of discovery.

Recognized exceptions to the statute of limitations and even to the statute of repose vary significantly from state to state. For example, most states recognize "disability" of a person as an exception to the statute of repose. Disability can include minority (i.e., the patient is under the age of majority) or mental incapacity. In cases of incapacity, the term of the statute of limitations usually begins to run when the disability is removed (i.e., when the person reaches majority or is no longer mentally incapacitated). For example, children may be considered under a disability when they sustain an injury but are under the age of majority. The term of the statute of limitations does not commence until a child reaches the age of majority, at which time the young adult has the normal term of the statute of limitations in which to file a suit. Disability might also exist when an adult patient suffers brain damage following a seizure resulting from failure to diagnose and treat pregnancy-induced hypertension in a timely manner. After 2 years and significant rehabilitation, the patient may be able to think and function independently once more. Arguably, the term of the statute of limitations would begin to run at that time. Sometimes the "disability" is considered removed when a legal representative is appointed for the individual with the disability. Military service outside of the United States is also considered a disability that prevents the running of the term of a statute of limitations.

When the patient is a minor and thus has significantly more time to file a lawsuit, there is a potential for a protracted claim. Some states have a specific statute addressing the time limits for filing suit (i.e., if the injury is the result of a birth-related incident or the child is very young at the time of the injury). For instance, a child injured at birth because of the negligence of the neonatal nurse practitioner who failed to intubate and suction (in the presence of 3+ meconium) may have 6 years after birth before the 2-year term of the statute of limitations would commence. The justification for this special rule of law limiting the minority exception is an equitable one. The rule allows the potential defendant(s) time to preserve facts and retain records before this evidence (which forms the basis for the action) becomes stale, forgotten, or lost.

Finally, justice requires an exception to the limitation period, particularly regarding the statute of repose, when the reason for the delay is not under the control of the claimant. Examples of these exceptions include fraudulent concealment, foreign object, and continuing treatment. In these situations, the patient does not have an opportunity to discover the injury. In a fraudulent concealment case, the provider has information that professional negligence occurred but intentionally misinforms the patient about the incident. The patient's reliance on the truth of the professional's statement has delayed legal action. In a case of a foreign object (e.g., a sponge left inside the patient's body after surgery), the patient may not become aware of the existence of the foreign object for many years. Continuing treatment might extend the state of repose or limitation until the last day of care, regardless of when the negligent act actually took place.

Legal Terminology and Definitions

The maternal-child nurse can be found liable in a civil action based on a tort. A tort is a legal wrong, not involving a breach of contract, that causes injury to another and for which the person committing the wrong can be held liable for damages in a civil suit. Professional negligence is the legal wrong most often resulting in damages to the patient and exposure of the maternal-child nurse to liability. For a patient to be successful in a suit predicated on the professional negligence of a nurse, the patient must prove each of three elements: (a) negligence, duty and breach of duty; (b) causation; and (c) damages.

A civil action based in tort is distinct from a criminal action. Although the tort and the crime may share certain similar characteristics, the key distinction "lies in the interests affected and the remedy afforded by the law" (Prosser, 1984, p. 7). A crime is an insult to the state and the people it represents. The purpose of a criminal action is punishment of the wrongdoer and deterrence from repeated offensive conduct. In contrast, a civil action for a tort is brought by the patient or the patient's representative for the purpose of obtaining monetary compensation for injuries and damages suffered. The two actions are tried in different courts, before different juries, and with different standards of proof.

Negligence

Negligence is defined as "the omission to do something which a reasonable person guided by those ordinary considerations which ordinarily regulate human affairs, would do, or the doing of something that a reasonable and prudent person would not do" (*Schneider v. Little Company*, 1915). Every person has an obligation to act as a reasonably prudent person would act under the same or similar circumstances. This standard is called the *reasonable per-*

son rule. A caregiver may be liable for negligence when she fails to perform an act that she had a duty to perform, and that failure results in injury to the person to whom the duty is owed. The duty owed depends upon the existence of a relationship and the nature of the relationship in the given circumstances. For example, in an action based on an automobile collision, the plaintiff (injured party) claims that the defendant owed plaintiff a duty to drive safely and that the defendant breached that duty, causing plaintiff to sustain injury.

Professional Negligence

Malpractice has traditionally been used to describe professional negligence (i.e., misconduct by a professional). When a maternal-child nurse establishes a relationship with the patient (i.e., the pregnant woman and her fetus, the newborn or infant, or the child), she owes the patient "due care" in diagnosing and treating. The special nature of this relationship transforms the reasonable person rule used in the definition of simple negligence to the reasonably prudent maternal-child nurse acting under the same or similar circumstances. Thus, the maternal-child nurse is required to possess the same degree of skill and knowledge that is customary in other maternal-child nurses practicing in the same area under the same or similar circumstances. The practitioner must practice within this broad standard of care. The degree of care required of the practicing maternal-child nurse is not the highest degree of care possible but, rather, only that degree of care practiced by others in the profession. Professional negligence occurs when there is a lack of "ordinary" or "reasonable" care, resulting in injury to a patient. A nursing professional can be found liable for negligence when: (a) she fails to possess the requisite skill and knowledge (e.g., the nurse is unaware that an overdose of oxytocin causes tetanic uterine contractions and thus decreases blood flow to the fetus), (b) fails to exercise reasonable care (e.g., the nurse fails to perform a glucose screen on the infant of a diabetic mother), or (c) fails to use her best judgment (e.g., the nurse discharges within 24 hours after delivery a single, first-time mother and her infant, when the mother cannot speak English and has no support at home). The maternal-child nurse must also use her experience and knowledge to question any orders or practice that she believes may be harmful to the patient.

The maternal-child nurse is required not only to possess the requisite skill and knowledge but also to use her best judgment in exercising that skill and applying that knowledge (*Pike v. Honsinger*, 1898). Therefore, the practitioner may be liable for: (a) not knowing what to do when the reasonably prudent practitioner would have known what to do, (b) knowing what to do but not doing it, or (c) knowing what to do but doing it carelessly.

Professional negligence is generally not a crime. Criminal conduct is significantly more than just mistakes, inattention, or inexperience. However, acts of negligence that are wanton or done with malice may be considered criminal. Gross negligence, an aggravated form of negligence "usually accompanied by a conscious indifference to the consequences" or with reckless disregard for the rights and safety of others, can be a crime (Prosser, 1984,

p. 213). Generally, to be convicted of a crime, a person must be proved to have a state of mind and intent to do harm, as well as criminal conduct. For example, a crime has been committed when a nurse knowingly possesses a nonprescribed controlled substance for her personal use.

Duty

The maternal-child nurse is professionally accountable for her nursing practice. Her accountability is premised upon the concept of duty, an obligation to another to comply with particular standards of conduct. The nurse's professional duty is expressly set forth in nurse practice acts and is generally based upon the foreseeability of harm to others as a result of the acts or omissions of the nurse. The maternal-child nurse is duty bound not only to her patient but also to the public, to her employer, and the nursing profession (ANA, 1985).

Duty to the Patient Based on her knowledge, skill, education, and experience, the maternal-child nurse is expected to perceive a patient's needs and risks to a degree that the average layperson would not perceive. The maternal-child nurse must exercise reasonable care to avoid conduct that can foreseeably cause injury to the patient. The nurse's duty to the patient includes affirmative action and disclosure. A breach of the maternal-child nurse's duty to her patient can result in liability for any subsequent harm resulting from that breach.

Duty to the Employer Although the maternal-child nurse is always responsible for her own negligent acts and omissions, her employer (e.g., hospital, clinic, home health agency) may be called upon to answer for the nurse's conduct as well. This concept of derivative liability is termed vicarious liability (i.e., "let the master speak for its servant"). Legally, an employer may be held responsible for the negligent acts of its employee or agent but generally not those of an independent contractor. The key element of an employment relationship is the extent of control the employer exercises over the nurse (i.e., does the employer control not only the work done but also the manner in which it is done?) (Jenkins, 1994). Supervision of the maternal-child nurse usually implies the right to control, which is generally sufficient to establish the employer-employee relationship. The employer can be found liable when the nurse employee's act or omission (which gives rise to the claim) occurred within the course and scope of employment. For instance, a hospital may be found liable for the nurse's professional negligence based upon the inappropriate manner in which she gave a patient injection. However, the hospital is not liable when the nurse causes an automobile accident while she is away from the hospital on lunch break.

Apart from the hospital's liability arising out of acts or omissions of its employees, a hospital can be found independently negligent under the doctrine of hospital corporate negligence. This theory of negligence includes a hospital's duty to screen, select, and retain only qualified and competent staff

(*Bleiler v. Bodnar,* 1985; *Darling v. Charleston Community Memorial Hospital,* 1966). A hospital may be found liable for hiring an inadequately trained nurse to work in the newborn nursery. A hospital may also be found individually negligent for not having a supervising nurse specially trained and capable of determining if an emergency exists warranting a call to a physician (*Northern Trust Co. v. Louis A. Weiss Memorial Hospital,* 1986).

Duty to the Profession In the interest of the health, safety, and welfare of the public, the state exercises its regulatory power over the practice of nursing through the state board of nursing. In every state, the lawful practice of professional nursing requires a valid nursing license, which bestows on the nurse the right to practice her profession. Nursing licenses are issued by the board of nursing, which has the power to modify and enforce the requirements for licensure.

The board can take action against the nurse's license by means of the grievance procedure, an administrative rather than a court proceeding. The board has the power to revoke, suspend, or limit the nurse's license to practice upon *proof* that the nurse has acted inconsistently with the standards of nursing practice. Action against a nurse's license is justified for: (a) negligent practice, (b) reckless practice, (c) physical or mental disabilities, (d) false procurement of a license to practice, (e) ethical violations, and (f) criminal conduct.

Standard of Care

The standard of care within which the maternal-child nurse must practice is defined in numerous ways (i.e., national, state, local, and institutional) and is based on factors such as the practice setting or available equipment. The standard of care is established by defining what the reasonably prudent practitioner would do in the same or similar circumstance. The maternal-child nurse will be held to the standard of care of a nurse practicing in that particular specialty service (*Ewing v. Aubert,* 1988). Professional care providers must be aware that the standards of care for a specialty area are constantly changing through research and technology. A professional requirement exists to remain competent and continually updated on the standards of care and practice (ANA, 1991).

National

Previously, the health care community was small, and available resources were limited. In today's mobile society, with advances in telecommunications, the maternal-child nursing standard of care is generally considered a national standard. In other words, the standard of practice is the same no matter where in the United States the maternal-child nurse is practicing. This standard is national because most accredited schools have a similar core curriculum and use the same textbooks. In addition, nurses throughout the country read the same journals and attend similar continuing education forums.

In areas of specialty practice such as maternal-child nursing, standards of practice are established by the practitioner's peer associations (see Chapter 6). Association publications offer recommendations and general guidelines rather than strict rules of practice and are intended to be adapted to the specific practice situation. However, expert witnesses frequently rely on these same recommendations and guidelines as establishing the standard of care in a professional negligence case.

State

The standard of practice is further defined by each state's nurse practice act. The nurse practice act, mandated by the state's legislature, creates a board of nursing to regulate nursing conduct (including licensing, discipline, and parameters of practice). Generally, the nurse practice act outlines the activities within the scope of practice for a given level of nurse (i.e., licensed practical/vocational nurses, registered nurses, and advanced practice nurses). For example, most nurse practice acts require a registered nurse to perform an assessment and formulate a nursing diagnosis based on the data collected on each of her patients. The nurse may not delegate this nursing action to any other assistive personnel who are unqualified to perform a task for which a license is required (ANA, 1994b). For example, measuring the vital signs of a patient in labor may be within the scope of a licensed practical nurse or vocational nurse (LPN/LVN), but performing a sterile vaginal examination is not. In addition, some states have established perinatal care councils and regional boards to articulate and disseminate appropriate standards of care for the maternal-child nurse.

Local and Institutional

The standard of care is also delineated in a hospital's policies, procedures, and protocols. As outlined in a hospital protocol, a particular method of treatment may be more complete than that required by the standard of care. However, once such a protocol has been approved by hospital personnel and applicable practice committees within the hospital, a presumption is created that the protocol is the standard of care that should be followed, at least within that particular hospital. In order for a hospital policy, procedure, or protocol to be considered the standard of care, it must reflect the national and state standard of care. Policies, procedures, and protocols must also: (a) be periodically updated and dated (JCAHO, 1995), (b) be prepared by a qualified committee with the collaboration of physicians and nurses who practice in the area, (c) refer to current professional literature, (d) be archived by the hospital for the length of liability, and (e) be accessible and familiar to the staff.

Standards of care are not limited to one course of treatment. Where alternative methods of treatment exist, the nurse may use her best judgment in determining the appropriate course of treatment. Generally, a nurse is not liable, under the law, for a mistake in judgment or an unfortunate outcome, as long as the nurse exercises reasonable care in making that judgment.

The maternal-child nurse's deviation from the usual and customary standard of care for a nurse practicing in the same specialty under the same or similar circumstances can be considered professional negligence. Proving that the nurse deviated from the standard of care generally requires a nurse expert to articulate what that standard of care is. An expert nursing opinion requires: (a) expertise in the area of maternal-child nursing based upon clinical experience in the specialty, (b) knowledge of the applicable professional literature, and (c) knowledge of the standards set forth at the national, state, local, and institutional levels. In addition, the standards referenced must have been applicable at the time the incident occurred.

Causation

Before a maternal-child nurse specialist can be found liable for professional negligence, the plaintiff (the patient's attorney) must prove that the negligent act or failure to act actually caused the patient harm. A nurse cannot be held responsible for the patient's damages if the damages sustained were not the result of the act of negligence forming the basis for the claim. For instance, even though a labor and delivery nurse did not recognize the late decelerations on the fetal monitor and report her findings to the physician, the nurse should not be found liable in a civil action for professional negligence if the child is born without complication or if it can be shown that the injury occurred prior to the labor. Causation must be established to a reasonable degree of medical probability or certainty (defined as greater than 50%) by an expert witness who is competent and qualified to render such opinion (usually a physician or an advanced practice nurse).

Potential Liability Within Each Step of the Nursing Process

The practice of professional nursing encompasses the performance of activities within the scope of nursing practice, including independent, interdependent, and dependent functions. Professional nursing includes the prevention, diagnosis, and treatment of diseases, injuries, and conditions within the parameters of the nurse practice act and the standard of care. The nurse carries out her duties by using the nursing process. The nursing process is premised on systematic, concurrent, and recurrent (a) patient assessment, (b) nursing diagnosis, (c) planning of nursing care, (d) implementation of the care plan, and (e) evaluation. Each step in the process is designed to meet the needs of the patient, and opportunity for error exists at each step of the nursing process (Table 4-1).

Assessment

The maternal-child nurse specialist must collect data about the status of the health of the patient. A nurse must use the skills and knowledge within the scope of her practice to evaluate the patient and has a duty to observe signs,

Table 4-1 Most Common Allegations in Nursing Malpractice

Nursing Process	Nursing Errors
Assessment	Failure to take appropriate steps to gather information Failure to recognize the significance of information gathered Failure to communicate/document
Diagnosis	Failure to identify the correct nursing diagnosis Overdiagnosis or diagnosis of a nonexistent health care problem
Plan	Incomplete care—omission Inappropriate commission of care
Implementation	Patient identification Patient safety (e.g., falls, unsafe environment, failure to follow policy/protocol) Failure to respond to patient/family request/input Medication errors Equipment failure
Evaluation	Failure to review, revise, and alter the plan of care

symptoms, and changes in the condition of the patient and to report to appropriate persons and document accordingly. Data are obtained by interview, examination, observation, and review of the medical records of the patient. Errors in this phase of the nursing process include: (a) failure to take appropriate steps to gather information, (b) failure to recognize the significance of the information that is gathered, and (c) failure to communicate or document.

Failure to Take Appropriate Steps to Gather Information In assessing patients, maternal-child nurses use numerous techniques and various tools to gather relevant data and information. They collect subjective data by interviewing patients, reviewing history (e.g., antenatal, perinatal, medical, psychosocial), and asking questions related to the current condition. When dealing with a newborn, infant, or child, the nurse cannot obtain subjective data directly from the patient. Because the parent is the nearest and most reliable source of subjective information about the child, professionals must interview, question, and heed parental observations and assessments (Whaley & Wong, 1995). Since the subjective data from pregnant women about fetal movement are reliable data regarding fetal well-being, professionals should inquire about and follow up on any information given by the mother (see Chapter 8).

When collecting objective data from mothers and children, nurses use the physical assessment skills of inspection, palpation, percussion, and auscultation. Maternal-child nurses also use specialized assessment technology (e.g., internal and external fetal monitors and invasive and noninvasive neonatal-pediatric monitors). Assessment and interpretation of laboratory data is a nursing responsibility that includes: (a) understanding normal lab values, (b) determining if lab results are normal or abnormal, (c) determining if immediate notification of the physician is necessary, (d) knowing what intervention is required by the standard of nursing and medical care, and (e) advocating for appropriate intervention (NAACOG, 1991).

Unlike the verbal adult, the nonverbal infant or child communicates needs primarily through behavioral clues. Through objective observations and evaluations, the neonatal-pediatric care provider interprets this behavior to gather information about the condition of the infant or child (Lepley, Gardner, & Lubchenco, 1993). The licensed professional nurse who is educated and skilled in physical assessment and whose scope of practice includes initial and ongoing assessment is the preferred nursing care provider for the neonate in a level I, II, or III nursery (NAACOG, 1990). Maternal-child nurses must not delegate to other care providers (e.g., LPNs/LVNs or unlicensed assistive personnel—UAPs) any task that "requires professional nursing knowledge, judgment, or skill" (ANA, 1994b, p. 12). Delegation of assessment tasks must include supervision but does not and must not include total responsibility for patient assessment (ANA, 1994b; NAACOG, 1990, 1991). In the field of maternal-child nursing, assigning LPNs/LVNs or UAPs to take vital signs and perform physical assessments may be illegal (i.e., in violation of state nurse practice acts) as well as unethical (i.e., in violation of nursing code of ethics) (ANA 1985) unless those assessments are corroborated by a registered nurse (ANA 1994).

Assessing psychosocial concerns and developmental factors of the individual child and family is essential in predicting patient and family responses and planning interventions to achieve specific goals. To plan effective care, the nurse must consider the influence of society, culture, and developmental tasks upon the child and family. Information about previous coping strategies and current support systems provides clues in identifying pertinent psychosocial nursing diagnoses. Assessment of patient and family knowledge about health care problems is crucial in assessing learning needs for assumption of individual and family care.

The frequency of patient assessment is legally defined by the physician's orders; the institution's policies, procedures, and protocols; and the national standard of care. If a previous assessment is reliable, properly communicated, and not outdated, the nurse does not need to reassess. However, if the nurse suspects an earlier assessment is incomplete, inaccurate, or outdated because the patient's condition has changed, a reassessment is necessary. Deterioration of a patient's condition will give rise to the question of whether more frequent assessment by the nurse could have prevented this deterioration. Neither physician orders nor institution protocols will protect a nurse from liability when reasonable, professional nursing judgment would require more frequent assessment (ANA, 1985; *Darling v. Charleston Community Memorial Hospital*, 1966; *Lunsford v. Board of Nurse Examiners*, 1983). Some patients (e.g., fetuses during second-stage of labor; sick neonates; nonverbal pediatric patients at risk for apnea, seizures, and vomiting and aspiration; and children receiving pain medications) require continuous rather than intermittent observation.

Failure to Recognize the Significance of Gathered Information Specialized assessment technology is only one means of assessing the overall patient status, and the data obtained is only as good as the professional who interprets it. Many nurses working in obstetrics "lack skills in pattern recognition, interpretation of ominous fetal tracings, and basic electronic fetal monitoring concepts" (McRae, 1993, p. 419). The licensed professional nurse has a responsibility to understand the significance of the gathered information within the limits of ordinary prudent nursing knowledge. In the age of specialization and technology, nurses with expertise in one area of specialized nursing are not qualified to perform skills in another specialized area of nursing (see Chapter 3). Yet in many institutions nurses are often expected to "cross-train" and "float" to any area of the hospital where critical staffing needs exist. This practice increases the risks of legal liability for both the individual nurse and the institution as employer, since both share the responsibility and accountability to ensure safe, quality nursing care (ANA, 1985; Florida Nurses Association, 1989; Massachusetts Nurses Association, 1983). Practicing out of one's area of specialization and expertise increases the risks of not understanding the significance of assessment data, failing to make timely observations, and failing to respond appropriately to the assessment data. Assessment errors also include failure to compare current to previous data to detect changes and failure to identify the significance of these changes.

Failure to Communicate Steps Taken A part of patient assessment is the responsibility to communicate information, both orally and in writing. All professionals involved in the patient's care must be told pertinent data that the nurse obtains when conducting the admission interview, when monitoring patient status, and when assuming all or part of patient care. For example, at change of shift, an oral report from nurse to nurse, either in person or tape recorded, must cover all pertinent changes in patient status that the new nurse must know to assume and continue care. When patients are transferred to another unit, home care agency, or another health care institution, oral as well as written communication is essential. Failure to notify the physician in a timely manner is a critical omission, a breach of the nurse's duty to the patient, in liability cases (McMullen, 1990). The professional nurse is expected to distinguish normal from abnormal data to determine whether nursing care is a sufficient intervention or whether medical care is required. The nurse is then responsible for timely notification of the physician. If the nurse decides that medical care is needed, she must then decide how quickly it is needed (e.g., in 5 minutes or 5 hours). The nurse not only has a duty to notify the physician promptly but must also intervene if physician action is not prompt enough.

The nurse's failure to report is not excused by her belief that the physician is not likely to respond. Repeated physician notification is more likely to result in action than a single notification that is discounted with comments such as, "Let's watch the patient; I'll see him in the morning" or "He was OK when I saw him this morning." However, the need not to waste valuable nursing time and to intervene in a timely manner poses limits on repeated physician notification. If a professional nurse is concerned enough about the patient's condition to notify a physician, she should know: (a) what medical intervention she is seeking, (b) how soon the medical intervention must be obtained, and (c) what institutional chain of command to follow to obtain care for the patient (*Darling v. Charleston Community Memorial Hospital,* 1966).

The maternal-child nurse's duty to the patient includes maintaining accurate records: written documentation of the patient's condition, course of treatment, and response to treatment. Documentation standards are derived from federal, state, peer association, and institutional policies and procedures. The primary purpose of patient records is to communicate information about a patient's status among health care providers. Patient records also become primary evidence in defense of a claim arising from allegations of professional negligence or inappropriate care. The maternal-child nurse's charting should always include more rather than less information and be complete and accurate. See Charting Tips box on p. 38.

Nursing Diagnosis

The North American Nursing Diagnosis Association (NANDA), a group of professional nurses who identify and research nursing diagnostic labels, has formulated a taxonomy of nursing diagnoses that professional nurses are educationally and legally competent to treat. NANDA meets every 2 years to add new diagnoses and refine the taxonomy; nursing diagnoses currently approved by NANDA are listed in Appendix A.

Nursing diagnosis is the identification of actual or potential human response to health problems that the professional nurse is educated, licensed, and legally responsible and accountable to treat (independently or in collaboration with other health care providers). The nurse practice acts in most states require the licensed professional nurse to formulate nursing diagnoses for the patient. Various state boards of nursing have developed specific definitions for nursing diagnoses. For example, the Colorado Nurse Practice Act defines nursing diagnosis as "the use of professional nursing knowledge and skill in the identification of, and discrimination between, physical and psychological signs and symptoms to arrive at a conclusion that a condition exists for which nursing care is indicated or for which referral to appropriate medical or community resources is required" (Colorado Nurse Practice Act, C.R.S. Section 12-38-103(5)).

The professional nurse is responsible for the nursing and not the medical diagnoses of the patient (Table 4-2). Because the medical diagnosis identifies the disease and the nursing diagnosis identifies the patient's response, the medical and nursing diagnosis must be congruent to facilitate optimal patient care.

The maternal-child nurse specialist is obligated to collect and analyze the facts regarding the patient's condition in order to determine the nursing diagnoses and plan of care. As the patient's condition changes, nursing diagnoses are re-evaluated and modified. Nursing diagnoses should be congruent with the professional diagnoses of other health care providers. When nursing diagnosis is inadequate or inaccurate, it is impossible to develop a relevant care plan that includes measurable goals, actions, and evaluations. Diagnostic errors include failure to identify the correct nursing diagnosis and

Charting Tips

- Record only factual information (what is seen, heard, felt, or done).
- Notes should be legible, concise, and accurate.
- Notes should be dated, timed, and signed.
- Use consecutive lines without spaces between.
- Use only acceptable institutional abbreviations.
- Chart in black ink.
- Chart all assessments, interventions, and responses.
- Note orders completed.
- Document all treatments, how patient tolerated them, and results.
- Document lack of treatment and reason why not done.
- Chart all physician visits and examinations.
- Note all inquiries with physicians (when, what was told, and response).
- If physician does not respond or cannot be reached, institute and document the chain of command.
- If a deviation in practice occurs, note what happened and why.
- Do not chart judgmental or personal remarks regarding the patient or other care providers.
- Note admission time, mode, and condition.
- Chart all transfers, mode, and patient's condition.
- Document discharge teaching done and patient's understanding and response.
- Chart discharge instructions given, mode of instruction, and condition on discharge.
- When charting pain, describe location, severity, accompanying factors, interventions, and accompanying response.
- Medications: document name, route, site, time, response, and adverse reactions.
- If abnormal finding, describe and note action taken and chart response to that action.
- Check hospital policy for frequency of charting.
- Don't chart for anyone else.
- Read all notes before cosigning.
- Telephone orders must be appropriately written (i.e., T.O., V.O.) and signed.
- Errors: draw a single line through, date, time, and initial.
- Addenda: date, time, and sign.
- Never remove anything from the chart.

overdiagnosis or diagnosis of a nonexistent health care problem (Potter & Perry, 1993).

Plan

A nursing care plan is the collaborative establishment of patient goals and outcomes, based upon the nursing assessment and diagnosis, to maximize the patient's functional capacity. Goals must be prioritized, realistic, and col-

Table 4-2 Common Goal: Preservation and Restoration of Health

	Nursing Diagnosis	Medical Diagnosis
Definition	Identification of actual or potential human response to health problems	Identification of a disease condition based on evaluation of history, signs and symptoms, and laboratory data
Focus	"Care": psychosocial orientation with the goal of reaching maximum level of function and wellness	"Cure": physical disease
Obstetrical Example	Alteration in tissue perfusion: uterine related to blood loss secondary to placenta previa	Placenta previa
Neonatal Example	Ineffective gaseous exchange related to prematurity	Respiratory distress syndrome
Pediatric Example	Ineffective airway clearance related to airway edema and increased production of mucus	Asthma

laboratively planned with the client and family. The plan should include: (a) independent, interdependent, and dependent nursing actions, (b) methods for carrying out physician orders, and (c) educational needs of the patient and family. The care plan must include observable, measurable, mutual, and realistic evaluation criteria along with a timetable for ongoing evaluation of interventions.

Failure to develop comprehensive, individualized, and specific care plans results in incomplete patient care. For the maternal-child nurse specialist, this failure may lead to acts of omission in the implementation or evaluation phase of the nursing process. An incomplete plan may result in an inappropriate commission of patient care.

For those licensed professional nurses who supervise others (i.e., UAPs, LPNs/LVNs, and other RNs) planning decisions regarding allocation of staff time may result in liability (ANA, 1985). The needs of the patient, as outlined in the nursing care plan, must be met by a care provider with the education and skill to provide safe care (ANA, 1985; Florida Nurses Association, 1989; Massachusetts Nurses Association, 1983). Assignment of unqualified staff leading to injury or harm to the patient results in liability for the supervising nurse as well as the institution as her employer (Florida Nurses Association, 1989; Massachusetts Nurses Association, 1983).

Implementation

Implementation is the carrying out of the plan of care. Actions carried out by the nurse should be consistent with the plan of care. Implementation of the care plan by the licensed professional nurse requires affirmative action (i.e., the nurse owes a duty to the patient to take the proper steps to provide care). Affirmative action requires the nurse to take positive, even assertive, steps if she assesses a deterioration in the patient's condition. The legal precedent establishing the duty of nurses to take affirmative action was set in the 1960s.

In the Darling case (1966) nurses were found liable for failing to advocate for the patient by using the chain of command to ensure that the patient received proper medical care for a "too-tight" cast.

The scope of professional nursing practice encompasses independent, interdependent, and dependent functions and actions (Table 4-3). Providing a safe physical environment, whether in the hospital, clinic, or home, is one example of an independent nursing function. Collaboratively written protocols delineating interdependent nursing practice must be reviewed, revised, and updated according to the recommended schedule of accrediting agencies (e.g., JCAHO, State Board of Nursing). Regardless of whether the nurse is a staff nurse or an advanced nurse practitioner (i.e., certified nurse-midwife, nurse practitioner, or clinical nurse specialist), each time the nurse enacts an interdependent protocol, she must record the date, time, and reason for using the protocol and an evaluation of the patient's response.

Carrying out physician orders is a dependent nursing action. However, the physician's order does not excuse the nurse from the duty to ensure proper care for patient safety (*Bulala v. Boyd*, 1990). The nurse has a duty to interpret and carry out physician orders safely and properly. To fulfill this duty, the nurse needs knowledge and information about the drugs, treatments, and procedures ordered by the physician. The nurse may carry out physician orders that are within her scope of practice.

Although the nurse has a legal duty to carry out physician orders, she has no legal duty to carry out orders that are: (a) illegible, (b) erroneous or ambiguous, or (c) second hand. If a handwritten order is unreadable, the nurse should not guess at its content and meaning. An illegible order must be clarified and rewritten. An ambiguous, unreasonable, or erroneous physician order requires nursing action: clarification from the physician who wrote the order. An obviously erroneous order must be questioned, clarified, or challenged by the licensed professional nurse in her capacity as an advocate for the patient (ANA, 1985). If the ordering physician is unresponsive to

Table 4-3 Scope of Professional Nursing Practice

Functions/Actions	Definition
Independent	Aspects of nursing practice contained in state nurse practice acts that require no supervision or direction. Formulation of nursing diagnosis and application of the nursing process are independent nursing functions required by statute of the licensed professional nurse.
Interdependent	Aspects of nursing practice performed in collaboration with other health care professionals. Collaboratively written institutional protocols delineate the conditions and treatments the nurse is permitted to administer.
Dependent	Aspects of nursing practice dependent on the written order of another professional. The physician prescribes medications; the nurse administers the prescribed medication. The nurse also is responsible for independent actions: (a) knowing the proper medication, dosage, and route, (b) safe administration, (c) monitoring effects and adverse responses, and (d) advocating for the patient regarding proper medication, dosage, route.

the nurse's concern or if the nurse is not satisfied after discussion with the physician, she has a duty to invoke the chain of command (determined by institutional policy) to obtain other action. Pending review, the nurse has the right and responsibility to decline to carry out the order, notify the physician, and document the refusal and other actions taken in the patient's record. As the patient's advocate, the nurse has a duty to the patient that cannot be superseded by hospital policy or physician's order (ANA, 1985; *Lunsford v. Board of Nurse Examiners,* 1983).

The nurse has no duty to follow an order that was correctly written but becomes erroneous because of a change in the patient's condition. There is no duty to carry out second-hand orders (*Mahmoodian v. United Hospital Center,* 1991). Orders should be received directly from the patient's physician. Orders written by advance practice nurses or physician assistants must be delineated in advance-practice protocols. The nurse has no duty to carry out orders written by mid-level practitioners that are beyond the scope of written, collaboratively developed protocols.

Verbal orders are an efficient method of relaying instructions but are fraught with additional risks for the nurse and the institution. The nurse should know and adhere strictly to institutional policy on verbal and written orders. Safeguards for accepting verbal orders include: (a) the order is clear and understood, (b) the nurse requests immediate clarification for questions or concerns, (c) the nurse repeats verbal order to physician, (d) the nurse documents the order, including date, time, and form of communication as soon as possible, and (e) the nurse refuses to accept verbal orders from a third party (Carson, 1994).

Implementation of nursing care is carried out by nursing care personnel (i.e., advanced practice nurses, staff nurses, LPNs, LVNs, UAPs) in a nursing care delivery system (Table 4-4). Changes in the health care environment (e.g., health care reform, managed care, outpatient versus inpatient services) have resulted in hospital redesign and restructuring to cut labor costs. Redesigned work environments rely more on lower-paid UAPs. UAPs are defined by ANA as "individuals who are trained to function in an assistive role to the registered professional nurse in the provision of patient/client care activities as delegated by and under the supervision of the registered professional nurse" (ANA, 1994b, p. 2). Since the UAP has no authorization for practice as defined by the state nurse practice acts, only professional and practical nurses have legal scope of practice and authority to perform nursing actions. Responsibility lies with the nursing profession and the individual nurse "to control the training, practice, and utilization of UAPs involved in the provision of direct patient care" (ANA, 1994b, p. 4). Institutional policies about the utilization of UAPs must conform to: (a) minimum standards and scope of nursing practice defined by state nurse practice acts, and (b) professional standards of practice established by professional nursing organizations, e.g., *Code for Nurses* (ANA, 1985), *Standards of Clinical Nursing Practice* (ANA, 1991), *Nurse Providers of Neonatal Care* (NAACOG, 1990), *Registered Professional Nurses and Unlicensed Assistive Personnel* (ANA, 1994b).

Table 4-4 Nursing Care Delivery System

Type	Definition	Advantages	Disadvantages
Functional nursing system	Patient care divided into series of tasks that are delegated to lowest level of personnel having skill and competence to complete task.	Uses cheaper, less skilled personnel*	Poor continuity of care because numerous personnel perform specific tasks on all patients on the unit. Emphasis on tasks rather than patient needs. Professional nursing time used in delegating, coordinating, and communicating among personnel and patient care tasks rather than in direct patient care.
Team nursing system	Small group of personnel supervised by a licensed professional nurse provides care for a number of patients.	Uses cheaper, less skilled personnel*	Fragmented care because personnel provide individual patient care (rather than tasks) over one shift. Professional nursing time used in delegating care, coordinating team efforts, planning time for team conferences, and updating care plans.
Total patient care	A caseload nursing system in which a nurse is responsible for complete care of a number of patients throughout a shift.	Care totally individualized because a single nurse provides all aspects of care. Professional nursing time used in direct care, coordination of care with other professionals, and updating of the care plan. No delegation; individual nurse gives care and is responsible for care plan.	Poor continuity of care if nurses are not assigned to the same patients each shift. All professional nursing staff†
Primary nursing system	Primary nurse responsible for all aspects of patient care (24 hours/day from admission o discharge). Associate nurse assumes responsibility for care when primary nurse is off duty.	Primary nurse formulates care plan, delivers direct patient care, delegates care to associate nurses, and coordinates activities to ensure continuity of care.	Poor continuity of care if activities are not delegated, communicated, and coordinated between primary and associate nurses. All professional nursing staff†

*Seen as an advantage by administration interested in cost containment
†Seen as a disadvantage by administration interested in cost containment who do not understand that the research data shows the following: (a) Hospitals employing fewer RNs have longer lengths of stay associated with poor patient monitoring, omissions or delays in treatments, and an increase in medication errors and accidents. (b) Mortality rates rise with a reduction in quality of nursing care and ratio of RNs to all nursing staff. (c) Patient satisfaction is correlated with increased ratio of RNs on intensive and critical care units and patient care models such as case management, collaborative practice, and decentralized management. (d) Higher job satisfaction results in lower absenteeism and turnover rates as well as better patient outcomes. (e) Skill mix of providers is correlated with shorter patient stay, lower morbidity, fewer complications, and higher patient satisfaction. Lewin-VHI, Inc. (1995). *The nursing report card for acute care.* Washington, DC: American Nurses Association.

Although a nurse may delegate the performance of certain tasks in the patient's care plan, she may not delegate legal accountability or responsibility to UAPs (Table 4-5). The task being delegated by the nurse must: (a) be within her scope of practice, (b) be able to be properly and safely performed by the delegatee (as predetermined before delegation by the nurse), (c) not involve substantial risk of harm to the patient. The nurse is responsible for determining and providing an appropriate level of supervision. A licensed professional nurse may not delegate a task that requires nursing judgment (Table 4-6). The nurse may delegate the administration of medications only to a provider authorized to administer medications. Physical assessment of a child may not be delegated to a UAP when the state nurse practice act prohibits LPNs/LVNs from doing total body physical assessment (Colorado State Board of Nursing, 1990–91). Errors in the implementation of the nursing care plan often occur in these areas: (a) patient identification, (b) patient safety, (c) medication errors, and (d) equipment failures. Failure to check patient identification has resulted in administration of the wrong medication and the wrong blood, and the discharge of families with the wrong newborn. The nurse and institution have a duty to provide a safe environment for all patients, especially minors. Patient falls (e.g., a newborn who fell from weight scales; a 19-month-old who climbed over the bed rails, fell on his head, went into seizure, developed obstructive hydrocephalus, and had a ventriculoperitoneal shunt inserted; a sedated adult who fell from bed with the siderails up) result in institutional and professional liability. Improper positioning (as in a 1982 Minnesota case where an RN was charged with

Table 4-5 Roles and Responsibilities of Registered Nurses Toward Unlicensed Assistive Personnel

Concept	Definition	Comments
Supervision	Directing, guiding, and influencing the outcome of an individual's performance of an activity.	Types: **Onsite:** supervisor is physically present or immediately available while activity is being performed. **Offsite:** direction provided through written/verbal communication. Supervisor able to control activity: stop inappropriate act, review measures taken, regain control, and complete activity.
Delegation	Transfer of responsibility for performance of an activity from one individual to another, with the former retaining accountability for the outcome.	Delegator (RN) retains accountability for the process and outcome of the task. RN uses professional judgment in deciding which patient care task may be delegated, to whom, and under what circumstances. Professional judgment is framed by state nurse practice act and national standards of nursing. Institutional policies cannot contradict state law.
Assignment	Downward or lateral transfer of both responsibility and accountability of an activity from one individual to another. Transfer must be made from an individual with similar skill, knowledge, and judgment and must involve tasks or activities within the individual's legal or regulatory scope of practice.	Responsibility and accountability are transferred. Assignment cannot occur with UAPs.

Adapted from: American Nurses Association (1994). *Registered nurses and unlicensed assistive personnel.* Washington, D.C.: Author, pp. 9–15. Adapted with permission.

Table 4-6 Nursing Actions Not to Be Delegated

Nursing Process	Comments
Assessment	Initial and any subsequent assessment that requires professional nursing knowledge, judgment*, and skill.
Diagnosis	Nursing diagnosis and delineation of nursing goals.
Plan	Development of nursing plan of care.
Implementation	An intervention that requires professional nursing knowledge, judgment*, and skill.
Evaluation	Of the patient's progress or lack of progress in relation to the nursing care plan.

*Nursing judgment is the intellectual process that a licensed professional nurse utilizes in forming an opinion and reaching a conclusion by analyzing the ata.

From: American Nurses Association (1994). *Registered nurses and unlicensed assistive personnel.* Washington, D.C.: Author, p. 12. Reprinted with permission.

improperly positioning a neonate for a spinal puncture that resulted in a cardiorespiratory arrest leading to a semicomatose state) also results in litigation. Heightened concern about infant abduction has resulted in installation of elaborate security systems on MCN units as well as proactive preventive staff education (Beachy & Deacon, 1991; Johnston, 1989; Mead Johnson Laboratories, 1991; Rabun, 1991; Spadt & Sensenig, 1990; Webster, 1987). Unfortunately, prevention of sexual assault of older children in hospitals has not received the same proactive, preventive approach.

Medication Errors A medication error is defined as "a deviation from the physician's medication order as written on the patient's chart" (Allan & Barker, 1990, p. 555). The rate of medication errors is difficult to determine but is estimated to be one per patient per hospital day (Allan & Barker, 1990). The boxes on page 45 list types of medication errors and common causes of medication errors. The American Society of Hospital Pharmacists (ASHP) has developed 59 recommendations for preventing medication errors by (a) organizations/departments, (b) prescribers, (c) pharmacists, (d) nurses, and (e) patients and personal caregivers. See the box on page 46 for recommendations for nurses.

Product Liability Manufacturers of medical devices are regulated by the United States Food and Drug Administration (FDA) to provide safe, quality products (Food and Drug Administration, 1987). The Safe Medical Devices Act of 1990 extends the FDA's regulatory control from preproduction and quality assurance to postmarket surveillance (Koehler, 1993). The act requires facilities that use devices (e.g., hospitals, nursing homes, outpatient centers) to advise the FDA and the manufacturer whenever there is reasonable suspicion that a medical device has caused or contributed to serious injury, illness, or patient death. Since 82% of all device-related incidents are discovered by nurses and physicians, employing institutions must develop policies and procedures for employees regarding how to report problems with devices and what to report (Koehler, 1993). The FDA tabulates and analyzes these

Types of Medication Errors

- Prescribing error
- Omission error
- Wrong time error
- Unauthorized drug error
- Improper dose error
- Wrong dosage form error
- Wrong drug preparation error
- Wrong administration-technique error
- Deteriorated drug error
- Monitoring error
- Compliance error
- Other

From: American Society of Hospital Pharmacists (1993). ASHP guidelines on preventing medication error in hospitals, *American Journal of Hospital Pharmacy, 50,* p. 306. Reprinted with permission.

Common Causes of Medication Errors

- Ambiguous strength designation on labels or in packaging
- Drug product nomenclature (look-alike or sound-alike names, use of lettered or numbered prefixes and suffixes in drug names)
- Equipment failure or malfunction
- Illegible handwriting
- Improper transcription
- Inaccurate dosage calculation
- Inadequately trained personnel
- Inappropriate abbreviations used in prescribing
- Labeling errors
- Excessive workload
- Lapses in individual performance
- Medication unavailable

From: American Society of Hospital Pharmacists (1993). ASHP guidelines on preventing medication error in hospitals, *American Journal of Hospital Pharmacy, 50,* p. 307. Reprinted with permission.

reports, and protects the public's health and safety by publishing warnings, and removing defective devices from the market.

Just as professionals are insured by professional liability insurance, manufacturers of medical devices are insured by product liability insurance. However, product liability protection does not apply to: (a) the distribution

Recommendations for Nurses for Preventing Medication Errors

- Become familiar with system for ordering and using medications.
- Review medications for desired patient outcomes, therapeutic duplications, and possible drug interactions. Access adequate drug information.
- Verify drug orders prior to administration; compare order to dispensed medication; check identity and integrity of drug.
- Verify patient identity prior to and observe patient after the administration of medication.
- Administer at scheduled times; do not remove from packaging or remove label until time of administration; document administration as soon as it is completed.
- Dosage calculations, flow rates, and mathematical calculations should be checked by a second professional.
- Do not circumvent drug distribution system (i.e., "borrow").
- Verify medication order when large volume or number of dosage units is needed for a single dose.
- Understand medication administration devices, their operation, and potential for error.
- Communicate with patients and caregivers regarding their understanding, observations, or special precautions that are indicated.
- Listen to patient and family objections regarding a drug to be administered; double-check medication order and product dispensed prior to administration.

Adapted from: American Society of Hospital Pharmacists (1993). ASHP guidelines on preventing medication error in hospitals, *American Journal of Hospital Pharmacy, 50,* pp. 310–311. Adapted with permission.

or sale of products for purposes unauthorized by the manufacturer, (b) a change made in the condition of any product if that change is not authorized by the manufacturer, (c) the relabeling of a product by a third party not authorized to do so by the manufacturer, (d) the use of the product as a container, part, or ingredient of anything else not authorized by the manufacturer, and (e) items rented to others, which are no longer considered the manufacturer's. Manufacturers and distributors of medical equipment can be found liable under strict or products liability if they fail to provide adequate warnings or if the products are found to be unreasonably dangerous. Once the manufacturer has provided instructions and warnings, the legal burden shifts to the professional care provider to follow the manufacturer's directions, to use the equipment for its intended use, and to avoid altering the device (FDA, 1987; Health Industry Manufacturer's Association, 1984).

The maternal child nurse may be responsible for errors that result from equipment failure. A nurse may be held responsible when errors occur because she is unfamiliar with the equipment or uses the equipment incorrectly. If the nurse uses equipment that is obviously unfit for its intended use (e.g., a thermometer with a broken tip; a gavage or suction tube with a melted, sharp tip), she violates the standard of nursing practice to provide a safe environment (ANA, 1983, 1991). The nurse is also legally accountable if she continues to use equipment that she knows is malfunctioning or if she has knowledge of a continuing problem and a patient is subsequently injured or harmed by its use.

In its position statement on the reuse and single use of medical devices, the Health Industry Manufacturer's Association (HIMA) raises quality assurance concerns regarding reuse and cites numerous case reports of patient harm resulting from reuse (HIMA, 1984). The position statement identifies 11 issues that health care institutions and professionals should consider and resolve before reusing and reprocessing single-use devices. Disregarding a manufacturer's label can have serious consequences, since both the institution and the individual professional bears financial responsibility for injury and harm (FDA, 1987; HIMA, 1984).

To prevent the spread of serious infection, single-use devices and intimate care devices (e.g., trainer devices for nursing mothers) should not be reused (e.g., rented, loaned, or shared by patients) (Gardner, O'Donnell, & Weisman, 1993). Although reuse of single-use equipment by hospitals and care providers is primarily an economic issue, patient safety should be the primary concern. If the hospital or individual practitioner is unable to ensure product quality control (as required by equipment manufacturers), the hospital or practitioner assumes the risks of product liability if harm or injury occurs (FDA, 1987; HIMA, 1984).

Disposable-grade materials (e.g., glass baby bottles, polyethylene and polychloride tubing, single-dose vials) are labeled by the manufacturer as single-use only. Because these devices are not made of durable-grade (i.e., reusable) materials, the manufacturer cannot recommend reuse or resterilization.

In maternal-child care, devices have been used for other than their intended purpose. Use of makeshift pacifiers from bottle nipples has resulted in fatal aspiration (Millunchick & McArtor, 1986). In infants less than 1 year of age, use of honey in formula or on pacifiers or nipples is associated with infant botulism (American Academy of Pediatrics, 1981; Arnon, Midura, Damus, Thompson, Wood, & Chinn, 1979; Centers for Disease Control, 1979). Medicine droppers, syringes with gavage tubes, and rubber ear irrigators are sometimes used and recommended to parents for enticing infants to suckle. All these devices expel fluid via positive pressure into the infant's mouth. This practice is hazardous for two reasons: Fluid is not delivered under the infant's control and thus it can be forced or aspirated into the lungs, and delivery of fluid under pressure fails to elicit oral-motor responses, thereby causing, exacerbating, or continuing aberrant non-nutritive suckling (Avery, 1985). Because these devices are not intended by the manufacturer to foster suckling, the nurse who uses or recommends such devices assumes liability for any resultant injury or harm (FDA, 1987; HIMA, 1984).

Evaluation

The patient's progress or lack of progress toward established goals must be repeatedly evaluated and revised. Evaluation is the comparison of observed results with the outcome criteria (Potter & Perry, 1995). Relief of pain after narcotic injection is a positive evaluation of the effectiveness of the nurse's intervention. A negative evaluation—lack of pain relief—indicates that the intervention was not effective. Because the problem is unresolved, modifications in the plan are needed, and the entire nursing process sequence is reactivated. If nursing interventions are not positively affecting patient outcomes, evaluation directs a change in nursing practice (ANA 1983, 1985, 1991; NAACOG, 1990, 1991). Failure to evaluate the patient's ongoing status prevents the ongoing reactivation of each step of the nursing process.

Conclusion

The maternal-child nurse must master the basic skills and knowledge of her profession and be aware of the scope and limits of her permitted practice. She must realize the duty owed to the patient, public, profession, and employer. She must perform her activities and tasks with at least the care that the ordinary and reasonably prudent nurse would take in the same or similar circumstances. The maternal-child nurse must recognize that she is responsible for her acts and omissions, which render her liable for professional negligence, make her employer liable, subject her to a grievance procedure, and possibly expose her to criminal sanctions. The more the maternal-child nurse knows about her legal responsibilities, the better she can serve both the patient and her profession.

References

Allan, E., & Barker, K. (1990). Fundamentals of medical error research. *American Journal of Hospital Pharmacy, 47*, 555–571.

American Academy of Pediatrics (1981). *Honey and infant botulism.* Washington, D.C.: Author.

American Nurses Association (1983). *Standards of maternal-child nursing practice.* Washington, D.C.: Author.

American Nurses Association (1985). *Code for nurses.* Washington, D.C.: Author.

American Nurses Association (1991). *Standards of clinical nursing practice.* Washington, D.C.: Author.

American Nurses Association (1994a). *Guidelines on reporting illegal, unethical, and incompetent practice.* Washington, D.C.: Author.

American Nurses Association (1994b). *Registered nurses and unlicensed assistive personnel.* Washington, D.C.: Author.

American Society of Hospital Pharmacists (1993). ASHP guidelines on preventing medication errors in hospitals. *American Journal of Hospital Pharmacy, 50*, 305–314.

Arnon, S., Midura, T., Damus, K., Thompson, B., Wood, R., & Chin, J. (1979). Honey and other environmental risk factors for infant botulism. *Journal of Pediatrics, 94,* 331–336.

Avery, J. (1985). *Position statement on use of hazardous aids for breastfeeding.* Athens, TN: Lact-Aid International, Inc.

Beachy, P. & Deacon, J. (1991). Preventing neonatal kidnapping. *Journal of Obstetrical, Gynecological, and Neonatal Nursing, 21,* 12–16.

Bleiler v. Bodnar, 65 N.Y. 2d, 65, 479 N.E. 2d 230, 489 N.Y.S. 2d 885 (1985).

Bulala v. Boyd, 239 Va. 218, 389 S.E. 2d 670 (1990).

Carson, W. (1994). What you should know about physician verbal orders. *The American Nurse, 26* (3), 30–31.

Centers for Disease Control (1979). Honey and infant botulism. *Morbidity and Mortality Weekly Report, 28,* 73–74.

Colorado Nurse Practice Act, C.R.S. Section 12-38-101 et. seq.

Colorado State Board of Nursing (1990–1991). *Annual Report.* Denver. Author.

Darling v. Charleston Community Memorial Hospital, 33 Ill. 2d 326, 211 N.E. 2d 253 (1966).

Ewing v. Aubert, 532 S. 2d 876 (Lo. App. 1988).

Florida Nurses Association (1989). *Guidelines for registered nurses in giving, accepting, or rejecting a work assignment.* Orlando, FL: Author.

Food and Drug Administration (1987). *Compliance policy guidelines: Devices.* Washington, D.C.: author.

Gardner, S., O'Donnell, J., & Weisman, L. (1993). Breastfeeding the sick newborn. In G. Merenstein & S. Gardner (Eds.). *Handbook of neonatal intensive care,* 3rd ed. St. Louis: Mosby-Yearbook.

Health Industry Manufacturer's Association (1984). *The reuse of single-use medical devices.* Washington, D.C.: Author.

Jenkins, S. (1994). The myth of vicarious liability: Impact on the barriers to nurse-midwifery practice. *Journal of Nurse Midwifery, 39* (2), 98–106.

Johnston, J. (1989). Preventing abduction of hospitalized infants. *Pediatric Nursing, 21,* 33–35.

Joint Commission on Accreditation of Healthcare Organizations (1995). *Manual on Hospital Accreditation.* Oakbrook Terrace, IL: Author.

Koehler, C. (1993). Implementing the safe medical devices act. *The American Nurse, 25* (3), 13.

Lepley, C., Gardner, S., & Lubchenco, L. (1993). Initial nursery care. In G. Merenstein & S. Gardner (Eds.). *Handbook of neonatal intensive care,* 3rd ed., St. Louis: Mosby-Yearbook.

Lewin VHI, Inc. (1995). *The Nursing Report Card for Acute Care.* Washington, D.C.: American Nurses Association.

Lunsford v. Board of Nurse Examiners, 648 S.W. 2d 391 (Tex. App. 3 Dist. 1983).

Mahmoodian v. United Hospital Center, 185 W. Va., 59, 404 S.E. 2d 750 (1991) cert. den. 112 S. Ct. 185, 116 L. Ed. 2d. 146 (1991).

Massachusetts Nurses Association (1983). *Mechanisms to support nurses' abilities to exercise their right to accept or reject an assignment.* Canton, MA: Author.

McMullen, P. (1990). Liability in obstetrical nursing, *Nursing Connections, 3* (2), 61–64.

McRae, M. (1993). Litigation, electronic fetal monitoring and the obstetrical nurse. *Journal of Obstetric, Gynecologic, and Neonatal Nursing, 22* (5), 410–419.

Mead Johnson Laboratories (1991). *Safeguarding their tomorrows.* Evansville, IN: Author.

Millunchick, E. & McArtor, R. (1986). Fatal aspiration of a makeshift pacifier. *Pediatrics, 77* (3): 369–370.

Northern Trust Co. v. Louis A. Weiss Memorial Hospital, 143 Ill. App. 3d 479, 493 N.E. 6 (1986).

Nurses Association of the American College of Obstetrics and Gynecology (1990). *Nurse providers of neonatal care.* Washington, D.C.: Author.

Nurses Association of the American College of Obstetrics and Gynecology (1991). *Standards for the nursing care of women and newborns.* Washington, D.C.: Author.

Olsen v. St. Croix Valley Memorial Hospital, 55 Wisc. 2d 628, 201 N.W. 63 (1972).

Pike v. Honsinger, 49 N.E. 760 (N.Y. 1898).

Planned Parenthood of Northwest Indiana, Inc. v. Vines, 543 N.E. 2d 654 (Ind. App. 1989).

Potter, P. & Perry, A. (1995). *Basic nursing theory and practice,* 3rd ed. St. Louis: Mosby-Yearbook.

Prosser, W. (1984). *The law of torts,* 5th ed. St. Paul, MN: West Publishing Co.

Rabun, J. (1991). *Guidelines in preventing abduction of infants from the hospitals.* Arlington, VA: National Center for Missing and Exploited Children.

Renslow v. Mennonite Hospital, 67 Ill. 2d 348, 367 N.E. 2d 1250 (1977).

Schneider v. Little Company, 151 N.W. 587 (Mich. 1915).

Spadt, S. & Sensening, K. (1990). Infant kidnapping: It can happen in any hospital. *American Journal of Maternal Child Nursing, 15,* 52–54.

Teeters v. Currey, 518 S.W. 2d 512 (Tenn. 1974).

Webster, M. (1987). How secure is your hospital? *Nursing Life, 7,* 25–30.

Whaley, L. & Wong, D. (1995). *Nursing care of infants and children,* 5th ed. St. Louis: Mosby-Yearbook.

5

Risk Management and Continuous Quality Improvement

Lynette A. Ament, RN, CNM, MSN, PhD(c)

Risk management is intrinsic to all activities of daily living and is particularly important in maternal-child nursing. The concept of risk management involves making conscious decisions to act in a manner known to decrease risk. In maternal-child nursing, these decisions can be difficult, particularly when they involve vulnerable patients, or when institutions implement technological advances before research data are available to substantiate and validate their use. Nurses must face daily risks that increase with each new technological advancement and change, particularly changes in the mix of personnel (e.g., the use of unlicensed assistive personnel), the increased trend toward advanced nursing practice, and the shift in settings for health care from inpatient to outpatient and home care settings.

History of Risk Management in Health Care

Risk management was not a new concept when the health care industry adopted this stance in the 1970s. The insurance industry originally developed risk management strategies to decrease business-claim losses. The concept evolved in health care in response to a sharp rise in the frequency and severity of malpractice claims. As a result, the insurance industry was unable to predict the frequency of claims or to adequately price malpractice insurance (Korleski, 1990).

In 1971, the Nixon administration conducted one of the first studies to determine the extent of the "malpractice crisis" (Korleski, 1990). This study found that malpractice claims were mainly the result of injuries or adverse responses to medical treatment (Department of Health, Education, and Welfare, 1973). The 1977 American Bar Association Commission on Medical Professional Liability published similar findings and made recommendations to the health care industry to develop ways to prevent avoidable medically related injuries to patients (American Bar Association, 1977).

Other groups also responded to the "malpractice crisis." State legislators enacted laws attempting to restrict the amount of awards and set up arbitration standards. Some laws required risk management in hospitals. In response, the American Hospital Association (AHA) defined risk management as the scientific identification, evaluation, and treatment of financial risk and loss (Dankmyer & Groves, 1977). Also, in 1980 the American Society for Healthcare Risk Management (ASHRM) was formed within the AHA in response to the need for a professional association for the growing numbers of hospital risk managers (Korleski, 1990). In 1985 the US General Accounting Office conducted a study of medical malpractice claims and recommended that risk-management programs be expanded and strengthened (US General Accounting Office, 1987). The "malpractice crisis" continued into the 1990s.

Definitions of Risk Management

Other organizations besides the AHA have developed definitions of risk management. The 1989 Joint Commission on Accreditation of Healthcare Organizations' (JCAHO) accreditation manual for hospitals defined risk management as those activities which, in health care organizations, attempt to conserve institutional financial resources in risk of loss (JCAHO, 1989). The manual also states that risk-management functions relate to activities designed to identify, evaluate, and reduce risk of patient injury associated with care (JCAHO, 1989).

The American Society for Healthcare Risk Management (ASHRM) defines health care risk management as a discipline regulating insurance and quality control and comprising activities designed to minimize adverse effects and loss upon a health care organization's human, physical, and financial assets (ASHRM, 1982). ASHRM identified four basic components of risk management:

1. risk identification, which includes the organization's claims history, incident or event reporting, occurrence screening, and other input sources (patient representatives and quality assurance [QA] and utilization review [UR] activities)

2. risk management/analysis, promoting data collection and information systems, clinical and managerial expertise, and confidentiality of information

3. risk treatment, including loss prevention and reduction, risk avoidance, and risk financing

4. risk evaluation, an ongoing process of reviewing and evaluating incident reporting, policies and procedures, staff education, and communications (ASHRM, 1982)

These definitions focus on reducing the financial impact of malpractice claims within the institution; however, the overall goal of risk management is the protection of both the professional and patient.

Nursing and Risk Management

The American Nursing Association defines nursing as "the diagnosis and treatment of human responses to actual or potential health problems" (ANA, 1980). Like nursing, risk management addresses actual or potential problems. Nursing and risk management also have a common goal: to provide patient care which will promote the best possible outcome. A poor outcome may or may not become a risk concern depending on the quality of the nurse's caring, communication, and actions.

Luquire (1989) stated that one of the most commonly overlooked methods of keeping litigation costs at a minimum is through holistic health care, which she believes combats impersonal care. She includes in holistic care the care of the patient's family. If the family is involved with the patient, and if family members are treated with respect, caring, and understanding, the family and patient may be less likely to file a malpractice claim should a poor outcome occur.

Risk Management and Standards of Care

The essence of nursing's art and science is the safe care of patients, which can be defined best through its code of ethics and standards of care. Webster's Dictionary (1996) defines a standard as "something established by authority, custom or general consent." Nursing diagnosis identifies specific patient problems and their etiologies and aids the nurse in developing patient goals and interventions. These goals and interventions should reflect the standard of care. However, risk may occur regardless of whether the nurse has adhered to appropriate standards of care.

Standards are broad, measurable, patient-focused, and achievable (NAACOG, 1990). Standards have three components: structure, process, and outcome. Structural criteria are the desirable conditions needed to provide good patient care. Examples include: nursing staffing patterns, physical layout, and policies and procedures. Process criteria involve the concurrent review of nursing actions (NAACOG, 1990). Process allows for swift action in problem resolution. Outcome criteria describe end results and define measurable change in the patient population as a result of certain nursing activities (NAACOG, 1990).

There are three sources of standards: voluntary, involuntary, and regulatory. Voluntary standards are generated by the practitioners themselves. An example of voluntary nursing standards would be NAACOG's *Standards for the Nursing Care of Women and Newborns* (NAACOG, 1991) or ANA's *Standards of Clinical Nursing Practice* (ANA, 1991). Involuntary standards are insurance-generated and contain certain structures and procedures required by the hospital's professional liability carrier (e.g., reporting forms). Regulatory standards include professional and governmental regulations and statutes, such as JCAHO criteria for accreditation and state board of health requirements for staffing ratios.

Standards can be very positive for a profession. In nursing, standards based on scientific knowledge have the potential to contribute to improved care, and they inform clinicians about appropriate practice. Standards also address the expectations of health care consumers and promote a positive image of the profession among consumers. Lastly, if standards are observed, they serve as a defense in malpractice claims and may contribute to decreased malpractice premiums for the hospital.

Tan (1991) posed that using practice guidelines and standards in risk-management programs is essential in avoiding poor outcomes and the resultant payouts. Standards can be used to enhance continuing education efforts, identify occurrence screens and clinical indicators, focus quality-improvement and prevention efforts, and benefit credentialing (Tan, 1991). There may be a flaw with Tan's model, however. She recommends evaluating malpractice claims to develop standards, a form of retrospective rather than prospective risk management. In the practical world of maternal-child nursing, standards should be developed prospectively (i.e., proactively) rather than retrospectively to: (a) improve patient outcomes, and (b) decrease malpractice claims.

Outcomes of risk management ideally would eliminate all preventable risks (i.e., all risks that had previously been identified and through which standards of care had been created). Thus, risk management promotes the development and refinement of standards of care.

Assumptions of Risk Management

Four assumptions must be explored in any discussion of risk management. The first assumption is that bad things happen. In other words, every situation has risks; some are controllable and some are not. The domain of risk management is to focus on those risks that can be identified and controlled by the agent in question, which in this context is nursing.

The second assumption is that risk management is both a process and an outcome. Neither can be separated from risk management. Both must be examined when identifying untoward events and developing standards to prevent their occurrence or recurrence.

The third assumption is that risk management occurs in a collegial, collaborative setting. Health care does not exist in a vacuum and neither does risk management. A multitude of professionals may be involved in a single patient's care. Each component of each professional's caregiving plays a role in that patient's outcome. Components may overlap each other. The most obvious example is the care of a patient by a nurse, obstetrician, and pediatrician. If a poor outcome occurs, a collaborative effort between professionals is essential in preventing recurrence. Although no one can go back and reverse the outcome, a non-accusatory discourse among team members may result in positive change.

The fourth assumption is that health care risk management occurs in a variety of settings—wherever care is provided. These settings include hospitals, physicians' offices, birthing centers, outpatient centers, or patients' homes. Every contact with a patient presents a dynamic opportunity for risk management as part of the nursing process.

Quality Assurance

Florence Nightingale was first to recognize the importance of quality assurance in nursing. Nightingale (1859) was not only a nurse but a statistician who proposed a method for health care evaluation. In 1900, Codman, a physician, introduced a system called "end result analysis" at Massachusetts General Hospital to collect and evaluate large numbers of patient outcomes (Christoffel, 1976). In 1917, the American College of Surgeons established and published the *Minimum Standards for Hospitals*, which contained the first formal requirements for the review and evaluation of quality of patient care (Weitzman, 1990).

Webster's Dictionary (1996) defines quality as "an agreed upon level of excellence." The aim of quality in health care is to promote, preserve, and restore health (Weitzman, 1990). According to Blum (1974), the quality of health care has four components: (a) the patient's health status and attitudes on entry to care, (b) the suitability of the structure of care, (c) the processes of care, and d) the outcomes of the processes of care.

Quality assurance within healthcare guarantees a level of excellence in patient care. Quality assurance is both a retrospective and prospective process. By examining patient events that occurred in the past, nursing staff can learn from prior care experiences and improve future care. Nursing quality assurance is very similar to the nursing process. Collecting and evaluating data is similar to the assessment phase, identifying problems is like the diagnosis phase, identifying potential solutions and developing a philosophy of quality assurance are comparable to the planning phase, developing standards of care and practice is similar to the implementation phase, and reviewing effectiveness of actions is comparable to the evaluation phase (NAACOG, 1990). NAACOG's *OGN Nursing Practice Resource on Quality Assurance* is an excellent reference on the implementation of quality-assurance programs (NAACOG, 1990).

Risk management handles errors while quality assurance seeks excellence; coordinating the efforts of both reduces malpractice claims and improves patient care (Fiesta, 1991). The objective of a quality-assurance program is to evaluate the level of care provided to the health care consumer (NAACOG, 1990). While quality assurance is not unique to health care, JCAHO became involved in overseeing minimum standards in 1951. In the 1970s, quality-assurance programs became mandatory in the health care industry.

There are three general approaches to quality assurance: licensing, accreditation, and certification (Weitzman, 1990). Licensing is a legal procedure and pertains to both individuals and institutions. In health care, states license individual health care providers, as well as hospitals, nursing homes, and pharmacies. Licensing is a very minimal form of quality assurance. An individual qualifies for licensure after successfully completing an educational program and a licensing exam, testing a basic knowledge level. An individual may maintain licensure by simply paying a scheduled fee. This process does not confirm an individual's knowledge since an individual may maintain licensure for twenty years or more with no further education.

The second general approach to quality assurance is accreditation of institutions. Accreditation is voluntary and is not a legal procedure. It occurs when a group of similar institutions establish standards and evaluate members at regular intervals (Weitzman, 1990). JCAHO is a well-recognized accrediting body in health care. Nursing schools are accredited by the National League of Nursing.

The third general approach to quality assurance is certification, which applies to individuals. Like accreditation, certification is voluntary and is not a legal procedure. Certification tests basic education and achievement within a specialty area (e.g., obstetrics, neonatal, and pediatric nursing) (Weitzman, 1990). Certification is recognized by third-party payers, by employers, and consumers. In nursing alone, there are a minimum of twenty possible certifications.

JCAHO Ten-Step Process

In 1990, JCAHO introduced the ten-step process for quality-assurance monitoring and evaluation. The ten-step process, an outgrowth of JCAHO's *Agenda for Change* (1986), places an emphasis on the role of leadership and expands the scope of assessment and improvement beyond strictly clinical areas. The 1996 *Accreditation Manual for Hospitals* (JCAHO, 1996) presents a model for assessing quality that illustrates the relationship of dimensions of performance, important functions, and a range of patient populations and services (Figure 5-1). The quality cube is intended to stimulate thought about and focus measurements to improvement priorities.

Total Quality Management

Deming (1986) rejected the concept of total quality management (TQM) stating that it was undefined. Instead he proposed the term management for improvement of quality and instituted this model into the Japanese industry after World War II. At that time, his ideas were poorly received in the United States. After corporations in the US realized the extent of Deming's contributions to the Japanese market, competitive pressures led many to adopt his concepts, which are well known in the health care industry today.

Deming's work focuses on proactivity: employees build quality into the product or service rather than inspect for errors and assume that error removal will lead to quality (Kirk, 1992). The box on page 58 lists the 14 points of Deming's model, which differs from quality assurance in that TQM is a "management" framework; it must come from administration first before it can affect staff performance. TQM does not occur in a few days; rather, it is a process that develops slowly and may not be completely developed even after years. Furthermore, TQM promotes a holistic approach to management, including the concept of continuous quality improvement, which takes the concept of planning from the initial design through implementation.

Continuous quality improvement (CQI) is a management system for continuously improving performance at every level of the organization. CQI is accomplished by focusing on meeting or exceeding customer satisfaction. CQI differs from traditional systems for quality assurance in its emphasis on:

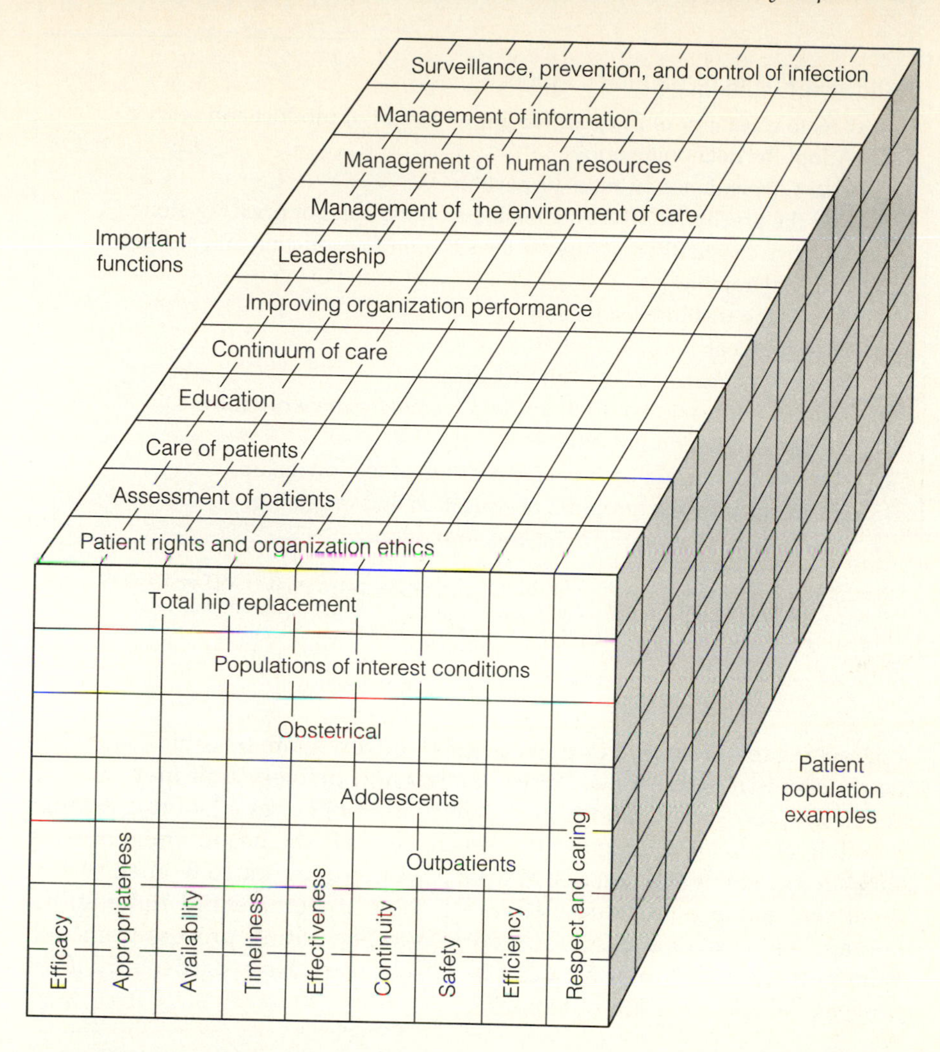

Figure 5-1 The quality cube: a model for assessing the quality of health care.

SOURCE: *Accreditation manual for hospitals*. Vol. I: Standards. Oakbrook Terrace, IL: Joint Commission on Accreditation of Healthcare Organizations, 1996, p. 25. Reprinted with permission.

prevention rather than detection; proactivity rather than reactivity; systems causes rather than individual causes; responsibility of many rather than responsibility of a few; and problem-solving by employees at all levels, rather than problem-solving only by authority figures.

Quality of care can be improved. The organization must focus on key activities, coordinate efforts among its members, develop effective performance measures, and use these measures appropriately. The measures must include not only outcomes, but also processes. Nurses should not attempt to

Fourteen Points of Deming's Model

1. Create constancy of purpose for improvement of product and service.
2. Adopt the new philosophy.
3. Cease dependence on mass inspection.
4. End the practice of awarding business on the basis of price tag alone.
5. Improve constantly and forever the system of production and service.
6. Institute training.
7. Adopt and institute leadership.
8. Drive out fear.
9. Break down barriers between staff areas.
10. Eliminate slogans, exhortations, and targets for the work force.
11. Eliminate numerical quotas.
12. Remove barriers that rob people of pride of workmanship.
13. Institute a vigorous program of education and retraining.
14. Take action to accomplish the transformation.

Reprinted from *Out of the Crisis* by W. Edwards Deming by permission of MIT and The W. Edwards Deming Institute. Published by MIT, Center for Advanced Educational Services, Cambridge, MA 02139. Copyright 1986 by The W. Edwards Deming Institute.

separate process from outcome, since good outcomes are possible even when the process is flawed. For example, a labor and delivery unit may be short staffed and have more laboring women than nurses. Yet a laboring woman may deliver a healthy infant in this setting, even if she has minimal nursing care. On the other hand, a nurse may be present throughout a woman's labor, but if that nurse is not knowledgeable about maternal-child nursing, the woman may deliver a compromised infant. Separating process from outcome in the evaluation of data can be falsely reassuring, particularly if the nurse examines only poor outcomes.

Integration of Risk Management and Quality Assurance

In 1989, JCAHO added a quality assurance standard to its *Accreditation Manual*. The standard stated that "there are operational linkages between the risk management functions related to the clinical aspects of patient care and safety and quality assurance functions" (JCAHO, 1989). The integration of risk management and quality assurance is logical, given the nature of the transactions in health care.

Several areas of overlap exist between risk management and quality assurance. Both systems involve the identification of problems leading to adverse events, and both focus on intervention to reduce the likelihood of recurrence. Also the overall focus of both quality assurance and risk management is and will always be patient-oriented.

Risk management and quality assurance also share several systems functions. Both require comprehensive monitoring that includes data gathering and genetic-outcome screening. Information analysis is an essential component to the success of both systems. In order to work efficiently and effectively, both systems require a budget and adequate financial support.

A "people component" is also necessary for both aspects to function. Employees in risk-management and quality-assurance positions must possess both clinical and managerial expertise. Within most organizations, these positions consist of vertical authority, not horizontal. The ability to communicate with members of all levels of the organization is essential. This includes patient and family, environmental services, nursing and medical staff, administration, and the governing board.

A study funded by the National Center for Health Services Research and Health Care Technology Assessment (USHHS, 1988) validated the need for communication skills. The study examined medical malpractice claims for seven years, and found certain characteristics associated with better claims experiences: (a) a policy specifying who had responsibility for informing the patient or family of errors, (b) a policy to notify clinical chiefs of adverse medical incidents, (c) governing board receipt of risk management reports on a regular basis, and (d) educational efforts focused on the responsibilities of nurses and physicians in quality assurance and risk management.

Certain job functions are unique to risk management and do not affect quality assurance. Besides a patient care component, risk management must also address physical plant and property preservation and protection issues. The risk manager is also involved in worker's compensation and employee benefits, general liability, professional liability, and directors' and officers' liability insurance. The risk manager must manage past, current, and potential claims and decide how to provide sufficient risk financing.

Proactive Strategies for Risk Management and Quality Assurance

Incident Reports

In recent years, incident reports have taken on a variety of other names such as occurrence screens or critical events screens. Whatever their name, incident reports traditionally have been a retrospective form of risk management. More recently, as risk management has assumed a proactive role, incident reports are triggering investigations of the circumstances of events and promoting changes necessary to prevent recurrence. Incident reports also serve as tracking devices for risk-management issues.

Because incident reports are part of a hospital risk- and claims-management program, in many states they are protected from discovery by attorney/client privilege and the attorney work-product rule. However, inappropriate preparation or handling of incident reports may make them admissible in a legal action. In *Bernard v. Community Hospital Association*, 1968, the Colorado court ruled that incident reports not prepared exclusively for the hospital's risk manager or attorney are not privileged communication and are, therefore, discoverable. To protect incident reports from discovery or admissibility at trial, professionals and the organization should: (a) treat incident reports as confidential and mark as such, (b) limit distribution of copies of the reports, (c) refrain from placing a copy in patient record or unit file, (d) limit content of report to facts, not conclusions or assignments of blame, (e) address report to hospital attorney or risk manager by name, and (f) use same care to fill out incident reports as is given to medical records (Mahoney, 1987).

When completing incident reports, health care professionals should record details in objective terms. The incident report should describe only what was seen or heard, and it should be completed by the person who witnessed or participated in the event. If no health care personnel witnessed the incident, and it is subsequently recorded as hearsay, the account of events should be documented in the words of the witness and the witness' name recorded.

An incident report should never admit to error or place blame. These reports should not include suggestions on how to avoid the incident in the future or how the incident could have been avoided. The report should include actions that were taken at the time of the incident to provide care. The time of the incident and the names of all personnel notified should be recorded. It is unnecessary to record the names of health care personnel who were witnesses but did not participate in the event.

Objective details of the incident should be documented in the progress notes. These notes should describe the event in factual terms, including the patient's response to the incident, any treatment given, and follow-up care. The progress notes may include statements by the patient regarding the incident. *Do not write "incident report filed" in the progress notes.*

A nurse's personal records of incidents are discoverable by the plaintiff's attorney during deposition. Upon questioning, a defendant nurse would be compelled to produce any personal notes related to the incident in question. Therefore, these notes, like incident reports, should contain only factual data, not personal interjections. To maintain patient confidentiality, personal documents should not contain the patient's full name.

Opinions differ as to whether a nurse should keep her own personal record of incidents. Theoretically, all facts surrounding the event should be documented in the incident report and the patient chart. For example, if the event occurred during a time of short staffing, an incident report should reflect patient acuity and staffing ratios. If a physician states that he will respond to fetal bradycardia after office hours, the nurse should not only invoke the chain of command, but also document the response of the physician as a quotation in the incident report and chart.

The filing of an incident report does not indicate that malpractice occurred. Cases are reviewed to determine whether standards of care were or were not maintained. In reviewing cases through screening, a list of exceptions should also be used for concomitant review. If there is an exception (e.g., when there is a rational explanation for the occurrence, and standards of care were followed), there needs to be no further review of the case. Otherwise, the case is forwarded for further review and corrective actions to

Sample Occurrence Screens in Maternal-Child Nursing

- Newborn with an APGAR score less than or equal to six in the delivery room
- Elective induction of labor
- Primary/repeat cesarean section
- Failed vaginal birth after cesarean section (VBAC)
- Eclampsia
- Excessive maternal blood loss (i.e., HCT less than 22)
- Maternal length of stay more than four days
- Term infant admitted to the NICU
- Transfer of a neonate to NICU at another institution
- Maternal or infant death
- Birth not attended by physician/certified nurse midwife (CNM)

risk management and quality assurance. Each unit should have its own list of incident reports, including labor and delivery, postpartum, newborn nursery, and pediatrics. If an event listed on the screen occurs, an unusual occurrence report is completed. The accompanying box lists sample incident reports.

Many hospital professional liability carriers require the completion of an incident report, or an unusual occurrence screen, when a potentially compensable event occurs. These are events that would not be expected to occur in the normal course of care; in other words, they are poor outcomes. The goal of such screens is to: (a) deal with the identified situation while the patient is still hospitalized, and (b) serve as a source of risk identification and trending to determine if these events are preventable.

Competency-Based Practice

Technology and knowledge are continually changing, especially in the area of maternal-child health. Staff, including nurses, have a professional obligation to be aware of relevant new information. Even so, professional obligation does not guarantee that nurses seek or complete continuing education. To protect society, which has given professionals the sanctions to practice, health care institutions must guarantee, to the best of their ability, that practitioners meet practice standards. This trend has led to such terms as competency-based practice.

Ament (1993) discussed the pros and cons of competency assessment versus credentialing in promoting professional nursing practice. Whatever system is used, hospitals are required to maintain documentation of the training and special knowledge of its professionals. Each nurse should also maintain her own documentation, which may include: (a) copies of the orientation skills checklist, (b) certificates of continuing education programs, and (c) all in-hospital inservices. Copies of information presented at these sessions should also be included.

Staff nurses should be certified in CPR every year, and some institutions are requiring NALS, PALS, or ACLS for nurses in specific maternal-child areas. Neonatal resuscitation certification should be maintained every two years, and staff should participate in mock codes at least once a month. Nurses responsible for fetal monitoring should have continuing education once a year and monthly fetal-monitoring strip updates. These reviews are then documented on the individual's continuing-education record.

There is now another avenue for establishing competency of health care professionals. In the 1980s the Health Care Quality Improvement Act created the National Practitioner Data Bank. The data bank is a national source of information about health care professionals who have had malpractice payouts made on their behalf or who have had action taken against their professional license. All hospitals and health care employers, state licensing boards, and insurance companies are required to report certain information about nurses and other health care professionals. Suits that have been filed without payment are not reported.

Information that must be reported includes malpractice payments made by or for the nurse, as a result of judgments, arbitration settlements, and out-of-court settlements. Licensure actions that must be reported include revocation, suspension, reprimand, censure, and probation. The data bank was established to decrease the numbers of practitioners who move from state to state with poor professional records. The data bank is federally funded, and hospitals, other health care employers, professional societies, and even plaintiffs' attorneys have access to this information.

Hospitals must query the data bank every two years for each nurse and physician on staff (NSO Risk Advisor, 1992). Hospitals must also check the data bank prior to granting privileges to an applicant. Professionals may also request information that pertains to themselves. Prior to being listed in the data bank, the professional receives a copy of the report to review, and has sixty days to dispute the report (NSO Risk Advisor, 1992).

Communication Issues

Communication issues in risk management can be divided into two categories: peers and patients. Peer communication (i.e., to nurses, physicians, and other health care professionals) occurs in verbal and written forms. If the nurse needs to notify a peer of an event, follow-up documentation of the communication should include: (a) reason for the notification, (b) person notified, and (c) response received. It is not acceptable to document "Dr. X notified of FHR decelerations." This recording does not state what type of decelerations were occurring, what nursing interventions were performed in response to the decelerations, how the decelerations responded to nursing interventions, if Dr. X was notified by phone or in person, time of notification or what the nurse requested (physician notification or physician response). If a sufficient or acceptable response is not received, all nurses (i.e., staff, advanced practice nurses, or administration) have an obligation to the patient to proceed further with the communication through the chain of command. If this process does not yield satisfactory results, or a poor outcome occurs, the nurse files an incident report. Nurses have a professional and ethical obligation to act in the best interests of the patient (i.e., as the patient advocate) (ANA, 1985).

The second type of communication involves the patient. If the patient communicates dissatisfaction concerning care issues or comments about the potential for a lawsuit, the nurse documents the patient's comments in the progress notes and reports them to the immediate supervisor within the organization. This is a prospective process to avoid a future claim, but more importantly, it may help to rectify a situation of patient unhappiness or frustration.

Telephone communication/triage is a vital portion of patient care, and standardization is a major risk-management strategy. This begins with the staff developing a standard response to the most common calls and documenting all calls. Each unit must maintain a telephone log next to the unit phone. The log may contain a variety of information, but at a minimum should contain: (a) date and time of call, (b) name of the person calling, (c) reason for the call, (d) staff response, (e) caller's response to information received (e.g., verbalizes understanding), (f) name and credentials of staff giving information, and (g) follow-up, if necessary. While it cannot eliminate difficulties entirely, this type of system reduces significantly the number of problems occurring as a result of patient non-response. In specific patient situations (e.g., four hours after phone advice, a woman with vaginal bleeding appears with abruptio placenta and denies that she was instructed to come immediately to the hospital), documented staff advice serves as evidence. While some may argue that it is one person's word against another, established protocols and consistent telephone documentation strengthen the staff's position in the event of litigation. Use of a telephone log is not only a risk-management strategy, but also a quality-assurance tool. The log can be reviewed for consistency, follow-up, and outcomes.

The importance of good communication skills is illustrated in a study reported by Hospital Risk Management (1992). Over 100 mothers with closed malpractice claims were surveyed to determine why they sued. The results may be a surprise: 15% were advised to sue by someone in the medical profession; 70% were upset that no one provided them with information that their infant might have permanent problems or die; 48% said the physician attempted to mislead them; 32% said the physician would not talk with them; and 13% said the physician would not listen to them.

Protocols

Inherent in the previous discussions of various risk-management and quality-assurance strategies is the assumption that protocols for these strategies exist. Protocols provide instruction on standardized practice, focusing on problem-solving and decision-making skills. Certain components, such as personnel, equipment, outcomes, and references, need to be included in all protocols (NAACOG, 1991). The protocol should delineate what categories of personnel may perform the procedure and any special knowledge or skills the person must possess prior to performing the procedure. For example, oxytocin (Pitocin) infusions must be performed by an RN who has completed a fetal-monitoring course and is credentialed for Pitocin administration. Protocols need to contain supportive data such as: (a) ambiguous term definitions, (b) special equipment needed for performance of the protocol, (c) expected outcomes, and (d) references. Protocols should be reviewed yearly and updated as technology and knowledge change.

Conclusion

One common difficulty with both risk management and quality assurance is eliciting nursing-staff participation. With increasing patient acuity and decreasing staff numbers, patient care and documentation can be overwhelming. Nevertheless, it is essential that nurses have a working knowledge of the concepts covered in this chapter. Administration must encourage staff involvement, establish structure, and define criteria. Strategies used to educate nurses to the concepts of risk management should include new and ongoing inservices and formal and informal staff education (Ament, 1992).

While hospital staff have a peer-review process for quality assurance, a unit-specific incident-control team may increase the participation of staff nurses while decreasing risks to patients, families, and staff. The team may consist of: (a) a risk manager, (b) quality assurance coordinator, (c) medical representative, and (d) nursing representative. A committee meeting should be held immediately after a poor outcome occurs to discuss resolutions to the incident and options to assist the patient and family. The committee should not wait until the poor outcome results in litigation.

Nurses should receive the necessary knowledge and skills in their educational program to provide safe, quality care. With the assistance of adequate systems support, educational programs, and risk-management resources, nurses are able to decrease the number of poor patient outcomes.

References

Ament, L. (1992). Educating the RN: The risk manager's role. *Perspectives in Healthcare Risk Management, 12*(1), 29–30.

Ament, L. (1993). Competency assessment versus credentialing: Promoting professional nursing practice. *Journal of Nursing Staff Development, 9*(3), 157–159.

American Bar Association. (1977). *Report of the commission on medical professional liability.* Chicago, IL: Author.

American Nurses Association. (1980). *Nursing: A social policy statement.* Washington, D.C.: Author.

American Nurses Association. (1985). *Code for nurses.* Washington, D.C.: Author.

American Nurses Association. (1991). *Standards of clinical nursing practice.* Washington, D.C.: Author.

American Society for Healthcare Risk Management. (1982). *Definition of healthcare risk management.* Chicago, IL: Author.

Bernardi v. City and County of Denver, No. 166 C.V. 280, 443, P2d.708, Colorado Supreme Court (1968).

Blum, H. (1974). Evaluating healthcare. *Medical Care, 12,* 12.

Christoffel, T. (1976). Medical care evaluation: An old idea. *Journal of Medical Education, 51,* 2.

Dankmyer, T. & Groves, J. (1977). Taking steps for safety's sake. *Hospitals,* 51, 60.

Deming, E. (1986). *Out of crisis.* Cambridge, MA: Massachusetts Institute of Technology Center for Advanced Engineering Study.

Fiesta, J. (1991). QA and risk management: Reducing liability exposure. *Nursing Management, 22*(2), 14–15.

Joint Commission on Accreditation of Healthcare Organizations. (1986). *Agenda for change.* Chicago, IL: Author.

Joint Commission on Accreditation of Healthcare Organizations. (1989). *Accreditation manual for hospitals.* Chicago, IL: Author.

Joint Commission on Accreditation of Healthcare Organizations. (1996). *Accreditation manual for hospitals.* Vol. I: Standards, Oakbrook Terrace, IL: Author.

Kirk, R. (1992). Total quality management and continuous quality improvement. *Journal of Nursing Administration,* 22(4), 24–31.

Korleski, D. (1990). The emergence of a profession. In B. Youngberg (Ed.), *Essentials of hospital risk management.* Rockville, MD: Aspen.

Luquire, R. (1989). Nursing risk management. *Nursing Management, 20*(10), 56–58.

Mahoney, D. (1987). *The chart as a legal document.* Paper presented at St. Francis Hospital, Colorado Springs, CO.

Nightingale, F. (1859). *Notes on nursing: What it is and what it is not.* London: Harrison and Sons.

NSO Risk Advisor. (1992). *How to stay out of the malpractice data bank.* Trevose, PA: Author.

Nurse's Association of the American College of Obstetrics and Gynecology. (1990). *Obstetrical and gynecological nursing practice resource: Quality assurance.* Washington, D.C.: Author.

Nurse's Association of the American College of Obstetrics and Gynecology. (1991). *Standards for the nursing care of women and newborns.* Washington, D.C.: Author.

Tan, M. (1991). Using practice guidelines and standards in quality assurance and risk management programs. *Journal of Quality Assurance,* March/April, 22–24.

US Department of Health, Education, and Welfare. (1973). *Report of the secretary's commission on medical malpractice.* DHEW No. (OS) 73-88. Rockville, MD: US Government Printing Office.

US Department of Health and Human Services. (1988). Do hospital risk management programs make a difference? *Malpractice claims: The Maryland experience, 1977–1985.* Rockville, MD: Author.

US General Accounting Office. (1987). *Medical malpractice: A framework for action.* Washington, D.C.: Author.

Weitzman, B. (1990). The quality of care: Assessment and assurance. In A. Kovner (Ed.), *Health care delivery in the United States.* New York: Spring Publishing Company.

Webster's new collegiate dictionary. (1996). Springfield, MA: Merriam.

6

A Model for Professional Nursing Practice

Mary I. Enzman Hagedorn, RN, PhD, CNS, CPNP
Sandra L. Gardner, RN, MS, CNS, PNP
Marcia Garman Laux, RN, MSN
Georgia L. Gardner, RN, BSN, MS

Professionalism requires accountability and professional accountability means that one is answerable to more than the self.
Curtin, 1982

In *Notes on Nursing,* Florence Nightingale defined nursing as a profession separate from medicine. Her definition included the key aspect of environment and its impact on health. Since that time, nurses have continued to refine the definition of nursing as a profession. The Congress on Nursing Practice defined nursing as "the diagnosis and treatment of human response to actual or potential health problems" (ANA, 1980, p. 8). Anderson, Anderson, and Glanze (1994) defined a nurse as "a person educated and licensed in the practice of nursing; one who is concerned with the diagnosis and treatment of human responses to actual or potential health problems" (p. 1087).

Current nursing theorist Watson and nurse philosopher Gadow identified caring as the moral imperative of nursing practice. Caring is the core of nursing (Gadow, 1984, 1989; Watson, 1985). Watson (1985) views caring as "the moral ideal of nursing where there is utmost concern for human dignity and preservation of humanity" (p. 63). Preservation and advancement of human care becomes a critical issue for nursing in our depersonalized society. "Caring requires a personal, social, moral, and spiritual engagement of the nurse and a commitment to oneself and other humans, nursing offers the promise of human preservation in society" (Watson, 1985, p. 29). Through caring relationships, the nurse protects, enhances, and preserves a person's humanness. She helps the person to find meaning in illness, suffering, pain, and existence and to gain knowledge, control and self-healing (Watson, 1985). Further, Gadow (1980, 1984, 1989) interprets nursing as existential advocacy. This philosophical foundation poses that the nurse's participation within a caring relationship assists the patient in determining "the unique meaning which the experience of health, illness, suffering, or dying has for the individual" (Gadow, 1980, p. 81). Embodying a caring philosophy, the nurse is able to promote autonomy and empowerment for patients and families (Gadow, 1984, 1989).

Characteristics of Nursing as a Profession

A profession is defined as a practice domain characterized by a unique "body of knowledge derived from experience (leading to expertise) and research (leading to theoretical foundations of knowledge)" (Leddy and Pepper, 1993, p. 4) and derived through university-based education. As nursing has evolved over the past century, it has come to exhibit more and more characteristics of a profession.

Unique Body of Knowledge

When Florence Nightingale wrote *Notes on Nursing* in 1859, she identified key constructs that separated nursing from medicine. Nightingale saw nursing's role as having "charge of somebody's health" (Nightingale, 1859, p. 24). Although Nightingale herself was university educated, she developed and implemented nursing education through hospital-based training programs. Through her writing, educational efforts, and service in the Crimean War, changes in the image of nursing emerged. "She made public opinion perceive, and act upon the perception, that nursing was an art, and must be raised to the status of a trained profession" (Kjervik and Martinson, 1979, p. 22). Thus, Nightingale's contributions helped nursing enter the modern era. The principles of nursing education and practice developed by Nightingale are woven into all aspects of nursing education and practice today.

The focus of nursing as a professional discipline with a unique body of knowledge has emerged over several decades. As nursing developed information and experience about patients' responses to human health conditions, a distinct body of knowledge emerged. Nursing knowledge was derived from a belief and value system concerned with social commitment, the nature of services delivered, and an area of responsibility (Newman, Sime, & Corcoran-Perry, 1991). "Nursing's body of knowledge includes caring and the human health experience" (Newman et al., 1991, p. 3).

The essential question of the discipline of nursing "has something to do with how nurses facilitate the health of human beings" (Newman, 1990, p. 234). Newman (1990) asks "What is the quality of relationship that makes it possible for the nurse and patient to connect in a transformative way?" (p. 234). Phillips (1990) stated that "nursing research should focus . . . on the study of people's experiencing of their health, the sense of interconnectedness with others, and how health emerges from a mutual process" (p. 103). Nurses conduct research to further refine the art and science of nursing, and this in turn leads to increased specificity of knowledge within practice. Through theory and research, nurses have developed models that provide a basis for curricula, scope of practice, and further nursing research.

Mastery and use of theoretical knowledge occurs through specialized nursing education. Historically, nursing education followed a format similar to medicine, based on a systems approach, that limited the scope of nursing practice to the identification of diseases. Today, nursing education focuses on teaching the art and science of nursing (i.e., human caring). In the early 1970's, nursing identified a process of data collection, diagnosis, planning, treatment, and evaluation of human responses to health and illness. With evolution and refinement of the nursing process, nurses established distinct nursing diagnoses separate from medical diagnoses. Since the mid 1970's, a growing taxonomy of nursing diagnoses has been established (North American Nursing Diagnosis Association [NANDA], 1995). A complete list of NANDA-approved nursing diagnoses is provided in Appendix A.

Unlike other professions that have established a singular educational program, nursing has a variety of educational options for entry into practice, including hospital-based diploma programs and associate- and baccalaureate-degree programs. The variety of educational programs poses confusion not only for nurses, but also for other professionals not associated with nursing and for the public (Table 6-1). Educational programs should prepare the nursing student for a scope of practice that includes independent, interdependent, and dependent functions. Professional nursing practice is also characterized by critical thinking and specialized skills (ANA Commission on Nursing Education, 1975; Leddy & Pepper, 1993). Although all nursing graduates are licensed by individual states as registered nurses after successful completion of the NCLEX/CAT-RN, "professional organizations agree that baccalaureate education is the minimum education necessary for professional nursing practice" (Leddy & Pepper, 1993, p. 57).

The confusion surrounding nursing education is compounded by the presence of vocationally trained personnel who enter nursing to augment patient care at the bedside. These licensed practical or vocational nurses (LPN/LVN) are educated in nine- to twelve-month programs awarding a certificate at completion. These students are then entitled to licensure as a practical or vocational nurse after successful completion of a licensure examination. The LPN or LVN is unable to practice independently and requires ongoing supervision by a registered nurse when providing care. An LPN or

Table 6-1 Educational Nursing Programs

Program	Type of Degree	Description
Basic	Associate Degree	Two-year program located in community/technical college.
	Diploma	Three-year program located in hospitals and affiliated with universities.
	Baccalaureate (BSN)	Four-year university-based program awarding a Bachelor's degree.
	Nursing Doctorate (ND)	Five-year university-based program (post-baccalaureate degree in another field) awarding a nursing doctorate (ND).
Advanced	Master's	One- to two-year graduate program awarding a Master's degree with special emphasis in clinical practice (e.g., clinical nurse specialist, nurse practitioner, or nurse midwife), administration, generalist, or education.
Doctoral		Five- to seven-year post-graduate program awarding a Doctor of Philosophy (PhD) or a Doctor of Nursing Science (DNSc) degree. The PhD focuses on research and theory development; the DNSc focuses on advanced clinical practice and research.

LVN cannot: (a) independently perform initial assessment of patient condition/status, (b) formulate nursing diagnoses, (c) independently carry out steps of the nursing process, or (d) independently provide care to the patient without RN supervision.

Service to Public/Society

Nursing provides a key public service: the promotion, maintenance, and restoration of health. Public acceptance of the need, value, and worth of this service is a prerequisite for the nursing profession's existence, autonomy, and self-governance. Nurses serve others with respect for basic human rights, within the context of personal and professional integrity and within a credentialing system (i.e., licensure and certification) that ensures competence. State nurse practice acts and regulatory agencies provide the structure for the protection of society against incompetent, unethical, or negligent practice.

Autonomy and Accountability

Autonomy, the ability to function independently, includes the concepts of self-regulation, self-determination, and self-control. Autonomy and decision-making within practice have been difficult for nursing to establish. Traditionally, nurses have practiced predominantly in institutional settings as employees of the organization. Instead of developing "political power and professional credibility through technical competence and specialized knowledge," nurses have sought status "through increased rank in the hierarchy rather than through expert practice" (Leddy & Pepper, 1993, p. 10). Often the roles, responsibilities, and functions of nursing are defined by non-nurses (e.g., administrators, physicians, other health care providers). The development of advanced practice nursing, direct third-party reimbursement, and community-based nursing services are advancing autonomous nursing practice.

Accountability and responsibility for nursing actions and judgments accompany autonomy. Accountability includes not only responsibility, but also "answerability, the necessity of offering answers and explanations to certain others" (Leddy & Pepper, 1993, p. 271). Professional nurses are accountable to: (a) self, (b) client/public, (c) the profession, and (d) the employer (ANA, 1985).

Professional Organizations/Societies

Professional organizations/societies are among the most visible and powerful means by which a group demonstrates its professional status in society (Leddy & Pepper, 1993). Professional organizations/societies deal with problems and issues that affect the profession. The American Nurses Association (ANA) represents nursing through lobbyists active at the federal level, maintains a code of ethics, evaluates nursing education, promulgates standards, and promotes other interests for the good of the profession. The National League for Nursing (NLN) is a coalition of individuals and agencies that focus primarily on nursing education and practice to improve the quality of health care. By establishing a code of ethics, standards of practice, and stan-

Moral Principles Guiding Nursing Practice

Respect—for persons and for human dignity
Autonomy—self-determination
Beneficence—doing good
Nonmaleficence—avoiding harm
Veracity—truth-telling
Confidentiality—respecting privileged information
Fidelity—keeping promises; commitment
Justice—fairness, equality
Privacy—freedom from intrusion

Adapted from: American Nurses Association. (1985). *Code for nurses with interpretive statements.* Washington, D.C.: Author, p. 1. Reprinted with permission.

dards of care, the profession through its organizations/societies autonomously defines and attempts to enforce that for which its members are accountable.

Code of Ethics A code of ethics defines principles by which a profession functions—a standard of behavior accepted by all members of the profession. Development of a code of ethics is an essential activity of a profession and enables self-regulation and autonomy (ANA, 1985). Nursing's code of ethics includes "general principles to guide and evaluate nursing actions" (ANA, 1985, p. ii). On entering the profession, each nurse is obliged to adhere to the profession's code of conduct and maintain ethical practice. Both personal and professional integrity can be guaranteed only if individual nurses are committed to the profession's code of conduct (ANA, 1985). The accompanying box lists moral principles guiding nursing practice.

The *Code for Nurses with Interpretive Statements,* which the ANA adopted in 1950, and revised in 1976 and 1985, is "a collective expression of nursing's conscience and philosophy" (ANA, 1985, p. iii). Used as a framework for ethical decision-making, the Code authorizes nursing's accountability to the public, to others on the health care team, and to the profession (ANA, 1985). In the introduction, ANA warns that the Code "is not open to negotiation in employment settings, nor is it permissible for individuals or groups of nurses to adopt or change the language of the Code" (ANA, 1985, p. iv). Eleven points of the ANA's Code for nurses are listed in the box on page 72.

Although "requirements of the Code may often exceed those of the law" (ANA, 1985, p. iv), violation of any parameter of the Code constitutes unethical practice (ANA, 1994). In some states all or part of the Code has been incorporated into the nurse practice act; thus, violation constitutes not only unethical, but also illegal practice (ANA, 1994). Since the Code requires nurses to "maintain competence in nursing" (ANA, 1985, p. 9), incompetent practice that violates the standards of care and the standards of practice also

Code for Nurses with Interpretive Statements

1. The nurse provides services with respect for human dignity and the uniqueness of the client, unrestricted by considerations of social or economic status, personal attributes, or the nature of the health problems.
2. The nurse safeguards the client's right to privacy by judiciously protecting information of a confidential nature.
3. The nurse acts to safeguard the client and the public when health care and safety are affected by the incompetent, unethical, or illegal practice of any person.
4. The nurse assumes responsibility and accountability for individual nursing judgments and actions.
5. The nurse maintains competence in nursing.
6. The nurse exercises informed judgment and uses individual competence and qualifications as criteria in seeking consultation, accepting responsibilities, and delegating nursing activities to others.
7. The nurse participates in activities that contribute to the ongoing development of the profession's body of knowledge.
8. The nurse participates in the profession's efforts to implement and improve standards of nursing.
9. The nurse participates in the profession's efforts to establish and maintain conditions of employment conducive to high-quality nursing care.
10. The nurse participates in the profession's efforts to protect the public from misinformation and misrepresentation and to maintain the integrity of nursing.
11. The nurse collaborates with members of the health professions and other citizens in promoting community and national efforts to meet the health needs of the public.

From: American Nurses Association. (1985). *Code for nurses with interpretive statements.* Washington, D.C. : Author, p. 1.

constitutes unethical practice (ANA, 1994). The ANA Code (and most state nurse practice acts) requires the nurse to act to safe-guard the client/public from incompetent, unethical, or illegal practice. Appropriate action includes: (a) expressing concern to the professional performing the questionable practice, (b) reporting and documenting concern to the appropriate administrative person within the agency, and when practice is not rectified within the agency, (c) documenting and reporting to appropriate authorities (e.g., practice committee of professional organization, licensing and regulatory agencies, etc.) (ANA, 1994).

In 1994, ANA's Center for Ethics and Human Rights conducted a survey of 934 nurses attending the annual ANA convention (Scanlon, 1994a). Respondents represented all 50 states, and the majority: (a) had a baccalaureate (37%) or master's degree (40%), (b) worked in a hospital as staff or manager, and (c) had from 1–20 years of nursing experience (59%) (Scanlon,

1994a). Even though these nurses confronted ethical issues or problems daily or weekly, the majority did not receive sufficient ethics content in their education (Figures 6-1 and 6-2). When asked to identify the most frequently occurring ethics and human-rights issues, more than 50% identified: (a) cost containment, (b) end-of-life decisions, (c) confidentiality breaches, and (d) incompetent, unethical, or illegal practices of colleagues (Figure 6-3). Although most respondents identified resources for nurses with ethical problems, including (a) literature/journals (44%), (b) ethics committees (42%), and (c) continuing education (39%), eleven percent could identify no available resources (Scanlon, 1994a).

Standards Standards are "authoritative statements by which the nursing profession describes the responsibilities for which its practitioners are accountable" (ANA, 1991a, p. 1). Professional nursing organizations have a responsibility to members and to the public/society to develop standards of practice (ANA, 1991a, 1991b). Reflecting professional values and priorities, standards provide: (a) a direction for professional nursing practice, (b) a framework for practice evaluation, (c) a definition of professional accountability, and (d) a definition of professional responsibility for client outcomes (ANA, 1991a).

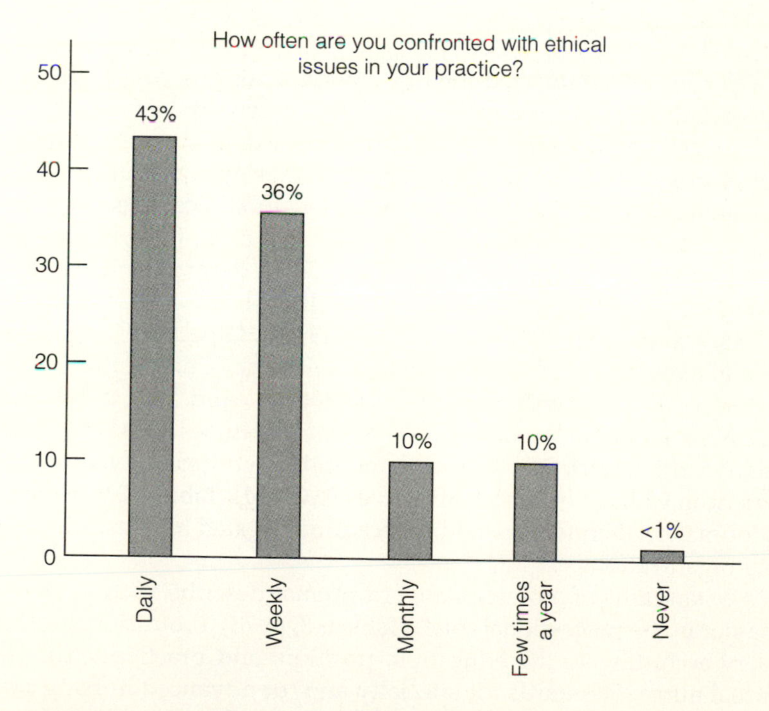

Figure 6-1 Ethical issues in nursing practice.

From: Scanlon, C. (1994a). Survey yields significant results. *American Nurses Association Center for Ethics in Human Rights Communique*, 3 (3), 3. Reprinted with permission.

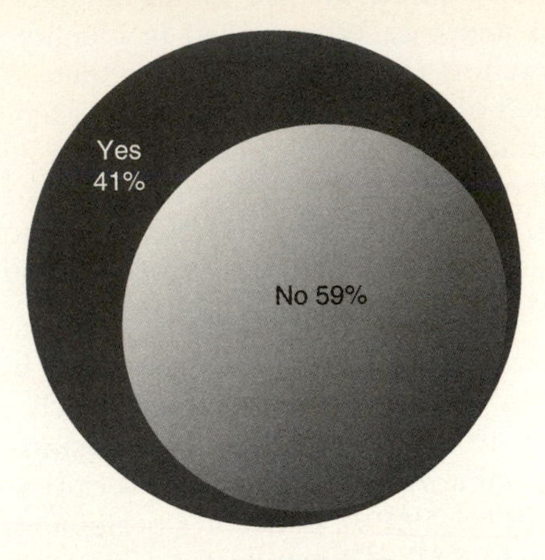

Figure 6-2 Ethical content in nursing education.

From: Scanlon, C. (1994a). Survey yields significant results. *American Nurses Association Center for Ethics in Human Rights Communique, 3* (3), 3. Reprinted with permission.

In 1973, the ANA published the first standards of practice for the nursing profession (ANA, 1973). The initial standards, based on the nursing process, pertain to general nursing practice. The revised document, *Standards of Clinical Nursing Practice,* includes standards that apply to all professional nurses "engaged in clinical practice, regardless of clinical specialty, practice setting, or educational preparation" (ANA, 1991a, p. 1). Specialty professional organizations and subcommittees of ANA define standards for specialty and advanced practice nurses (e.g., clinical nurse specialists, nurse-midwives, and nurse practitioners) (ANA, 1991a). "Specialty" organizations devoted to maternal-child nursing include: Maternal-Child Council of ANA, Association of Women's Health, Obstetrics and Neonatal Nurses (AWHONN), National Association of Neonatal Nurses (NANN), National Association of Pediatric Nurse Associates and Practitioners (NAPNAP), and the American College of Nurse-Midwives (ACNM). Table 6-2 presents standards for maternal-child nursing practice promulgated by these professional nursing organizations.

ANA's standards of professional performance describe a "competent level of behavior in the professional role" (Table 6-3, p. 78). Professional role activities vary according to the education, position, and practice setting of the individual nurse. Standards for specialty and/or advanced nursing practice may be an elaboration of the professional roles listed in the table and are promulgated by specialty organizations and advance-practice councils (ANA, 1991a). Professional nursing practice is also enhanced by: (a) membership in a professional nursing organization, (b) specialty practice or certification,

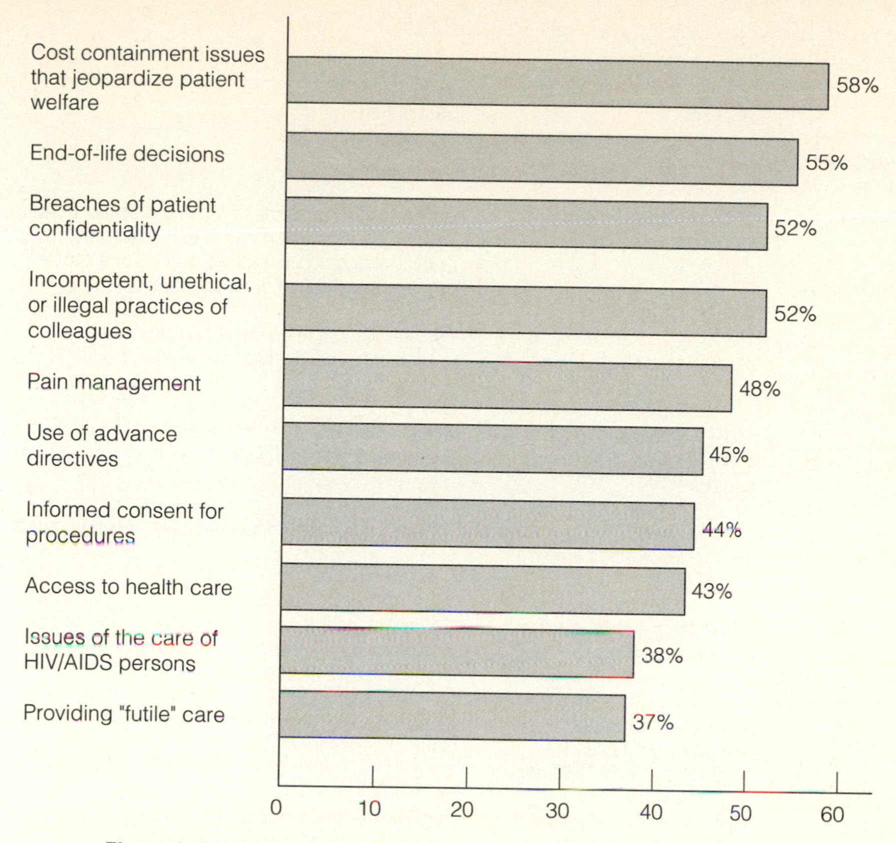

Figure 6-3 Ten most frequently occurring ethics and human rights issues confronting nurses in their practice.

From: Scanlon, C. (1994b). Ethics survey looks at nurses' experiences. *American Nurse, 26* (10), 22. Reprinted with permission.

and (c) advanced academic education (ANA, 1991a). Measurement criteria, "key indications of competent practice," are included for each professional practice standard (ANA, 1991a, p. 3).

ANA's standards of care describe a "competent level of nursing care as demonstrated by the nursing process, involving assessment, diagnosis, outcome identification, planning, implementation, and evaluation" (Table 6-4, p. 79). Used as the framework for nursing care, the nursing process "encompasses all significant actions taken by nurses in providing care to all clients and forms the foundation of clinical decision-making" (ANA, 1991a, p. 3).

Professional Liability Insurance

Demonstrating financial responsibility for nursing practice is essential because the public expects the professional to provide "remedy for any harm caused by error in the practice of the profession" (The American Association

Table 6-2 Maternal-Child Nursing Standards Promulgated by Professional Organizations

Organization	Standards	Description
American Nurses Association (ANA) • First nursing organization (1911) • First definition of professional nursing (1932) • Reorganized in 1966 into: practice, education, services, and economic and general welfare • First standards of nursing practice (1973) • Lobbies at local, state, and national level	*1980. Nursing: A social policy statement*	Defines basic standards of nursing practice; differentiates between standards of care and standards of professional practice. Defines nursing and clarifies the nature and scope of nursing practice.
	1980. A statement on the scope of maternal-child health nursing practice	Position statement on the scope of practice with childbearing and childrearing families.
	1980. A statement on the scope of high-risk perinatal nursing practice	Defines high-risk perinatal nursing, scope of practice, and nursing responsibilities.
	1983. Standards of maternal and child health nursing practice (out of print)	Defines standards of maternal-child nursing practice.
	1985. Standards of practice for the perinatal nurse specialist	Defines standards of practice for the perinatal nurse specialist (with advanced educational preparation at the master's or doctoral level).
	1985. Code for nurses with interpretive statements (revision of the 1976 edition)	Defines eleven components of the ethical code of conduct.
	1986. Standards of home health nursing practice	Defines standards of practice for organizations and nurses providing home health care across the lifespan.
	1988. Standards for organized nursing services	Defines standards for all settings where services are delivered; defines responsibilities and qualifications of nurse administrators.
	1991. Standards of clinical nursing practice (Revision of: *Standards of nursing practice* - 1973)	Defines basic standards for all types of nursing practice; differentiates between standards of care and practice.
	1994. Guidelines on reporting incompetent, unethical, or illegal practices	Defines incompetent, unethical, and illegal practices, addresses reporting responsibilities, and provides a model procedure for reporting.
	1994. Registered professional nurse and unlicensed assistive personnel	Discusses trends in the utilization of unlicensed assistive personnel. Presents guidelines for supervision, delegation, and assignment. Clearly presents what *not* to delegate.
Association of Women's Health, Obstetric, and Neonatal Nurses (AWHONN) • Founded in 1969 • Published first standards in 1974 • Independent organization in 1993	*1990. Nurse providers of neonatal care: Guidelines for educational development and practice*	Defines nursing roles, goals, and education for neonatal nursing specialization.

Table 6-2 Maternal-Child Nursing Standards Promulgated by Professional Organizations *(Continued)*

Organization	Standards	Description
Association of Women's Health, Obstetric, and Neonatal Nurses (AWHONN) (Continued)		
	1990. The obstetric-gynecologic/ women's health nurse practitioner: Role definition, competencies, and educational guidelines, 3rd edition	Describes roles, competencies, and education for advanced practice.
	1991. Standards for the nursing care of women and newborns, 4th edition (revision of 1974, 1981, and 1986 editions)	Describes specialty-specific practice standards for both inpatient and outpatient care.
	1991. Nursing practice competencies and educational guidelines: Antepartum fetal surveillance and intrapartum fetal heart monitoring, 2nd edition (revision of 1986 edition)	Defines competencies for use of electronic fetal monitors. Provides educational guidelines.
	1993. Nursing practice competencies and educational guidelines: Limited ultrasound examinations in obstetric and gynecologic/ infertility settings	Defines competencies and education required to perform ultrasound examinations.
	1993. Didactic content and clinical skills verification for professional nurse providers of basic, high-risk, and critical-care intrapartum nursing	Describes educational content and clinical skills verification for basic, high-risk, and critical-care intrapartum nursing.
	1994. Didactic content and clinical skills verification for professional nurse providers of perinatal home care	Describes educational content and clinical skills verification for perinatal home care.
National Association of Neonatal Nurses (NANN) • Founded in 1984 • Subspecialty interest groups (e.g., clinicians, practitioners, clinical nurse specialists, transport nurses, and educators) • Promulgates standards on practice and education • Plans, develops, and conducts conferences	*1990. Role definitions for advanced practice*	Defines advance-practice roles (e.g., clinical nurse specialist, neonatal nurse practitioner, and neonatal nurse clinician).
	1992. Neonatal nurse practitioners: Standards of education and practice	Defines neonatal nurse practitioner, educational requirements, professional practice, and roles.
	1993. Standards of care for neonatal nursing practice	Provides directives for minimum levels of care common to neonatal nursing practice.
	1994. Neonatal nursing transport standards and guidelines	Provides basic knowledge of transport patient problems and safety.

(Continued)

Table 6-2 Maternal-Child Nursing Standards Promulgated by Professional Organizations *(Continued)*

Organization	Standards	Description
National Association of Pediatric Nurse Associates and Practitioners (NAPNAP)		
• Founded in 1973 • Promotes child health care through education, research, and legislative action	*1987. Standards of practice for PNP/A's*	Defines the role of pediatric nurse practitioners (PNP) and the pediatric nurse associate in relation to standards.
American College of Nurse-Midwives (ACNM)		
• Founded in 1955 • Accredits educational programs • Establishes practice standards • Certifies nurse-midwives • Continuing education seminars and workshops	*1993. Standards of practice for ACNM's*	Ten-page brochure containing: (a) eight clinical practice standards, (b) code of ethics, (c) philosophy, and (d) guidelines for incorporating new procedures into nurse-midwife practice.

Table 6-3 Standards of Professional Performance

Standard	Statement
I. Quality of care	The nurse systematically evaluates the quality and effectiveness of nursing practice.
II. Performance appraisal	The nurse evaluates her own nursing practice in relation to professional practice standards and relevant statutes and regulations.
III. Education	The nurse acquires and maintains current knowledge in nursing practice.
IV. Collegiality	The nurse contributes to the professional development of peers, colleagues, and others.
V. Ethics	The nurse's decisions and actions on behalf of clients are determined in an ethical manner.
VI. Collaboration	The nurse collaborates with the client, significant others, and health care providers in providing client care.
VII. Research	The nurse uses research findings in practice.
VIII. Resource utilization	The nurse considers factors related to safety, effectiveness, and cost in planning and delivering client care.

From: American Nurses Association (1991). *Standards of clinical nursing practice.* Washington, D.C.: Author, pp. 13–17. Reprinted with permission.

of Nurse Attorneys, 1989, p. 1). Both the ANA and The American Association of Nurse Attorneys (TAANA) recommend that all nurses be insured against liabilities that may arise from their professional practice (ANA, 1991c; TAANA, 1989). While ANA recommends that each nurse purchase individual liability coverage, TAANA's brochure is presented in a form to assist the professional nurse in making an informed decision.

Table 6-4 Standards of Care

Standard	Statement
I. Assessment	The nurse collects client health data.
II. Diagnosis	The nurse analyzes the assessment data in determining diagnosis.
III. Outcome Identification	The nurse identifies expected outcomes individualized to the client.
IV. Planning	The nurse develops a plan of care that prescribes interventions to attain expected outcomes.
V. Implementation	The nurse implements the interventions identified in the plan of care.
VI. Evaluation	The nurse evaluates the client's progress toward attainment of outcomes.

From: American Nurses Association (1991). *Standards of clinical nursing practice.* Washington, D.C.: Author, pp. 9–11. Reprinted with permission.

Nationwide there is a trend toward increased nursing liability due to tort reform, the increased litigiousness of society, and increased professional accountability for nursing practice. According to ANA (1991c), the average liability award against nurses is around $40,000. However, claims for neurologically impaired infants are among the highest injury awards and out-of-court settlements ($250,000 to $900,000). If found liable for injury or harm to a patient, a nurse is responsible for financial compensation to that patient. If the judgment exceeds the limits of the insurance policy or the nurse is uninsured, payment may be collected from current and future assets, including savings accounts, inheritances, liens on properties, and garnishment of wages (TAANA, 1989). In some states, jointly owned property and assets may be protected from seizure by successful litigants. Understanding one's personal exposure—how much there is to lose—is crucial to the decisions made regarding liability coverage.

As mentioned in Chapter 4, obstetrical, neonatal and pediatric nurses have prolonged liability. This longer statute of limitations coupled with large settlements and jury awards make maternal-child nurses "high risk" for liability coverage. In 1985, certified nurse-midwives were dropped by the only insurance company still providing liability coverage. For a time in 1987, nurse practitioners had no coverage, and in 1988 nurses designated as "high risk" continued to have difficulty securing affordable coverage (ANA, 1991c).

Tort reform, and capping liability for each defendant, encourages naming multiple defendants, including nurses. ANA cites an increase in the number of nurses named as sole defendants in malpractice cases (ANA, 1991c). State nurse practice acts that delineate the independent functions of nursing (e.g., diagnosis, treatment, education, intervention, etc.) also increase the nurse's legal accountability and liability for exercising independent judgment and responsibility.

Understanding the limits and extent of nursing liability, the increased risk of the maternal-child specialty, and the influences of state laws enables the professional nurse to assess her personal exposure. Understanding the major types of insurance policies (Table 6-5) and the difference in coverage between an institutional and an individual liability policy (Table 6-6) enables the professional nurse to make an informed choice about being covered solely by the employer or about purchasing her own liability insurance.

Table 6-5 Types of Insurance Policies

Type	Characteristics
"Claims-Made"	Covers claims reported while policy is in force *only*.
	If policy is discontinued, future claims will not be covered unless the policy-holder purchases "tail" (a conversion from claims-made to occurrence coverage).
	Institutional policies typically are claims-made.
"Occurrence"	Covers acts or omissions rendered during the contract's policy period (even if claims are made after the policy period has ended).
	Individual policies typically are occurrence policies.

Adapted from: American Nurses Association (1991). *Liability prevention and you.* Kansas City, MO: Author, pp. 27–31 and The American Association of Nurse Attorneys, Inc. (1989). *Demonstrating financial responsibility for nursing practice.* Baltimore, MD: Author, pp. 4–8. Adapted with permission.

Table 6-6 Professional Liability Insurance Options

Type	Characteristics
Institutional liability policy	Employer purchased and provided.
	Typically "claims-made" coverage.
	Institution is primary insured party with fullest rights and responsibilities.
	Individual nurse as "additional insured" may have no right to separate defense.
	Covers specific professional activities (i.e., scope of nursing practice) while on the job (i.e., scope of employment).
	Institution may be able to sue nurse for all or part of money paid in settlement, judgment, and legal fees.
	Insurance company employs attorney; individual nurse may have no right to select counsel.
	Individual nurse has no right to refuse or authorize settlement.
Individual liability policy	Commercially purchased insurance or self-insurance.
	Typically "occurrence" coverage.
	Individual nurse is primary insured party; policy issued in individual name of insured nurse.
	Covers specific professional activities (i.e., scope of nursing practice) of the insured at any time and place (e.g., off-the-job).

Adapted from: American Nurses Association (1991). *Liability prevention and you.* Kansas City, MO: Author, pp. 27–31 and The American Association of Nurse Attorneys, Inc. (1989). *Demonstrating financial responsibility for nursing practice.* Baltimore, MD: Author, pp. 4–8. Adapted with permission.

Practice Discipline

Historically, the nursing profession has been described as a practice discipline. Nursing knowledge is derived primarily through clinical experience and nursing practice that stresses the importance of developing caring, personal relationships with patients. This is in contrast to the typical uniform, impersonal approach present in other practice disciplines (e.g., medicine, dentistry) (Bishop & Scudder, 1991). A practice discipline not only has a dominant moral sense that provides meaning, but also provides a sense of identity for its practitioners (Gadamer, 1981). This sense of identity comes from making choices for the inherent good of the patient (Gadamer, 1981). Consistent with Gadamer's approach to practice is MacIntyre's (1984) definition of practice as "any coherent and complex form of socially established cooperative human activity through which goods internal to that form of activity are realized in the course of trying to achieve those standards of excellence which are appropriate to, and partially definitive of, that form of activity, with the result that human powers to achieve excellence, and human conceptions of the ends and good involved, are systematically extended" (p. 187). This definition emphasizes the meaning of the whole and not of the particular skills involved in the practice. Newman et al. (1991) stated that a discipline is "distinguished by a domain of inquiry that represents a shared belief among its members regarding a reason for its being" (p. 1). A professional discipline is defined by its social, moral, and value orientations.

A Proactive, Professional Model for Nursing Practice

Models for professional nursing practice have emerged over the last two decades (e.g., ANA, 1980; Carpenito, 1993). Some of these models emphasize the use of a scientific process to analyze specific patient situations (i.e., the nursing process). In these models, the approach to the analysis of patient care situations is reactive (i.e., evaluating patient situations retrospectively). This approach recommends a uniform way of providing care (i.e., assessment, diagnosis, planning, implementation, and evaluation) and performing skills. "Standard care plans" focusing on disease processes (e.g., bronchiolitis, pregnancy-induced-hypertension, respiratory distress syndrome, etc.) and utilizing nursing diagnoses are derived from these models. These care plans can be helpful in the clinical setting to guide nursing actions. Unfortunately, in many instances, nurses do not individualize these standard care plans to the patient, but practice them as a "routine" approach to care (e.g., vital signs q 4 hrs, monitor patient condition q 2 hrs). Also, nurses may not include patients and families in the decision-making process. In some cases, nurses may not utilize critical thinking, communication, and individualized nursing therapeutics/skills as part of their problem-solving approach for care delivery.

Benner (1984) presented a practice-based model for nursing. In an interpretive study with practicing nurses, Benner uncovered 31 competencies of nursing practice which she grouped under seven domains: (a) the helping function, (b) the teaching/coaching function, (c) the diagnostic/monitoring function, (d) effective management of rapidly changing situations, (e) administering and monitoring therapeutic interventions and regimens, (f) monitoring and ensuring the quality of health practices, and (g) organization and work-role competencies. Benner poses a model for nursing practice that emphasizes not only functional aspects of nursing but the moral imperative for developing competency and therapeutic relationships with patients. In this model, she describes role development within nursing as a maturational process and skills acquisition from novice to expert.

Our model for nursing practice emphasizes proactive empowerment as a way to approach patient care. This model also integrates multiple patterns of knowing within nursing practice, including empirical, ethical, aesthetic, personal, and sociopolitical. In addition, several techniques of nursing practice are used, including critical thinking, communication, nursing therapeutics/skills, and the nursing process (Figure 6-4). We developed this model to teach practicing nurses to evaluate care as it is rendered, thus preventing patient injury/harm and subsequent litigation.

Proactive Empowerment

The practicing nurse experiences the conflict between empowerment and paternalism acutely because it is the nurse who must reconcile nursing's traditional alliance with the patient and its modern loyalty to medicine (Gadow, 1980). Although a paternalistic society has socialized women to accept powerless roles, in practicing their profession and advocating for patients, nurses must assume empowered roles. In fact, individual state nurse practice acts legally mandate empowered nursing practice. "The law generally assumes the same standard as does the profession" (Nosek, 1987, p. 41), and empowered nursing practice is also mandated by the *Code for Nurses* (ANA, 1985) and the *Standards of Clinical Nursing Practice* (ANA, 1991a).

The model in Figure 6-4 advocates proactive empowerment as the encompassing construct of professional nursing practice. Proactive means taking "the initiative and responsibility to make things happen" (Covey, 1989, p. 71). Proactive people recognize their ability to choose their response; their behavior is a product of their conscious choice (Covey, 1989). Proactivity is characterized by: (a) taking initiative, (b) focusing efforts on circumstances within one's control, (c) use of positive energy and attitudes to effect positive change, (d) acknowledging, correcting, and learning from mistakes, and (e) making and keeping commitments (Covey, 1989).

Empowerment is "the ability to enact one's own will and love for self in the context of love and respect for others" (Wheeler & Chinn, 1991, p. 2). The empowered nurse embodies control, confidence, credibility, competence, and confidence (see Figure 3-1) (Moores, 1993). When becoming empowered, the nurse moves developmentally through three phases: (a) reacting to

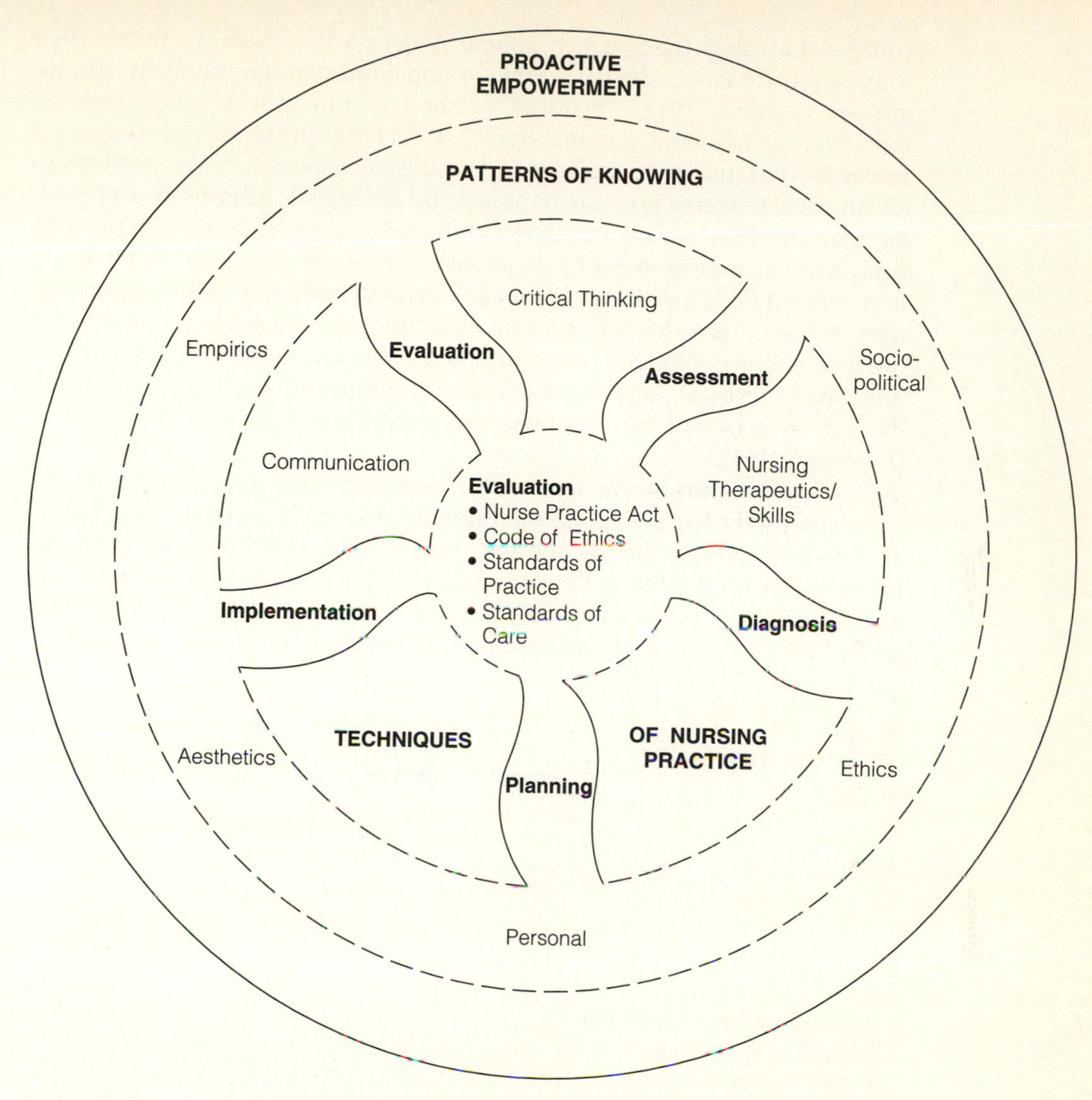

Figure 6-4 Proactive professional practice model.

threatening situations, (b) confronting nursing challenges, and (c) collaborating to resolve problems (see Chapter 3). The empowered nurse who practices proactively averts undesirable patient outcomes. Proactive problem-solving is a dynamic, ongoing process that occurs with every patient encounter. Empowered nurses assess, plan, implement, and resolve patient care issues *before* they become problems.

Empowered nursing practice is dependent not only on the individual professional but also on the support or lack of support provided by other professionals and the practice milieu. A supportive system provides the foundation for empowerment, while a nonsupportive environment disempowers (Moores, 1993). Institutions that integrate research into practice empower professional nursing staff. Keefe (1993) presented an integrated research-utilization model that promotes the collaboration of key institutional committees (nursing research, policy and procedure, education, and quality assurance) to develop a proactive risk management program (Figure 6-5). Proactive risk management by empowered nurses depends on the adoption of a supportive, proactive risk-management environment within an institution. A health care delivery system, expecting and supporting empowered nursing practice, benefits economically by preventing undesirable patient outcomes and legal liabilities. Professional status and autonomy also result in cost savings due to increased job satisfaction and nursing retention (Johnston, 1991).

Empowered nurses who take action are able to share power with patients and families by "approaching the nursing process as an enabling relationship, in which responsibility and accountability for health is shared with the client (patient)" (Leddy & Pepper, 1993, p. 392). A major role of the professional nurse is to act as a patient advocate (ANA, 1985, 1994). Gadow (1989) notes "advocacy typically has been understood as assistance to patients in

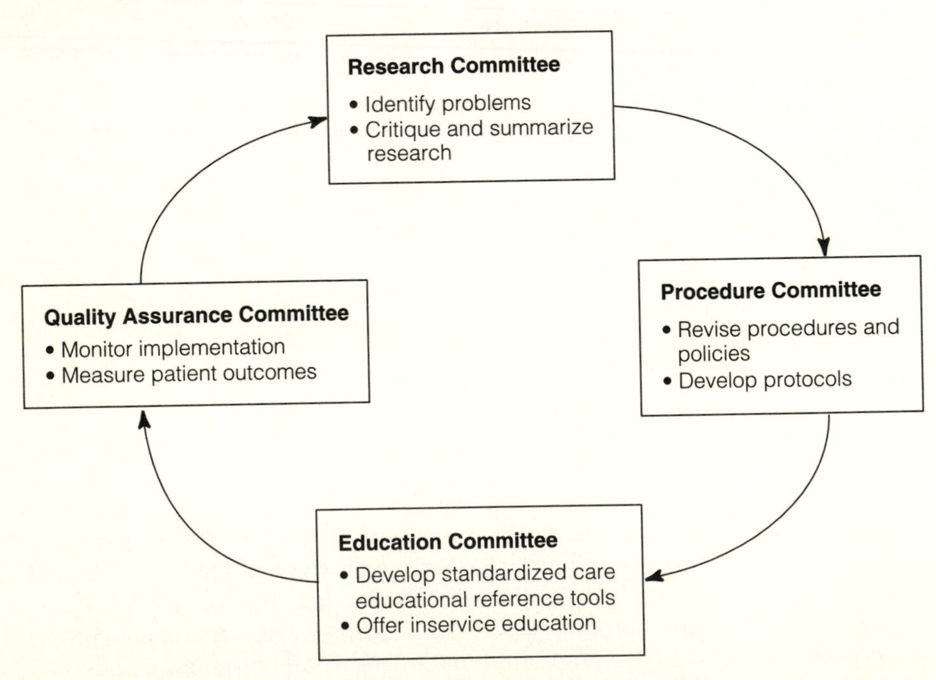

Figure 6-5 Integrated research-utilization model.

From: Keefe, M. (1993). An integrated approach to incorporating research findings into practice. *Maternal Child Nursing, 18,* March/April, (p. 66). Reprinted with permission.

giving voice to their values" (p. 541). Gadow's interpretation of nurses as existential advocates elaborates on a major theme of freedom of self-determination as the most fundamental and valuable of human rights. The nurse is an excellent existential advocate because she is situated between the patient, physician, and hospital bureaucracy. Empowered nurses are able to assist patients to become self-determining in ways that express "the full and unique complexity of their values" (Gadow, 1980, p. 97). This requires nurses to relate to patients as whole persons, bringing together the personal and professional and the lived body and the body object (Gadow, 1980). Gadow (1980) succinctly describes existential advocacy as "participating with the patient in determining the personal meaning which the experience of illness, suffering, or dying is to have for that individual" (p. 97). Gadow's contention lies in the call for nurses to assist patients to become self-determining whole human beings. The empowered nurse as advocate supports the patient, acts on the patient's behalf, and shares responsibility for decision-making with the patient (Leddy & Pepper, 1993).

Patterns of Knowing

A second construct within our proactive practice model utilizes Carper's (1978) and White's (1995) patterns of knowing, which may be defined as the ways in which nurses develop knowledge and evaluate patient situations (Table 6-7). Nursing's unique body of knowledge serves as the rationale for

Table 6-7 Carper's and White's Patterns of Knowing

Patterns of Knowing	Description
Empirics (the science of nursing) Describing, explaining, and predicting	Development of empirical knowledge by the scientific method (i.e., what is known is accessible through the senses).
Ethics (the moral imperative of nursing) Clarifying, valuing, and advocating	Making ethical judgments based on values, norms, formal codes, and principles.
Personal (self understanding/knowing) Experiencing, centering, and realizing	Inner experience; awareness of the genuine self.
Aesthetics (expressive aspect/art of nursing) Representing, interpreting, and envisioning	Moves beyond the immediate comprehension of meaning within a specific situation to the possibilities within the situation and actions taken to create those possibilities.
Sociopolitical (the sociopolitical context of nursing) Understanding the sociopolitical on two levels; the sociopolitical context of the person (nurse and patient), and of nursing as a profession Exposing, exploring, critiquing, and transforming	The sociopolitical context of the nurse-patient relationship fundamentally concerns cultural identity (through culture the self is intrinsically located). Cultural location influences each person's understanding of health and disease causation, language, identity, and connection to the land.

Adapted with permission from: Carper, B. (1978). Fundamental patterns of knowing in nursing. *Advances in Nursing Science, 1* (1), 13–23 and White, J. (1995). Patterns of knowing: Review, critique, and update. *Advances in Nursing Science, 17* (4), 73–86.

pratice that "serves as horizons of expectations and exemplifies characteristic ways of thinking about phenomena" (Chinn & Jacobs, 1987). The integration of Carper's and White's patterns of knowing into this model extends nursing knowledge and invites nurses to question critically what it means to know.

Techniques of Nursing Practice

A third construct within our proactive practice model is techniques of nursing practice. These techniques include: critical thinking, communication, and nursing therapeutics/skills.

Critical Thinking In today's practice milieu, nurses must be able to adopt a scientific approach to solving problems. Critical thinking is a creative, cognitive process based on reflective thought and a tolerance for ambiguity. Critical thinkers: (a) are self directed, (b) are oriented toward inquiry, analysis, and critique, (c) are multidimensional, multilogical problem-solvers, (d) generate options, and (e) make discriminating decisions (Beth El College of Nursing, 1996). Nurses who are critical thinkers exhibit an openness to change and an awareness of the diversity of values, behaviors, and social structures within patient-care encounters (Leddy & Pepper, 1993). Using critical thinking, the nurse evaluates information and makes judgments and decisions about the patient's plan of care.

Critical thinking in nursing practice includes use and articulation of a scientific or empirical basis for practice (Keefe, 1993). Often nursing practice is based on rituals and routines that do not have a research base. Research utilization incorporating or applying research findings in the delivery of patient care, results in research-based nursing practice (Figure 6-6) (Keefe, 1993). The Joint Commission on Accreditation of Health Care Organizations (JCAHO, 1995), as well as professional nursing organizations (ANA, 1985, 1991a;

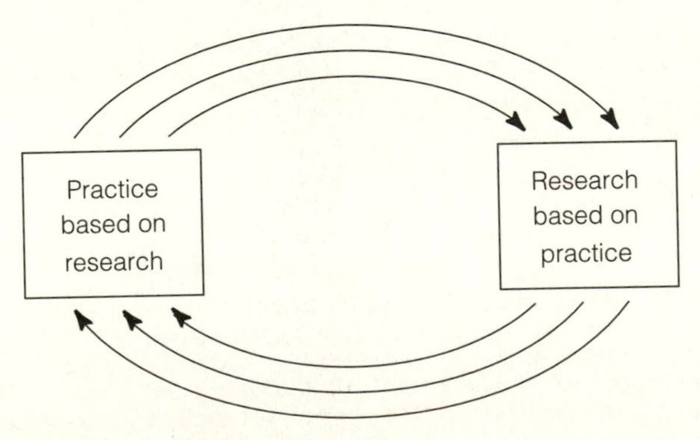

Figure 6-6 Influence of research on nursing practice.

From: Keefe, M. (1993). An integrated approach to incorporating research findings into practice. *Maternal Child Nursing, 18,* March/April, (p. 66). Reprinted with permission.

NAACOG, 1991), mandate the use of scientific knowledge (i.e., research findings) as the basis for nursing practice.

Communication Within the milieu of high technology and increased workload, nurses must develop new and effective communication skills. Commonly, nurses communicate information about the patient through verbal and nonverbal strategies and written documentation. On a daily basis nurses assess, inform, educate, and support patients. Through a nonjudgmental and compassionate approach, nurses plan and implement care while identifying each patient as a unique being.

Within the nurse-patient and/or family relationship, all participants undergo emotional experiences as a function of the communication process (Leddy & Pepper, 1993). The quality of communication between the nurse and patient and/or family depends on establishing a professional, caring relationship. Communication with the patient and/or family must be therapeutic. "Communication that is therapeutic is the outcome of behaviors that are purposeful, authentic, and consonant with an attitude of caring" (Hein, 1980, p. 17).

Human beings influence others primarily through communication. Communication is described as the "matrix for all thought and relationships between persons" (Murray & Zentner, 1979, p. 62). Four major purposes of communication include: (a) to inquire, (b) to inform, (c) to persuade, and (d) to entertain (Cecchio & Cecchio, 1982). The professional nurse may attempt to achieve any of these purposes with patients, peers, other health care personnel, and even herself. With a variety of communication techniques, the professional nurse hopes to create new situations with the patient or other health care providers in making decisions regarding care.

Messages are communicated verbally and nonverbally (Leddy & Pepper, 1993). Three sources of verbal/nonverbal communication exist within nursing practice: (a) nurse-to-nurse, (b) nurse-to-patient and/or family, (c) nurse-to-other professionals (e.g., physicians, therapists, pharmacists). Nurse-to-nurse communication often concerns patient status and needs or unit issues. Ideally, verbal communication concerning the patient's condition occurs in a quiet place where confidentiality is assured. Nurse-to-patient communication is an ongoing process in which the nurse conveys information concerning treatments, skills, and self-care. Nurses must introduce themselves as the providers of nursing care and develop communication strategies that convey respect and care. Successful therapeutic communication is based on credibility (i.e., the patient and/or family's belief in, or trust of, the nurse). The messages nurses give patients occur not only verbally but through non-verbal behaviors which either support or refute the verbal message (Table 6-8). Nurses also communicate with a myriad of other health care providers to facilitate optimum patient care.

Further, implicit in all models of communication is the concept that communication has two interacting components: (a) the content value of the

Table 6-8 Communication Techniques

Verbal Communication	Nonverbal Communication
Vocabulary: use of terms that the patient understands.	Appearance: physical appearance may convey messages about professional competence, concern, role model of health.
Denotative meaning: shared meaning of words between individuals.	Posture and gait: may indicate emotional state, self-concept, and overall health.
Connotative meaning: thoughts, feelings, or ideas conveyed through the use of words which cannot be easily misinterpreted.	Facial expression: may reveal certain emotions (e.g., surprise, fear, anger, disgust, happiness, and sadness).
Pacing (e.g., talking rapidly, using awkward pauses, or speaking slowly and deliberately) may convey messages that are unintended.	Eye contact: may signal a willingness to listen. Avoid looking down at the patient; sit at eye level. Lack of eye contact may be cultural.
Intonation: tone of voice that affects perceived meaning or is misinterpreted (e.g., as uncaring, condescending, indifferent).	Gestures: may convey a specific message through the use of hand motions or foot tapping.
Humor: stimulates the production and release of catecholamines and endorphins, creating feelings of well-being; improves pain tolerance; reduces anxiety; induces respiratory relaxation; enhances metabolism. With humor, patients and nurses interact more openly and honestly.	Touch: very personal form of communication which may convey concern, emotional support, and authenticity. The nurse must consider the client's attitude toward touching prior to its use.
Clarity and brevity: communication is simple, direct, and to the point. Stategies include using easily understood words, speaking slowly, and enunciating clearly. Use words that express an idea simply and directly.	Sounds: nonverbal inflections (e.g., crying, moaning, and sighing) may be interpreted as other than intended.
Timing and relevance: timely presentation of ideas using patient cues of readiness and relevance.	Space and territory: defined by distance between patient and nurse. Intrusion of personal space may elicit a defensive response, preventing effective communication. The distance separating the nurse from the patient is often determined by the nature of the interaction (i.e., intimate: 0 to 18 inches; personal: 18 inches to 4 feet; social: 4 to 12 feet; public: 12 feet or greater).

Adapted with permission from: Potter, P. & Perry, A. (1995). *Fundamentals of nursing: Concepts, process, and practice.* St. Louis: Mosby-Yearbook, pp. 308–316.

message, and (b) the interactional or perceptual value of the message and the communicators. Lack of congruence in verbal communication among nurse, peers, health care professionals, and/or the patient usually results from the nurse's inability to relay a coherent, valid message, to accurately transmit the intended message, or to achieve the outcome expected from communication of the issue. Nurses must strive to be clear, succinct, objective, and factual about the information to be communicated.

Nurses use verbal and written communication to convey pertinent information about the patient's condition. Standards established by the JCAHO (1995) require quality-improvement audits aimed at identifying and correcting actual or potential problems. Documenting patient care is a professional responsibility and must reflect the use of the nursing process (ANA, 1991a). The nurse supports each component of the nursing process by documentation included in the patient's medical record. This is a legal document, the key purpose of which is to communicate interdisciplinary care, treatments, and progress toward health restoration. In the event of litigation, the medical record documents the care rendered and, as a defense tool, demonstrates that the standard of care was met. Incompleteness of medical records can in turn implicate the providers of care. ("If it's not charted, it wasn't done.") Again, the nurse must document *all* components of the nursing process (see Chapter 4).

Therapeutics/Skills Nursing therapeutics/skills include actions, behaviors, and interventions the nurse uses to promote self-healing of the patients for whom she cares. These actions, behaviors, and interventions are elemental to a transpersonal caring relationship during the nurse/patient encounter. Nursing therapeutics/skills include: (a) implementation of clinical decision-making, (b) interventions critical to nursing practice, (c) theory-based nursing activities, and (d) interdisciplinary collaboration. A key concept in nursing therapeutics/skills is competence. Competence emerges as the nurse develops the knowledge-base critical to nursing practice and gains skills to successfully resolve patient and/or nursing issues. The *Standards of Clinical Nursing Practice* (ANA, 1991a) outlines several key skills a nurse must possess in practice, and *Code for Nurses* (ANA, 1985) states that the nurse must maintain competency within practice.

Nursing Process

The core, ongoing evaluation, of our proactive model and its emerging strands together convey the nursing process as a dynamic, changing, problem-solving method (see Figure 6-4). The strands which depict the components of the nursing process (assessment, diagnosis, plan, implementation, and evaluation) continually flow and are mutually interrelated to the patterns of knowing and the techniques of nursing practice. The components of the nursing process are interrelated, influence the whole, and are sequential, but not linear (Leddy & Pepper, 1993). To illustrate the separate, yet interrelated, nature of the activities of the nursing process, the strands are depicted as non-linear with open boundaries representing flow between the ways of knowing, the techniques of nursing practice, and ongoing evaluation.

The nursing process organizes specific information and data in an orderly manner, and represents a systematic approach for the pursuit of knowledge and the accomplishment of specified goals. Evolving from the scientific method, the nursing process is part of the model that nurses use to direct actions and achieve patient care goals (Table 6-9). The nursing process may be used in any patient care situation to: (a) assess the patient's health status or related needs, (b) formulate nursing diagnoses, (c) collaboratively plan with the patient and family to resolve identified needs, (d) implement nursing interventions, and (e) continuously evaluate outcomes (to determine the effectiveness of each of the previous activities and the need for further revision).

Table 6-9 Comparison of the Steps in the Scientific Method, a Problem-Solving Method, and the Nursing Process

Scientific Method	Problem-Solving Method	Nursing Process
Recognizing the problem Collecting data	Encountering problem Collecting data	Assessing
Formulating hypothesis	Identifying exact nature of problem	Formulating nursing diagnosis
Selecting plan for testing hypothesis	Determining plan of action	Planning
Testing hypothesis	Carrying out plan	Implementing
Interpreting results Evaluating hypothesis	Evaluation plan in new situation	Evaluating

From: Potter, P. & Perry, A. (1995). *Fundamentals of nursing*. St. Louis: Mosby-Yearbook, p. 148. Reprinted with Permission.

The nursing process consists of five components, depicted as wave-like strands in the model: (a) assessment, (b) diagnosis, (c) planning, (d) implementation, and (e) evaluation (ANA, 1980; Carpenito, 1993; Leddy & Pepper, 1993). Assessment includes data gathering, verification, and interpretation. The nurse collects and interprets the patient's history (e.g., physiologic, psychosocial, developmental, spiritual, and environmental data). Multi-disciplinary input is often necessary to formulate a comprehensive data base. Data must be accessible, communicated, and recorded (ANA, 1991a). Common errors in assessment include: (a) lack of complete data, (b) changing data, (c) inability to interpret data, and/or (d) inability to recognize the significance of information gathered (see Chapter 4). These errors result in erroneous or substandard assessments.

Diagnosis is the classifying of data into clusters or categories for labeling (Potter & Perry, 1995). Nursing diagnosis is defined as "a statement that describes the human response (health state or actual or potential altered interaction pattern) of an individual or group which the nurse can legally identify and for which the nurse can order the definitive interventions to maintain the health state or to reduce, eliminate, or prevent alterations" (Carpenito, 1992, p. 5). Nursing diagnoses are made up of three components: (a) the patient's actual or potential health problem, (b) the etiologic factor(s), and (c) supporting signs and symptoms (Gordon, 1982). An inability to incorporate data into appropriate nursing diagnostic terminology precludes professional nursing actions and interventions, resulting in unmet patient needs (see Chapter 4).

Planning, the third phase, initiates nursing management of patient care (Potter & Perry, 1995). Utilizing assessment data and nursing diagnoses, the nurse provides for continuity of care by prioritizing patient needs and goals. The nursing care plan: (a) gives direction and guidance to care providers, (b) provides a method of communicating, synchronizing, and organizing care activities, and (c) provides for continuity of care (Griffith & Christensen, 1982). Common errors occurring in the planning phase include failure to construct comprehensive, individualized, and specific care plans, resulting in acts of omission or commission (see Chapter 4).

Implementation, the action phase of the nursing process, includes independent, interdependent, and dependent nursing actions based on patient needs (see Table 4-3, Chapter 4). Diverse skills, including psychomotor abilities, teaching, leadership, management, and communication are essential in effective nursing interventions (Leddy & Pepper, 1993). Common errors in the implementation of nursing care include: (a) patient identification errors, (b) patient safety errors, (c) medication errors, and (d) product liability (see Chapter 4).

Traditionally, evaluation has been depicted as the final phase in the nursing process. In our proactive practice model, evaluation is the core and a recurring construct. According to this model, the practicing nurse proactively evaluates each activity of the nursing process as care is rendered. In order to practice professionally, the nurse must be: (a) knowledgeable about the scope of practice delineated in individual state nurse practice acts, (b) knowledgeable about the code of conduct delineated in the nursing code of ethics, (c) knowledgeable about standards for general, specialty, and/or advanced practice, and (d) knowledgeable about standards of care, including application of the nursing process in general, specialty, and/or advanced practice. With ongoing evaluation, the progress or lack of progress toward the achievement of patient goals is determined collaboratively by both nurse and patient. Evaluation continually reorders priorities, redirects assessments, develops new goals, and alters and revises the nursing care plan. Failure to evaluate results in failure to reassess, plan, diagnose, and intervene in new or alternative ways (see Chapter 4).

When the nursing process is not used or is used incorrectly, the result is substandard patient care. In a retroactive process, in which nursing care is evaluated during litigation or after harm has occurred, the outcome is analyzed to determine the point(s) at which negligent care was delivered. Retroactive evaluation often reveals that the undesirable patient outcome could have been averted if professional, proactive nursing practice had occurred.

Our professional nursing practice model proactively evaluates each activity within the nursing process according to the mandates of nursing practice, within the framework of proactive empowerment, and encompassing patterns of knowing and techniques of nursing practice. Chapters 7 to 14 of this book present actual nursing malpractice cases. Facts of the cases are followed by case commentaries divided into undesirable and desirable patient outcomes utilizing components of the nursing process. Evaluations of desirable patient outcomes cite nurse practice acts, code of ethics, and standards of practice and standards of care that, if followed, would have resulted in very different results for the patient, the defendant nurses, and their employers.

References

American Nurses Association. (1973). *Standards of nursing practice.* Kansas City, MO: Author.

American Nurses Association. (1980). *Nursing: A social policy statement.* Kansas City, MO: Author.

American Nurses Association. (1985). *Code for nurses with interpretive statements.* Washington D.C.: Author.

American Nurses Association. (1991a). *Standards of clinical nursing practice.* Washington DC: Author.

American Nurses Association. (1991b). ANA statement. In B. Barnum (Ed.). An interview with Carolyn Hutcherson. *Nursing and Healthcare, 12,* 244–247.

American Nurses Association. (1991c). *Liability prevention and you.* Kansas City, MO: Author.

American Nurses Association. (1994). *Guidelines on reporting incompetent, unethical, or illegal practices.* Washington D.C.: Author.

American Nurses Association Commission on Nursing Education. (1975). *Standards for nursing education.* Kansas City, MO: Author.

Anderson, K., Anderson, L., & Glanze, W. (Eds.). (1994). *Mosby's medical, nursing, and allied health dictionary,* 4th ed. St. Louis: Mosby-Yearbook.

Benner, P. (1984). *From novice to expert.* Menlo Park, CA: Addison-Wesley Nursing.

Beth El College of Nursing. (1996). *Conceptual practice model.* Colorado Springs, CO: Author.

Bishop, A. & Scudder, J. (1991). *Nursing the practice of caring.* New York: National League for Nursing Press.

Carpenito, L. (1992). *Nursing diagnosis and application to clinical practice,* 5th ed. Philadelphia: Lippincott.

Carpenito, L. (1993). *Nursing diagnosis and application to clinical practice,* (6th ed.). Philadelphia: Lippincott.

Carper, B. (1978). Fundamental patterns of knowing in nursing. *Advances in Nursing Science, 1* (1), 13–23.

Cecchio, J. & Cecchio, C. (1982). *Effective communication in nursing theory and practice.* New York: Wiley.

Chinn, P. & Jacobs, M. (1987). *Theory and nursing.* St. Louis: Mosby-Yearbook.

Covey, S. (1989). *The seven habits of highly effective people.* New York: Simon & Schuster.

Curtin, L. (1982). Autonomy, accountability, and nursing practice. *Topics in Clinical Nursing, 4* (1), 7–14.

Gadamer, H. (1981). *Reason in the age of science.* (F. Lawrence, trans.). Cambridge, MA: MIT Press.

Gadow, S. (1980). Existential advocacy: Philosophical foundation of nursing. In S. Spicker & S. Gadow (Eds.), *Nursing images and ideals.* New York: Springer.

Gadow, S. (1984). Touch and technology: Two paradigms of patient care. *Journal of Religion and Health, 23* (1), 63–69.

Gadow, S. (1989). Clinical subjectivity: Advocacy with silent patients. *Nursing Clinics of North America, 24* (2), 535–541.

Gordon, M. (1982). *Manual of nursing diagnosis.* New York: McGraw-Hill.

Griffith, J. & Christensen, P. (1982). *Nursing process: Application of theories, frameworks, and models.* St. Louis: Mosby-Yearbook.

Hein, E. (1980). *Communication in nursing practice,* 2nd ed. Boston: Little, Brown, & Company.

Johnston, C. (1991). Sources of work satisfaction/dissatisfaction for hospital registered nurses. *Western Journal of Nursing Research, 13,* 503–513.

Joint Commission on Accreditation of Healthcare Organizations. (1995). *Accreditation manual for hospitals.* Chicago: Author.

Keefe, M. (1993). An integrated approach to incorporating research findings into practice. *Maternal Child Nursing,* 18, March/April, 65–70.

Kjervik, D. & Martinson, I. (1979). *Women in stress: A nursing perspective.* Norwalk, CT: Appleton-Century-Crofts, p. 22.

Leddy, S. & Pepper, J. (1993). *Conceptual bases of professional nursing,* 3rd ed. Philadelphia: Lippincott.

MacIntyre, A. (1984). *After virtue,* 2nd ed. Notre Dame, IN: University of Notre Dame Press.

Moores, P. (1993). *Becoming empowered: A grounded theory study of staff nurse empowerment.* Ann Arbor, MI: UMI Dissertation Services. Order number 9401789.

Murray, R. & Zentner, J. (1979). *Nursing concepts for health promotion,* 2nd ed. Englewood Cliffs, NJ: Prentice-Hall.

Newman, M. (1990). Nursing paradigms and realities. In N. Chaska (Ed.), *The nursing profession: Turning points.* St. Louis: Mosby-Yearbook.

Newman, M., Sime, A., & Corcoran-Perry, S. (1991). The focus of the discipline of nursing. *Advances in Nursing Science, 14* (1), 1–6.

Nightingale, F. (1859). *Notes on nursing: What it is and what it is not.* London: Harrison and Sons.

North American Nursing Diagnosis Association (1995). *Nursing diagnosis: definition and classification.* Philadelphia, PA: Author.

Nosek, J. (1987). Expanded role liability in perinatal nursing. *Journal of Perinatal and Neonatal Nursing, 1* (2), 39–48.

Nurses' Association of the American College of Obstetricians and Gynecologists. (1991). *Standards for the nursing care of women and newborns.* Washington, D.C.: Author.

Phillips, J. (1990). The different views of health. *Nursing Science Quarterly, 3* (3), 103–104.

Potter, P. & Perry, A. (1995). *Fundamentals of nursing.* St. Louis: Mosby-Yearbook.

Scanlon, C. (1994a). Survey yields significant results. *American Nurses Association Center for Ethics and Human Rights Communique, 3,* (3) 1–3.

Scanlon, C. (1994b). Ethics survey looks at nurses' experiences. *The American Nurse, 26* (10), 22.

The American Association of Nurse Attorneys, Inc. (1989). *Demonstrating financial responsibility for nursing practice.* Baltimore, MD: Author.

Watson, M.J. (1985). *Nursing: Human science and human caring.* Norwalk, CT: Appleton-Century-Crofts.

Wheeler, C. & Chinn, P. (1991). *Peace and power: A handbook of feminist process,* 3rd ed. New York: National League for Nursing Press.

White, J. (1995). Patterns of knowing: Review, critique, and update. *Advances in Nursing Science, 17* (4), 73–86.

7

Low-Risk Obstetrical Care

Christine Sullivan, RN, MSN, CNM, CNAA, PhD
Mary A. Bowden, RN, MSN, WHNP
Sandra L. Gardner, RN, MS, CNS, PNP
Mary I. Enzman Hagedorn, RN, PhD, CNS, CPNP
Marcia Garman Laux, RN, MSN

Maternal-child health care practices and policies are undergoing dramatic changes in today's environment of cost containment and managed care. One significant change directly impacting maternal care is the implementation of early-discharge programs mandated by many third-party payers as a mode for cost containment. Health care organizations also are trying to lower their costs through the development of alternative care-delivery systems that incorporate unlicensed assistive personnel (UAPs), a move which "weakens the intricate web of safe, high-quality health care" (Phillips, 1995, p. 55). Phillips (1995) continues: "The fact remains that nurses, who are primarily women, are still seen as being dispensable in a male-dominated health care system, where they can be exchanged for less qualified persons to decrease health care costs" (p. 55). Over the last decade, low-risk maternal-newborn care has experienced several transitions, including the advent of mother-baby units and birthing centers, an increased use of advanced practice nurses (CNMs), and an increased number of early-discharge programs, all of which influence the number of professional versus unlicensed personnel providing health care services.

Low-risk obstetrical care is a misnomer. At any given moment, a low-risk situation can change to one of high risk. Designating a woman as low-risk (either prenatally or intrapartally) simply implies that she does not demonstrate key risk factors which often lead to poor outcomes for either a mother, a fetus, or both (see Appendix C). Twenty to thirty percent of low-risk pregnancies become high-risk cases intrapartally (Hobel, Hyvarinen, Okada, Oh, 1973). About 20% of pregnancies in the US are at some risk and about 5% are at very high risk. Clinicians identify 50% of these women antenatally and another 25% during labor. Low-risk pregnancy can become high risk postpartally as well (Benson & Pernoll, 1994). Therefore, obstetric nurses must at all times consider the unexpected and foresee the potential for maternal and/or fetal harm. Universal implementation of the nursing process, using critical thinking, anticipatory planning, and monitoring in all patient care situations, is critical to nursing competency and may reduce the risk of poor outcome for the mother or baby. Failure to utilize and individualize the steps of the nursing process to identify actual or potential risk factors results in serious nursing negligence.

Consumer demands have prompted efforts by hospitals and other health care institutions to provide a home-like environment for childbirth. This has resulted in a decreased use of invasive technology in many institutions. New technology, scientific advances, and research in obstetrics continue to challenge and change the standards of care and standards of practice. Unfortunately, health care administrators may not always incorporate these changes in practice into organizational policies to guide the nurse provider in her practice. Obstetrical risk management mandates the establishment of policies that ensure the nurse provider is properly oriented, trained, and credentialed to give obstetrical care. This is supported by the Joint Commission on Accreditation of Healthcare Organizations (JCAHO, 1995).

Obstetrical risk management should be a proactive process for all nurse providers, whether they are practicing in a small community hospital that does low-risk, low-volume obstetrics or a large teaching hospital that does high-risk, high-volume obstetrics. The continual rise in lawsuits involving obstetrics requires a thorough implementation of the nursing process in everyday practice. Managing obstetrical cases complacently, without attention to potentially ominous signs or preparation for unexpected adverse occurrences, increases liability for the nurse and the institution. Proactive measures to reduce the potential for harm include formulation of new institutional policies to guide nurses who engage in advanced practice and use advanced technology, as well as adherence to the current standards of practice defined by the institution, state nurse practice acts, and national professional organizations.

This chapter presents three low-risk obstetrical cases that developed complications. The first case demonstrates how a lack of communication and a failure to identify developing risk factors led to fetal demise. In the second case, a cross-training program without proper implementation and supervision resulted in maternal morbidity. The final case describes how an early-discharge program without appropriate policies and procedural guidance resulted in maternal death.

Case 1

Facts

In a small 99-bed community hospital, the maternity area consists of eight labor, delivery, and recovery rooms (LDRs) and a 20-bed postpartum-nursery unit. During office hours, obstetrical patients are assessed by their physicians unless they are in active labor, in which case they come to the labor and delivery area for assessment and triage by obstetrical nurses. At the time of the events described in this case, there were six patients in labor and four RNs on duty. One RN was assisting a patient who was complete and pushing. Another RN was admitting a patient in early labor and was also assigned to a second patient who was in active labor. A third RN, Nurse Stone, was assigned to the examination/admission room and assisting the other RNs as needed. A fourth RN, Nurse Poe, was assigned to two patients in active labor. Early in the evening, the following sequence of events occurred:

2000: Marianne Jones, a 28-year-old gravida (G) 2 para (P) 1 at 38 weeks gestation, called Labor and Delivery (L&D) and spoke to Nurse Poe informing her that she had been contracting every five to ten minutes for the past two hours. During the conversation, Nurse Poe asked Marianne if she had felt her baby move during the past day. Upon hearing that she had not felt fetal movement, Nurse Poe instructed Marianne to come to the hospital immediately.

2100: Marianne and her husband arrived at Labor and Delivery. Nurse Stone was unaware that Marianne had not felt fetal movement in 24 hours. Nurse Poe had failed to communicate the information shared in the phone call to any other nurse. Nurse Stone introduced herself to Marianne and began orienting her to the L&D unit. During the admission interview, Marianne revealed that she had had contractions for the past two hours and when she called was instructed to come to the hospital.

Nurse Stone placed the fetal monitor, took vital signs, began the assessment interview, and reviewed the prenatal chart, after obtaining a copy of the chart from the files. Marianne confirmed that she had not had any prenatal complications nor any leaking amniotic fluid.

2110: Marianne's vital signs were recorded as follows: T 98, R 20, P 78, BP 110/65. Vaginal examination revealed: 1–2 cm dilated, 80% effaced, and vertex –2 station. Nurse Stone informed Marianne that she was still in early labor and asked about the quality of her contractions. Marianne stated that she was not overly uncomfortable but hadn't been able to sleep through the night. Nurse Stone offered and Marianne accepted a sleeping pill. Nurse Stone informed Marianne that she could go home when her fetal heart rate (FHR) monitoring test was completed (in about 20–40 minutes).

2125: After completing vital signs, writing a progress note, and bringing Marianne juice and a blanket, Nurse Stone left to check another patient.

2150: Upon Nurse Stone's return, she evaluated (via fetal monitor strip) and documented that one FHR deceleration into the 90s for 1.5 minutes (not associated with a contraction) had occurred. Baseline rate was in the 130s with baseline variability at ±10 beats per minute (bpm). Immediately after the deceleration, one FHR acceleration (into the 170s, 15–20 seconds) was noted. Contractions were 6–10 minutes apart, lasting only 30–60 seconds. Nurse Stone explained that the FHR deceleration could be a sign that the umbilical cord was compressed for a short period of time. She asked

Marianne if in her absence, she moved. Upon confirmation, Nurse Stone explained that this deceleration was due to Marianne's movement. Nurse Stone said that she would continue the monitor for a little while longer, and left to care for her other patients.

2210: Upon her return, Nurse Stone evaluated the FHR strip and noted that no further decelerations or accelerations had occurred. Baseline rate remained in the 130 to 140s. Since there were no further decelerations, Nurse Stone decided to discharge Marianne. Marianne asked about the sleeping pill. Nurse Stone gave her a sleeping pill, secobarbital (Seconal), and instructed her to come back: (a) if her contractions became stronger and more frequent, (b) if her membranes leaked amniotic fluid, or (c) if she noticed decreased fetal movement. Marianne informed Nurse Stone that her baby hadn't moved all day. Nurse Stone reassured her that the monitor showed that her baby was all right. Upon learning that Marianne's next doctor's appointment was in two days, Nurse Stone reassured her that her doctor would check her then. Marianne was discharged with her husband.

Upon arriving home, Marianne took the Seconal and slept well throughout the night. The next morning Marianne had no contractions and went about her daily activities. Because her fetus had been monitored the night before, Marianne felt reassured that her baby was all right, although she did notice that her baby had not moved that day.

The following day, at her weekly doctor's appointment, the physician could not hear the FHR with a doptone. To confirm his findings, he performed an ultrasound examination which revealed: (a) no fetal heart beat, and (b) no fetal movement.

Outcome

Intrauterine fetal death.

Legal

This case is currently under litigation.

Case Commentary

Undesirable Patient Outcome

Assessment Failure to communicate information from one RN to another resulted in an inadequate assessment of risk. Nurse Poe, who received the phone call, should have informed Nurse Stone, who was assigned to the examination room, that: (a) Marianne had felt no fetal movement that day, and (b) she had instructed Marianne to come in for examination. Since Nurse Stone was unaware of this relevant information, she failed to ask about fetal movement, a gross indicator of fetal health. Her assessment focused solely on determining adequacy of contractions, cervical dilation, and effacement (i.e., if the patient's progress warranted admission).

Diagnosis No nursing diagnoses were formulated.

Planning Inadequate assessment for fetal well-being resulted in no formulation of nursing diagnoses, and no development of a plan of care. The nurse's only plan was that the patient keep her scheduled physician-appointment in two days.

Implementation Inappropriate and inadequate nursing interventions occurred as a result of faulty assessment, no formulation of nursing diagnosis, and lack of a nursing care plan.

Evaluation Nurse Stone performed no evaluation because no plan of care existed.

Desirable Patient Outcome

Assessment Nurse Stone's assessment of fetal status was deficient. Since fetal movement is an indicator of fetal well-being, it is a critical part of nursing assessment of the pregnant woman (Ehrstrom, 1979; Leader, Baillie, VanSchalkwyk, 1981; Moore & Piacauadio, 1989; Olds, London, & Ladewig, 1996; Pearson & Weaver, 1976; NAACOG, 1991). A mother's complaint of decreased fetal movement is significant (Connors, Natale, & Nasello-Patterson, 1988; Liston, Cohen, Mennuti, & Gabbe, 1982; Olds, London, & Ladewig, 1996; Patrick, Campbell, Carmichael, Natale, & Richardson, 1982; Valentin & Marshal, 1986). Moore and Piacauadio (1989) found that patients with ten fetal movements in one hour, at least once during the day, met the criteria for adequate fetal movement. Institutional nursing protocols must define adequate fetal movement and nursing interventions for inadequate movement (NAACOG, 1991).

The presence of a significant variable deceleration, indicative of cord compression, should have alerted Nurse Stone to a potentially ominous situation (Olds, London, & Ladewig, 1996). Since FHR acceleration occurred after deceleration, Marianne's FHR strip was nonreassuring. This nonreassuring pattern requires further evaluation with a biophysical profile (BPP) or contraction stress test (CST).

Nursing assessment of the laboring patient requires: (a) a review of the prenatal record, particularly the prior history and physical examination, (b) identification of current problems, (c) assessment of vital signs, and (d) a current history and physical examination related to presenting complaints (NAACOG, 1991). A thorough current history includes: (a) onset, frequency, and duration of contractions, (b) date, time, and onset of leaking amniotic fluid, (c) fetal movement activity, (d) signs of infection, including presence of fever, and (e) other patient complaints (e.g., cramping, spotting, urgency and frequency, etc.) (NAACOG, 1991; Olds, London, & Ladewig, 1996).

Communication of relevant information among providers is vital to ensure that an appropriate assessment is performed. Although it is common for any staff member to answer the telephone on L&D, the chances of a failure to communicate relevant information increase when a policy guiding the documentation of telephone communication is not in place. Prudent nursing practice requires the nurse to document and communicate all telephone contacts.

Diagnosis Appropriate nursing diagnoses for this mother and fetus include:

> ***Risk for Injury: Fetal***
> ***Knowledge Deficit: Maternal*** related to lack of information about signs of fetal well-being
> ***Risk for Altered Tissue Perfusion (uterine)***

Planning To meet the standard of care for the intrapartum patient and to facilitate the development of the nursing care plan, the following should occur: (a) assessing maternal history and fetal activity, including information on daily fetal movement, (b) consulting with the primary care provider about the necessity for further fetal assessment, and (c) collaborating with the primary care provider about the necessity for induction (NAACOG, 1991).

Implementation Continued monitoring was an inadequate intervention for Marianne's fetus, especially since no further accelerations had occurred. Although the nurse was concerned about the cord compression, she rationalized its occurrence as a consequence of a position change and reassured the patient instead of consulting with a physician. Fetal movement is an indicator of fetal well-being and a critical part of the nursing assessment of the pregnant patient (Olds, London, & Ladewig, 1996). The patient's complaint of decreased fetal movement was significant. Failure to heed the patient's comment about the lack of fetal movement resulted in Nurse Stone's failure to: (a) adequately interpret the FHR tracing, which showed variable late deceleration, acceleration, and baseline rate, (b) differentiate between nonreassuring and reassuring patterns, and (c) consult with the primary care provider. In some institutions, all patients who present with decreased fetal movement have an amniotic fluid index (AFI) or a biophysical profile (BPP) performed to assess fetal well-being. In some facilities, the woman is asked to return for a repeat nonstress test (NST) and AFI if active fetal movement does not resume within a few hours (or within 24 hours when a reactive NST, negative CST, or adequate BPP is obtained). Nurses need to be cognizant of the community and/or institutional standards which define "adequate fetal movement." Furthermore, the nurse needs to know the proper treatment for inadequate fetal movements (Olds, London, & Ladewig, 1996).

Failing to recognize a compromised fetus, Nurse Stone gave Marianne a sleeping pill (Seconal). Administration of Seconal, a central nervous system (CNS) depressant, to a patient with decreased fetal movement is contraindicated because this medication causes CNS depression of the fetus that further complicates detection of fetal movement and delays diagnosis of fetal distress (Bartram, Clewell, Kasnec, 1993). The indications for barbiturate use in the pregnant woman are: (a) false labor, or (b) early stages of beginning labor (Olds, London, & Ladewig, 1996).

No written policies or procedures existed in this institution to govern the specific criteria for: (a) assessing the patient in labor, (b) consulting with the primary care provider, (c) follow-up nursing actions (e.g., AFI or oxytocin challenge testing (OCT) with nonreassuring FHR patterns), (d) independent administration of sedatives, and (e) discharge of patients without notification or consultation with primary care provider. Clearly delineated written policies and procedures that reflect the national standard of care as well as institutional and local standards of care provide guidelines for nursing practice (NAACOG, 1991). Implementation of nursing standards of care and practice require that all staff be properly educated, oriented, and competent.

Nurse Stone should have performed the following nursing interventions: (a) fetal monitoring of significant length (i.e., 30–40 minutes [Puder & Sokol, 1994]) to assess for further FHR decelerations, (b) an AFI or BPP (if Nurse Stone was credentialed and competent to perform; otherwise a consultation with a credentialed colleague), (c) consultation with the primary care provider regarding the results of the nonreassuring FHR pattern and other fetal screening measures (CST, AFI, BPP), (d) preparation of the woman for induction of labor if further testing revealed that fetal well-being was at risk (Olds, London, & Ladewig, 1996). Had an institutional protocol been in place, the following nursing interventions could have been instituted: (a) provide explanation of intervention, (b) administration of oxygen per nasal cannula/mask, (c) repositioning of woman to left side, (d) maintenance of hydration (this may have required an IV), (e) monitoring of vital signs with B/P for detection of hypertension, (f) continued assessment of labor process, and (g) preparation for further medical intervention (e.g., fetal blood sampling; cesarean, etc.) (Olds, London, Ladewig, 1996).

Evaluation This intrauterine fetal death could have been prevented, because signs were evident that further assessment measures were required. Lack of further testing prevented earlier recognition of fetal distress and prompt induction of labor. Timely intervention could have been instituted to save this fetus in distress.

This institution did not evaluate its nurses' competency to assess, formulate nursing diagnoses, design a plan of care, implement interventions, or evaluate care of a pregnant woman. RNs were not required to complete an FHR monitoring program nor undergo periodic recertification in triage and care of a laboring patient (AWHONN, 1993). Credentialing and competency assessment of nurse providers requires a systematic process to ensure that all are cognizant of the requisite standards of performance. A skills inventory of all high-volume and high-risk nursing procedures and actions should be utilized to ensure proper orientation, education, and evaluation of continued competence (AWHONN, 1993).

Case 2

Facts

In a large, private hospital with 22 labor, delivery, recovery, and postpartum rooms (LDRPs), the monthly delivery rate averages 200. Staffing for the LDRPs includes L&D, postpartum, and nursery nurses who have been cross-trained to all nursing care responsibilities. Actively laboring women are assigned primarily to RNs who have demonstrated strong skills in labor and delivery. Postpartum and nursery nurses are then assigned postpartum patients. However, when the unit is busy, all nurses are expected to function in any role to meet patient needs.

During the night of May 19th, the census on the LDRP unit was 18 patients. Eight of these were in active labor, while the remaining ten were postpartum. Four of the postpartum patients were post-operative cesarean sections and the remaining six were vaginal deliveries. The unit was staffed with eight RNs, two LVNs, and two UAPs. At 0200 Jane Smith, a 22-year-old G3 P2 at 39+ weeks gestation with an uncomplicated prenatal course, presented in active labor. Jane's previous births were both spontaneous vaginal deliveries of infants weighing 8 lbs. 14 oz. (4026 grams) and 9 lbs. 2 oz. (4139 grams). Jane began regular contractions and ruptured membranes at 2400. Nurse Whitlow, who had eight years of experience on L&D, examined Jane and found: (a) 4–5 cm dilation, (b) complete effacement, (c) vertex –1 station, and (d) ruptured membranes. Contractions were 2–3 minutes apart, with a duration of 60 seconds. Vital signs were within normal limits and no risk factors were identified. After assessing Jane, Nurse Whitlow informed the physician, received approval for the requested epidural, and called anesthesia.

0300: An anesthesiologist arrived and a continuous epidural catheter was placed and anesthesia started. Jane was comfortable after insertion of epidural and FHR and contractions were within normal limits.

0400: Dr. Young, the obstetrician, arrived and examined Jane, who was 8–9 cm dilated, and vertex presentation, left occipital anterior (LOA) at +1 station. Since Jane felt the sensation to push and was having difficulty not doing so, the anesthesiologist was consulted and gave a bolus of epidural Marcaine (Bupivacaine) at 0415 to suppress her urge to push.

0515: Jane again felt like pushing. Dr. Young examined her and found her to be completely dilated with head presenting on the perineum.

0525: Over an intact perineum, Jane spontaneously delivered a viable female weighing 8 lbs. 13 oz. (3997 grams) with Apgars of 9 and 9.

0545: After an intact placenta spontaneously delivered, Dr. Young noted persistent uterine atony and ordered oxytocin (Pitocin) (40 units/1 liter) to be rapidly infused to sustain uterine hemostasis. After five minutes of continual fundal massage and rapid infusion of Pitocin, uterine bleeding decreased, although periodic gushes occurred. The cervix, vaginal walls, and perineum were examined for evidence of lacerations.

0555: On examination, Dr. Young noted that the lower uterine segment was still slightly boggy and periodically released gushes of blood. Physician orders included: (a) keep close watch on uterine bleeding, (b) follow the current IV with a second liter of fluid with 20 units of Pitocin, and (c) inform me if bleeding persists. Estimated blood loss was 500 ccs.

0615: Nurse Whitlow continued to assess the patient by taking vital signs and checking her lochia characteristics frequently. Occasionally, she vigorously massaged the fundus to ensure that clots were expelled.

0630: Two new patients were admitted, and Nurse Whitlow assumed the care of an additional patient who was 6–7 cm dilated and in active labor.

0645: Nurse Whitlow transferred Jane's care to Nurse Quick, a nursery nurse who was being cross-trained to the mother-baby unit. In report, Nurse Whitlow advised Nurse Quick about the epidural anesthesia, the episode of uterine atony and heavy bleeding, and the need to increase and continue the Pitocin administration. She also instructed Nurse Quick to inform Dr. Young and continue the IV Pitocin if heavy bleeding persisted.

0700: Upon assuming Jane's care, Nurse Quick noticed that the last assessment of vital signs was at 0645. Since the flowsheet indicated that the next vital signs were due on a 30-minute schedule, she waited until 0715 to evaluate the patient.

0715: Vital signs: P 100, B/P 90/60. Jane's perineum was bruised and swollen, her fundus was slightly above the umbilicus, and her lochia was moderate. Nurse Quick changed Jane's pad. After deciding that Jane was stable, Nurse Quick discontinued her IV fluids.

0745: Vital signs: P 102, B/P 92/54. Fundus was now 4 cm above the umbilicus, lochia was moderate, and the perineum remained slightly swollen.

0800: Vital signs: P 104, B/P 90/62. Fundus was now firm with the uterus 10 cm above the umbilicus and moderate to heavy lochia flow. After deciding that Jane was stable, Nurse Quick discontinued the Pitocin infusion. At change of shift report, Nurse Quick told Nurse Stark, a postpartum nurse with over 15 years of experience, "Jane delivered spontaneously at 0525, a girl, 8 lbs. 13 oz., no episiotomy. She has been fine; no problems since I have had her."

0815: Nurse Stark's first assessment revealed the following vital signs: P 130, B/P 80/40. Fundus was 4 cm above the umbilicus. After fundal massage, a large clot of approximately 400 ccs. was expelled. The fundus continued to be boggy with heavy lochia expressed during massage.

0815: Nurse Stark notified Dr. Young. She then felt Jane's bladder, which was quite distended.

0835: Instituting the protocol, Nurse Stark catheterized Jane and obtained 1000 ccs. of urine. Continuous massage of the uterus evacuated more large clots and lochia steadily continued.

0845: Vital signs: P 130, B/P 70/30; color pale and diaphoretic. Nurse Stark called the desk asking for help from the charge nurse.

0855: The charge nurse asked another obstetrician, Dr. Schwartz, who was making morning rounds, to evaluate Jane. After completing a vaginal examination, Dr. Schwartz noted persistent uterine blood flow and then initiated a bimanual uterine tamponade. Before transporting Jane to the operating room (OR), methylergonovine maleate (Methergine) (0.2 mg) IM and Prostin (Prostaglandin) were administered.

0910: In the OR, an IV with Pitocin (40 units) was restarted and rapidly infused. Despite another dose of Methergine and Prostin, Jane continued to bleed profusely and now her entire uterus was boggy.

0925: Uterine curettage retrieved only small membranous fragments, profuse bleeding continued, and the uterus would not contract.

0940: Profuse bleeding and decreasing blood pressure continued until the carotid pulse was barely palpable. An estimated 2 liters of blood were lost and Jane was now unconscious. The anesthesiologist began blood transfusions.

0950: General anesthesia and a hysterectomy were performed, 20 units of blood were transfused, and Jane was transferred to the intensive care unit.

Outcome

Postpartum hemorrhage, blood transfusions, and hysterectomy.

Legal

This case is currently under litigation.

Case Commentary

Undesirable Patient Outcome

Assessment When Nurse Quick assumed care of Jane, she failed to assess her bleeding adequately. In fact, she did not initially assess the patient until 30 minutes after receiving report. Due to her lack of knowledge, skill, and experience in postpartal maternity care, Nurse Quick did not consider the history of uterine atony, heavy bleeding, epidural anesthesia, and multiparity as risk factors for postpartum hemorrhage. Nurse Quick failed to recognize key assessment data; for example, she did not realize that fundal height above the umbilicus was indicative of: (a) full bladder, displacing the uterus, and/or (b) retention of intrauterine clots.

Diagnosis No nursing diagnoses were formulated.

Planning No nursing care plan was formulated based on nursing assessment and diagnosis.

Implementation Nurse Quick did not ensure that the patient's bladder was empty, either by encouraging the patient to void, by manual massage, or by catheterization. She did not thoroughly evaluate the fundus either by massage or by vaginal exploration of the lower uterine segment to determine if the uterus was firm and free of clots.

Evaluation Nurse Quick failed to evaluate the significance of tachycardia, hypotension, and increasing fundal height. Without evaluation criteria or consultation with a nurse colleague, Nurse Quick decided this patient was stable and (a) discontinued one IV infusion 15 minutes after assuming care, and (b) discontinued the Pitocin IV one hour after assuming care, even while noting a boggy uterus.

Desirable Patient Outcome

Assessment Assessment of the patient requires a thorough review of the patient's delivery history in addition to relevant information from the physical examination. The immediate postpartum physical examination requires thorough assessment of: (a) vital signs, (b) uterine tone (i.e. fundal checks), (c) characteristics and amount of lochia, (d) condition of perineum (e.g., bruising, lacerations, hematoma, episiotomy), (e) urinary elimination, and (f) level of pain (AWHONN, 1993; Olds, London, & Ladewig, 1996). Nurse Quick failed to realize the significance of gathered assessment data indicating a risk for postpartal hemorrhage, including multiparity, LGA infant, and epidural anesthesia. Nurse Quick failed to perform a thorough assessment of the uterus which includes: (a) fundal status, (b) quality and quantity of lochial flow, and (c) condition of the perineum. In assessing the involution process, it is imperative that the nurse assess the mother's voiding pattern, since a full bladder displaces the uterus and prevents adequate hemostasis.

Although Nurse Quick was an expert nursery nurse, she was not an expert in postpartum care, but was instead in the process of cross-training. Benner (1984) stated that nurses are not expert in all areas of nursing and in fact if placed in a new area of practice often assume the role of novice or proficient nurse. The accepted standard of nursing practice requires that obstetrical nurses be able to recognize major obstetrical complications (*Bendyck v. Shinde*, 1993). During a cross-training process, Nurse Quick should have been supervised by an expert postpartum nurse, since she was not competent to practice independently in postpartum care (ANA, 1985, 1991; NAACOG, 1991; Sullivan, 1994).

Diagnosis Appropriate nursing diagnoses include:

Altered Tissue Perfusion (uterine) related to multiple maternal risk factors including epidural anesthesia and delivery of LGA infant
Altered Urinary Elimination related to painful, bruised perineum secondary to delivery of LGA infant
Risk for Altered Tissue Perfusion (cardiac)

Planning Appropriate assessment and diagnoses should have resulted in a plan of care that included: (a) evaluation of uterus, including height, midline position, and firmness, (b) massage of uterus to determine firmness, indicating retained clots or persistent bleeding, (c) evaluation of urinary elimination (keep bladder empty to decrease potential for uterine displacement and atony), (d) increased frequency of assessments q 10–15 minutes, including vital signs and physical examination, (e) maintenance of Pitocin, and (f) consultation with physician for persistent uterine atony, inability to void, need for foley catheter placement, persistent bleeding, clot formation, and aberrant vital signs.

JCAHO (1995) stated, "The care, treatment, and rehabilitation planning process is designed to ensure that care is appropriate to the patient's specific needs and the severity level of his/her disease, condition, impairment, or disability . . . Qualified individuals plan and provide the care, treatment, and rehabilitation in a collaborative, and interdisciplinary manner, as appropriate to the patient" (p. 12). Planning for adequate staffing requires that nurses being cross-trained be assigned and supervised by a competent preceptor. In this case no preceptor was identified and Nurse Quick was allowed to perform independently a role for which she was not qualified.

Implementation In care of the postpartum patient, a competent nurse would have implemented the following actions: (a) continuation of IV Pitocin to facilitate uterine hemostasis, and (b) fundal massage to improve uterine tone and/or evacuate clots. Consultation with the physician to inform him of persistent uterine atony and numerous evacuated clots should have occurred much earlier. A dose of Methergine should have been obtained to potentiate uterine hemostasis and prevent persistent uterine bleeding. Nurse Quick should have insisted that the physician examine the patient to determine the need for further medical intervention such as uterine curettage.

Evaluation The adverse outcomes of postpartum hemorrhage, administration of blood, and hysterectomy could have been prevented. The substandard performance of one unsupervised RN, who assumed an assignment in which she was not qualified, resulted in an inadequate use of the nursing process. Nurses placed in or finding themselves in clinical situations requiring performance in a role for which they know they are not competent need to communicate these limitations to the appropriate charge nurse or nursing supervisor. Reassignment of patients to competent staff is an essential proactive measure which can prevent substandard performance and adverse outcomes (ANA, 1985; Florida Nurses Association, 1989; Massachusetts Nurses Association, 1983). The risk of "not knowing what one does not know" leads to an inadequate assessment which in turn contributes to deficiencies in all components of the nursing process.

Safe and competent care requires that skilled, appropriately trained nurses effectively utilize the nursing process. The individual nurse, the nurse manager, and the institution are all liable for ensuring that the nursing process is utilized and that competent staff provide care (ANA, 1985, 1988, 1991; NAACOG, 1991). As discussed in Chapter 3, an expert in one area of practice (e.g., Nurse Quick was an experienced nursery nurse) functions at the level of a novice in an unfamiliar specialty. "A nurse is not a nurse is not a nurse." In this era of specialized and highly technical care, nurses are not interchangeable units.

Nursing administration must ensure that processes are in place to adequately cross-train staff to attain role competency. Curtin (1994) stated, "Maintaining professional standards is at the heart of the profession's obligation to the public, and this obligation rests in a special way on the shoulders of nursing administrators. . . . By virtue of his or her position and authority, the nursing manager is responsible not only for the delivery of safe care, but also for the development of the profession and for the professional growth of the nurses" (p. 26).

Case 3

Early discharge (<24 hours) of mothers and babies began as a birth alternative in the birthing centers of the 60s and 70s (Day, 1963; Mehl, Peterson, Sikolosky, & Witt, 1976). Today, early discharge is often not voluntary but mandated by third-party payers. Early discharge raises both maternal and newborn concerns. Maternal concerns include rest, readiness to learn and assume self and newborn care, readiness to parent, and availability of support systems. Neonatal concerns include safety related to transition to extrauterine life, ability to feed and hydrate effectively, and development and early recognition of complications. The traditional model of medical-care delivery is being replaced by home- and community-based health care delivery. Care of mothers and babies must not cease at discharge from the hospital, but continue in the home and community. Early discharge must be based on: (a) maternal/neonatal criteria, (b) maternal knowledge and readiness to assume self and neonatal care, and (c) follow-up within 48 hours (NAACOG, 1991; AAP, 1992). When preparation and follow-up are assured, early discharge is safe and effective (as well as cost effective) (Brodish, McBride, & Bays, 1987; Evans, 1991; Lemmer, 1987; Norr & Nacion, 1987; Norr, Nacion, & Abramson, 1989; Williams & Cooper, 1993).

Facts

Mary Ellen is a 28-year-old G1 P0 accountant with a prenatal history of mild blood pressure elevation and occasional spotting. She was admitted to a level II metropolitan hospital, had a normal low-risk labor, and gave birth to an 8 lb. 9 oz. (3629 grams) infant at 1830 on August 10th. The baby's Apgars were 9 and 9, she bottle-fed well, and had a normal transition to extrauterine life. Because Mary Ellen's insurance company encouraged early discharge (i.e., within 24 hours) and her husband was in a hurry to get her home so that he could pack for a business trip, Mary Ellen was discharged at 0930 on August 11th. The postpartum nurse gave the couple brief discharge instructions about infant care and follow-up.

The following morning, Mary Ellen's husband departed for a week-long business trip. That afternoon, Mary Ellen was found dead in her shower in a pool of blood by a concerned neighbor investigating the incessant crying of Mary Ellen's infant.

Outcome

Maternal death.

Legal

A multi-million-dollar lawsuit has been filed by Mary Ellen's husband and infant son.

Case Commentary

Undesirable Patient Outcome

Assessment Mary Ellen's nurses documented all assessment data as "normal" for both mother and baby. They did not assess the family's home support system prior to discharge.

Diagnosis The nurses identified key nursing diagnoses related to low-risk maternal care:

Knowledge Deficit related to lack of information about self-care
Risk for Altered Tissue Perfusion (uterine)
Risk for Altered Patterns of Urinary Elimination
Risk for Constipation
Risk for Infection secondary to episiotomy

Planning The usual discharge teaching was abbreviated and centered primarily on infant care after discharge (e.g., circumcision care, feeding, care of umbilicus, follow-up care).

Implementation The nurses provided no discharge teaching about postpartum, maternal self-care, despite its identification in the list of nursing diagnoses.

Evaluation No evaluation of this primipara's knowledge-base regarding postpartal self-care was carried out prior to the decision to omit this aspect of maternal discharge teaching.

Desirable Patient Outcome

Assessment In the general nursing assessment, no physical, high-risk factors in either mother or baby were identified that would have precluded early discharge (AAP, 1992; Hurt, 1994; NAACOG, 1991). However, the nurses did not consider this mother's: (a) self-care assessment, (b) psychosocial assessment, or (c) ability to access and utilize health care resources (NAACOG, 1991). Since the father was leaving on a week-long business trip, the nurses should have assessed this mother's support system (i.e., "assistance with care by family members or support persons") (NAACOG, 1991, p. 46).

Diagnosis A key additional nursing diagnosis should have been:

Social isolation related to lack of support system or family nearby

Planning No hospital policies, procedures, or protocols delineated "criteria and procedure for early discharge and follow-up" (NAACOG, 1991, p. 61). Heightened concern about newborn health and safety in early discharge

(Conrad, Wilkening, Rosenberg, 1989) resulted in the plan to prioritize and focus solely on newborn content in abbreviated discharge teaching. No plan for follow-up with a home visit (Williams & Cooper, 1993), telephone call, or office visit (AAP, 1992) was formulated. Early discharge planning and follow-up should include at least one of the forementioned modes of contact.

Implementation Mary Ellen's nurses failed to give her either verbal or written instructions regarding self-care and complications. Postpartum instructions should have included: (a) postpartum recovery process, including lochial pattern and uterine involution, (b) breast, perineal, and bladder care, (c) care of hemorrhoids, (d) rest, exercise, and nutrition, (e) care of surgical incision (i.e., episiotomy or cesarean section), (f) medications, (g) emotional responses (e.g., grief, postpartal blues, depression, or parenting concerns), (h) availability of a support system, (i) recognition of complications, and (j) how to obtain emergency care (AAP, 1992; NAACOG, 1991). Since postpartum women have transient deficits in cognitive function, particularly in memory function, verbal instructions may be poorly remembered and should be augmented with written instructions (AAP, 1992; Eidelman, Hoffmann, & Kaitz, 1993). Verbal and written instructions about postpartum complications should include signs and symptoms of the top five causes of maternal death after live birth (Table 7-1).

As an advocate for the patient (ANA, 1985), the nurse has a duty to teach a new mother about self-care, the need for a support system at home, and a course of action for complications and emergencies. If the patient does not meet criteria for early discharge defined in the institution's protocol (NAACOG, 1991), the nurse as a professional care provider owes a duty to the patient to advocate for lengthened hospitalization (ANA, 1985; Hogue, 1988). If the institution has no protocol or has an inadequate protocol, the nurse still owes an independent duty to the patient that cannot be relieved by hospital policy or physician order (ANA, 1985; *Darling v. Charleston*

Table 7-1 Causes of Maternal Death After Live Birth*

Cause of Death	Percentage of Deaths
1. Pulmonary embolism†	27.1%
2. Pregnancy-induced hypertension†	22.5%
3. Hemorrhage†	18.3%
4. Other (e.g., pre-existing medical conditions such as cardiac, respiratory, liver disease, etc.)	16%
5. Infection	7.4%

*Retrospective data in the US from 1979 to 1986.
†From prospective data in the US from 1987 to present. Top three causes of maternal death remain the same as 1979–86 retrospective data (Berg, personal communication, 1995).

Adapted from Koonin, L., Atrash, H., Lawson, H., & Smith, J. (1991). Maternal mortality surveillance in the United States 1979–1986. *Morbidity and Mortality Weekly Report, 40,* 1–13.

Community Memorial Hospital, 1966; *Lunsford v. Board of Nurse Examiners*, 1983). In *Wickline v. State of California* as cited in Hogue (1988), the court ruled that providers must fulfill their "duty to protest" early discharge to third-party payers in order to shift liability to third-party payers. The court ruled that care providers who have the most direct knowledge of their patients' clinical needs must communicate that information to third-party payers, advocating for lengthier hospitalization when necessary. Professional actions on the patient's behalf, and the third-party payer's decision, should be documented in the patient's record. If the professional's request is denied, both care provider and third-party payer share liability for injury or harm resulting from premature discharge.

Evaluation Mary Ellen's nurses did not evaluate her understanding and readiness for self-care. In addition, no evaluation of the home environment or availability of a support system was done (AAP, 1992; NAACOG, 1991). The nurses did not provide the parents verbal or written instructions for accessing care in the event of complications or emergency (AAP, 1992; NAACOG, 1991). No provisions for follow-up by a home visit, telephone call, or office visit were made (AAP, 1992; NAACOG, 1991).

References

American Academy of Pediatrics-American College of Obstetricians and Gynecologists. (1992). *Guidelines for perinatal care*, 3rd ed. Washington, D.C.: Author.

American Nurses Association. (1985). *Code for nurses.* Washington, D.C.: Author.

American Nurses Association. (1988). *Standards for organized nursing services.* Washington, D.C.: Author.

American Nurses Association. (1991). *Standards of clinical nursing practice.* Washington, D.C.: Author.

Association of Women's Health, Obstetrics, and Neonatal Nurses. (1993). *Didactic content and clinical skills verification for professional nurse providers of basic, high-risk, and critical care intrapartum nursing.* Washington, D.C.: Author.

Bartram, J., Clewell, W., & Kasnec, T. (1993). Prenatal environment: Effect of neonatal outcome. In G. Merenstein & S. Gardner (Eds.), *Handbook of neonatal intensive care*, 3rd ed. St. Louis: Mosby-Yearbook.

Bendyck v. Shinde, 66 Ohio St. 3 d 573, 613 N.E. 2 d 1014 (1993).

Benner, P. (1984). *From novice to expert.* Menlo Park, CA: Addison-Wesley Nursing.

Benson, R. & Pernoll, M. (1994). *Handbook of obstetrics and gynecology.* New York: McGraw Hill.

Brodish, M., McBride, B., & Bays, S. (1987). Which mothers of newborns are most in need of home health followup? *Home Healthcare Nurse, 5*, 16–25.

Connors, G., Natale, R., & Nasello-Patterson, C. (1988). Maternally perceived fetal activity from twenty-four weeks' gestation to term in normal and at risk pregnancies. *American Journal of Obstetrics and Gynecology, 158*(2), 294–299.

Conrad, P., Wilkening, R., & Rosenberg, A. (1989). Safety of newborn discharge in less than 36 hours in an indigent population. *American Journal of Diseases in Children, 143,* 98–101.

Curtin, L. (1994). Ethics for, in, and about nursing administration. *Nursing Management, 25*(12), 25–28.

Day, G. (1963). Early discharge of maternity patients. *Nursing Outlook, 11,* 825–827.

Darling v. Charleston Community Memorial Hospital (1966). S0 Ill. App. 2d 253, 200 N.E. 2d 149.

Ehrstrom, C. (1979). Fetal movement monitoring in normal and high-risk pregnancy. *Acta Obstetrics and Gynecology Scandinavia,* (Suppl. 80), 6–32.

Eidelman, A., Hoffmann, N., & Kaitz, M. (1993). Cognitive deficits in women after childbirth. *Obstetrics and Gynecology, 81*(5), 764–767.

Evans, C. (1991). Description of a home follow-up program for childbearing families. *Journal of Obstetric, Gynecologic, and Neonatal Nursing, 20,* 113–118.

Florida Nurses Association. (1989). *Guidelines for the registered nurse in giving, accepting, or rejecting a work assignment.* Orlando, FL: Author.

Hobel, C., Hyvarinen, M., Okada, D., & Oh, W. (1973). Prenatal and intrapartum high-risk screening. *American Journal of Obstetrics and Gynecology, 117*(1), 1–9.

Hogue, E. (1988). Liability for premature discharge. *Pediatric Nursing, 14*(5), 421–423.

Hurt, H. (1994). Early discharge for newborns: When is it safe? *Contemporary Pediatrics, 11,* 68–88.

Joint Commission on Accreditation of Healthcare Organizations. (1995). *The Joint Commission Accreditation Manual for Hospitals.* Oakbrook Terrace, IL: Author.

Koonin, L., Atrash, H., Lawson, H., & Smith, J. (1991). Maternal mortality surveillance in the United States 1979–86. *Morbidity and Mortality Weekly Report, 40,* 1–13.

Leader, L., Baillie, P., & VanSchalkwyk, D. (1981). Fetal movements and fetal outcome: A prospective study. *Obstetrics and Gynecology, 57*(4), 431–436.

Lemmer, C. (1987). Early discharge: Outcomes of primiparas and their infants. *Journal of Obstetric, Gynecologic, and Neonatal Nursing, 16,* 230–236.

Liston, R., Cohen, A., Mennuti, M., & Gabbe, S. (1982). Antepartum fetal evaluation by maternal perception of fetal movement. *Obstetrics and Gynecology, 60*(4), 424–426.

Lunsford v. Board of Nurse Examiners. Texas App.3Dist.648S.W.2d391 (1983).

Massachusetts Nurses Association. (1983). *Mechanisms to support nurses' abilities to exercise their right to accept or reject an assignment.* Canton, MA: Author.

Mehl, L., Peterson, G., Sikolosky, W., & Witt, M. (1976). Outcomes of early discharge after normal birth. *Birth and the Family Journal, 3,* 101–106.

Moore, T. & Piacauadio, K. (1989). A prospective evaluation of fetal movement screening to reduce the incidence of antepartum fetal death. *American Journal of Obstetrics and Gynecology, 160*(5), 363–371.

Norr, K. & Nacion, K. (1987). Outcomes of postpartum early discharge, 1960-1986: A comparative review. *Birth, 14,* 135–141.

Norr, K., Nacion, K., & Abramson, R. (1989). Early discharge with home followup: Impacts on low income mothers and infants. *Journal of Obstetric, Gynecologic, and Neonatal Nursing, 18,* 133–141.

Nurses' Association of the American College of Obstetricians and Gynecologists. (1991). *Standards for the nursing care of women and newborns,* 4th ed. Washington, D.C.: Author.

Olds, S., London, M., & Ladewig, P. (1996). *Maternal-newborn nursing,* 6th ed. Menlo Park, CA: Addison-Wesley Nursing.

Patrick, J., Campbell, K., Carmichael, L., Natale, R., & Richardson, B. (1982). Patterns of gross fetal body movement over 24-hour observation intervals during the last 10 weeks of pregnancy. *American Journal of Obstetrics and Gynecology,* 142(4), 363–371.

Pearson, J., & Weaver, J. (1976). Fetal activity and fetal well-being: An evaluation. *British Medical Journal,* 1, 1305–1307.

Phillips, J. (1995). Homeless nurses and feeling homeless in nursing. *Nursing Science Quarterly, 8*(2), 55–56.

Puder, K. & Sokol, R. (1994). Clinical use of antepartum fetal monitoring techniques. In Dilts, P. & Sciarra, J. (Eds.), *Gynecology and obstetrics.* Philadelphia: Lippincott.

Sullivan, C. (1994). Competency assessment and performance improvement for healthcare providers. *Journal for Healthcare Quality, 16*(4), 14–19.

Valentin, L. & Marshal, K. (1986). Fetal movement in the third trimester of normal pregnancy. *Early Human Development, 14,* 295–306.

Williams, L. & Cooper, M. (1993). Nurse-managed postpartum care. *Journal of Obstetrics, Gynecologic, and Neonatal Nursing,* 22, 25–31.

8

High-Risk Obstetrical Care

Mary M. Lepley, RNC, MS, CNS, WHCNP
Sandra L. Gardner, RN, MS, CNS, PNP
Mary I. Enzman Hagedorn, RN, PhD, CNS, CPNP
Marcia Garman Laux, RN, MSN

The delivery of safe and effective perinatal care begins with the initial assessment, confirming pregnancy, and ends with the postpartum and newborn follow-up appointments. The goal of perinatal care is attainment of an optimal outcome for the family through early identification and prevention of actual or potential health problems associated with pregnancy. Early comprehensive risk assessment and intervention allows many high-risk women to deliver full-term neonates with no incidence—or decreased incidence—of conditions associated with morbidity and mortality. Risk assessment involves identifying those factors that "indicate a higher probability of adverse outcomes and help guide actions by the woman, her social support network, and her providers" (Committee on Perinatal Health, 1993, p. 28). Risk factors associated with morbidity and mortality for the mother and the newborn are listed in Appendix C.

High-risk obstetrical care may be required with any pregnancy, and early and ongoing risk identification enables the care provider to anticipate and plan for the worst scenario. All professionals working with obstetrical patients must be highly skilled and assertive. Nurses who are responsible for their actions and confident of their ability to recognize adverse signs and symptoms can avoid or alleviate problems. The nurse must then take the initiative as patient advocate to obtain the best care for both mother and baby (ANA, 1985).

Once risk factors are identified, the pregnant woman may be referred to and/or consult with a care provider who is a specialist in perinatal care. Antepartum, intrapartum, and postpartum management may proceed in collaboration with perinatal specialists, and may require care away from her primary physician or nurse-midwife, local hospital, and support system. Women who have their birth experiences in tertiary perinatal centers can expect a registered nurse to be in attendance at all times. The nurse must be educated and prepared in the specialty of maternity care to recognize and manage—using the nursing process—complications of labor and delivery.

Hospitals choosing to provide obstetrical care must meet the minimum standards of care in the delivery of obstetrical and neonatal services. Hospitals electing to provide level II and/or level III care must make a commitment to consumers, as well as staff, to facilitate the delivery of quality perinatal services.

The role of the obstetrical nurse is often different from other nurses' roles. Frequently, the OB nurse may be the only caregiver the patient has contact with until delivery. In many settings, the nurse assesses and determines whether a pregnant woman is in stable condition and can be discharged home undelivered. Obstetrical nurses must be knowledgeable, experienced, and committed to their role as patient advocate for both mother and fetus/newborn. The nurse must be determined and motivated to take positive, even assertive action to ensure the health of the mother and baby in all circumstances. This may require questioning the physician's orders, or even refusing to implement orders before examining the patient and assessing current fetal well-being. For patient advocacy and safety, the nurse must insist that the physician remain in the unit while some orders are implemented. If she believes the physician is putting mother or baby at risk, the nurse must be willing to initiate the institution's chain of command to ensure the safety of both patients.

This chapter presents cases of nursing liability related to lack of recognition and treatment of PIH and HELLP syndrome, lack of recognition of and intervention for fetal distress, and failure to advocate for the appropriate standard of medical care. The first case demonstrates nurses' failure to advocate, question, apply the nursing process, use the available chain of command, and practice within the standard of care for PIH and HELLP syndrome. The second case illustrates lack of competence in interpreting fetal heart rate (FHR) monitor tracings, deviation from the standard of care in nursing assessments during labor and delivery, and failure to initiate timely nursing interventions for fetal distress. The last case represents a failure of the obstetrical nurses to advocate for the standard of medical care for Group B streptococcal colonization, and for adequate neonatal care.

Case 1

Pregnancy-induced hypertension (PIH), the most common hypertensive disorder of pregnancy, is defined as "an increase in systolic blood pressure of 30 mm Hg and/or diastolic of 15 mm Hg over baseline" (Olds, London, & Ladewig, 1996, p. 493). Occurring in 6–8% of all pregnancies (Aumann & Baird, 1993), PIH is most often seen in the "last 10 weeks of gestation, during labor, or in the first 48 hours after childbirth" (Olds, et al., 1996, p. 494). PIH is more common in: (a) primigravidas, (b) African Americans, (c) patients with multiple gestation, (d) adolescents and older patients, (e) patients with a family history of PIH, and (f) patients with pre-existing disease. Hypertension accounts for 22.5% of maternal deaths (after live birth) (see Table 7-1). HELLP syndrome, associated with severe PIH, describes an alteration in hemolysis, elevated liver enzymes, and low platelet count. Cerebral hemorrhage, due to uncontrolled hypertension, is the most common cause of maternal death (Olds, et al., 1996).

Facts

On October 1 at 0355, 29-year-old Terri Keaton, a computer specialist and part-time aerobics instructor, was admitted to the birthing unit of a community hospital. A G1, P0, Terri's pregnancy was uncomplicated with a 24-pound weight gain, normal blood pressures (ranging from 100/60 to 130/70), and false labor two weeks prior to admission. Terri's membranes spontaneously ruptured at 0200 and she was 3 cm dilated, 90% effaced, and 0 station on admission. Admission vital signs were: T 37.2 C, HR 67, R 20, BP 159/74, and FHR 130.

During labor, Terri's BP readings ranged from 130/79 to 167/74, except for a 0615 reading of 143/81 and 0630 reading of 151/95. An epidural was inserted at 0455 with induction BP of 143/69 and a range of BPs from 143/69 to 160/84. At 0726, Terri delivered a 6 lb. 9 oz. (2977 grams) baby boy with Apgars of 8 and 9.

After delivery, Nurse Maroon cared for Terri from 0700–1000 and took eight BP readings. These ranged from 144/87 to 159/89, with six systolic values of 156–159 and seven diastolic values of 84–89. At 0940 Nurse Maroon called the mother/baby unit, gave Nurse Oxman report mentioning only a slightly elevated blood pressure and transferred Terri to the unit. Nurse Oxman, caring for Terri from 1000 to 1700, recorded the following BPs: (a) 150/98 at 1110; (b) 144/90 at 1200; and (c) 142/98 at 1610.

At 1700 Nurse Williams received report, including the BP values, from Nurse Oxman. At 1800, Nurse Williams gave Terri a Percocet (oxycodone) for complaints of pain and headache. At approximately 1850, Terri asked Nurse Williams if the pill that she took could cause "hard," "bad" pain in her stomach.

At 1900, Nurse Williams told Nurse Smith in report that Terri was having no problems except a minor complaint of stomach pain. In report, Terri's BPs during the shift were given. The documentations of Nurse Smith's care from 1930 to 0238 are in Table 8-1.

After countless readings of elevations in blood pressure, Terri arrested at 0244. On the cardio-pulmonary resuscitation (CPR) sheet, it was documented that the COR-O began at 0244 and ended at 0258 when Terri was transferred to the intensive care unit (ICU). In the ICU, neurosurgery and hematology were consulted, and laboratory and radiologic tests (including a CAT scan and EEG) were carried out. After these tests showed no brain activity, the ventilator was removed. Terri was pronounced dead at 0755 with her husband, parents, and parents-in-law present.

Outcome

Maternal death due to massive left intracerebral hemorrhage and acute hepatic necrosis as a consequence of hypertension and disseminated intravascular coagulopathy (i.e., HELLP syndrome).

Table 8-1 Nurse Smith's Care and Documentation

Original Chart Entry*	Altered Chart Entry†	Statements of Husband and Parents‡
1930: VS: T 37, P 118, R 20, BP 132/70 A/O abdomen soft, normal respirations, warm/dry skin, slightly swollen episiotomy,small amount lochia, fundus at umbilicus, soft breasts, ambulated in hall to nurses desk. C/O nausea and epigastric pain. To room, Mylanta tab given.	*1930:* Same entry as original.	Different nurses in and out of the room all day. Family never told about elevated BP. Electronic BP machine removed in Labor and Delivery at 0900.
1940: Emesis X 4. C/O severe epigastric pain. Pacing,unable to sit still. Call placed to Dr. Dale.	*1940:* Same entry as original.	Terri lying on her side in fetal position crying and screaming in pain. Terri described as stoic by family—this behavior highly out-of-character.
1950: Dr. Dale returned call. Pt. still c/o severe pain and nausea. Skin cold and clammy; c/o difficulty breathing.	*1950:* Same entry as original.	BP not monitored every 15 minutes throughout day. Terri stated she was dying. Parents described Terri as crying and screaming in pain and her stomach shaking like jello.
1955: Demerol (Meperidine) (50 mg) and Phenergan (25 mg) given IM. Lungs clear, BP 220/120. Respirations rapid.	*1955:* Same entry as original.	Nurse Smith told family pain could be food poisoning, gallstones, or uterus contracting. Terri's father suggested stomach pumping. Husband said, "No one else has food poisoning."
2010: Call placed to Dr. Dale; pt. still c/o severe pain.	*2010:* Same entry as original.	Nurse Smith's presence in room sporadic. Husband also asked nurse to get someone to look at his wife. Nurse said she was trying to get Dr. Dale.
2025: BP 170/110, R 28, respirations calmer, less rigid, still c/o epigastric pain.	*2025:* Same entry as original.	Wife talking to husband and family.
2030: Second call to Dr. Dale.	*2030:* Same entry as original.	Husband did not know about call to Dr. Dale at 1940.
2045: Dr. Dale returned call.	*2045:* Dr. Dale returned call. Late entry (untimed) notified of high BP.	Husband told Dr. Dale of wife's pain and said he didn't think it was gallstones or uterus, but might be food poisoning. Dr. Dale okayed an additional dose of Demerol.
2050: Demerol (Meperidine) (75 mg) IM medicated with an additional 75 mg of Demerol IM, Resp. 24, states pain is lifting "a little."	*2050:* Demerol IM per physician order. Medicated with an additional 75 mg Demerol IM, Resp. 24, states pain is lifting "a little."	Family believed Nurse Smith's attitude was, "Don't worry, it's OK; there's no problem." Family present for second Demerol dose.
2100: IV started in R hand with 22 gauge angio with D5.45NS at 125 cc./hr. Pt. states pain is decreasing; drowsy, denies nausea, R 20, BP 142/70.	*2100:* Same entry as original.	Nurses told family vital signs all normal, Demerol would relax her, help her sleep, and reduce amount of pain.
2120: Resting easier, states pain is decreasing.	*2120:* Skin warm & dry, IV checked, resting quietly on left side. States having only a "little pain."	Family remained with patient. Her eyes were closed, but she was not asleep.
2200: Appears asleep, Resp. regular.	*2200:* Appears asleep, Resp. regular, checked IV.	Husband believed wife OK and would be OK in AM. He went home at 2230. Terri's parents stayed all night. Parents helped Terri to the bathroom, noted increased vaginal bleeding, told the nurses who told them to change the pad and wash her underwear.

(*Continued*)

Table 8-1 Nurse Smith's Care and Documentation (*Continued*)

Original Chart Entry*	Altered Chart Entry†	Statements of Husband and Parents‡
2300: VS: T 37, P 108, R 18, & BP 140/70, urine q.s., up to BR with assist. Assisted with pericare, c/o headache and epigastric pain.	*2300:* Drowsy, respirations normal, skin warm & dry. Resting on right side, taking sips of water without nausea and vomiting, c/o slight headache.	Family repeatedly told that Terri was stable and that family was hysterical (at least ten times between 2230 and her death). Family unable to arouse Terri, found nurse and told her. She told them to let her sleep and to stop being so hysterical. Family states that the 2300 note is inaccurate; she wasn't coherent, so she couldn't deny pain/nausea, and she wasn't up to the bathroom.
2325: Demerol (50 mg) and Phenergan (25 mg) medicated with IM med for pain & nausea, emesis X 1.	*2325:* Demerol/Phenergan given per orders. Medicated for c/o headache and moderate epigastric pain with IM med. IV checked.	Family states she was unarousable to slapping of her face and hands after 2230.
2355: No documentation.	*2355:* T 37.5, P 68, R 18, BP 140/70, alert and oriented. Abdomen soft, normal respirations, skin warm & dry, slightly swollen episiotomy, small amount rubra lochia, fundus level at umbilicus, breasts soft, perineal care, up to BR, urine q.s., IV checked. Up to BR with assistance, steady on feet, voiding without difficulty. Assisted with pericare. Denied nausea, states pain med alleviating headache. Denies epigastric pain.	Family found nurse and brought her to Terri's room to show her a blood spot on pillow. Nurse said it was vomit and told family they were hysterical, that Terri was stable and to let her sleep; she'd be fine in the morning. Family states that no examination of abdomen, lungs, episiotomy, or stomach occurred. Terri did not go to the bathroom; she was comatose.
10/2 0005: Pt. resting, states h/a decreasing and epigastric pain minimal.	*0005:* No documentation.	Terri remained comatose.
0100: Pt. sleeping, difficult to arouse, and respirations regular and deep, P 68, R 20.	*0100:* No documentation.	Family saw another large spot of blood on Terri's pillow. Nurse never answered the call light, so family went to get a nurse to come to the room.
0115: No documentation.	*0115:* P 68, R 20, appears asleep. Respirations regular,heart rate regular, responds to verbal and tactile stimuli.When called by name, moans and pulls away.	Family disputes that Terri's vital signs were checked. They state that Terri could not respond to verbal or tactile stimuli or moan and pull away. Terri's father stated that she was in a "dying quiver."
0220: No documentation.	*0220:* P 120, R 10, BP 80/40, unresponsive. Blood on pillow case and side of mouth. Dr. Dale called.	Terri's father states he was screaming up and down the halls and finally got staff to come to Terri's room.
0225: No documentation.	*0225:* Narcan 0.4 mgm IV. Responsive to verbal command and "breathe Terri." Pt. responded by breathing.	Nursing supervisor called because family concerned about lack of responsiveness. Terri's father grabbed nursing supervisor as she was coming down the hall. Nursing supervisor entered the dimly lit room, saw Nurse Smith standing near the bedside but doing nothing. Nursing supervisor turned on the light, quickly assessed Terri, told Nurse Smith to call a COR-O, and suctioned Terri's mouth. When the COR cart arrived, she told Nurse Smith to start CPR.
0238: No documentation.	*0238:* No spontaneous respirations noted, COR-O called, CPR initiated.	

*Notes made *before* Terri Keaton was taken to the ICU

†Notes made *after* Terri Keaton was taken to the ICU

‡Sworn depositions of family members

Legal

Terri's husband and infant son filed a lawsuit against the nurses, physician, and hospital five months after her death for: (a) wrongful death, (b) outrageous conduct/punitive damages, and (c) violation of the consumer-protection act. One year after the case was filed, an out-of-court settlement was reached for an undisclosed amount. The hospital filed a lawsuit against the obstetrician to recover damages lost in the settlement. The obstetrician countersued the nurses and hospital for negligence and conspiracy. A jury trial has been scheduled.

Heath Care Finance Administration (HCFA) conducted an investigation of the hospital and found several deficiencies. After two versions of the medical record were discovered, HCFA requested the state health department to reopen its investigation. The state health department conducted two investigations of the hospital. It concluded that Nurse Smith did not summon the physician in a timely manner, and recommended that criminal charges be filed against the hospital for tampering with medical records.

The state board of nursing investigated five of the RNs involved in Terri's care and recommended disciplinary action for all of them:

- Nurse Smith was suspended from nursing until completion of classes in obstetrics and ethics.
- Nurse Maroon was admonished for not notifying the obstetrician of Terri's abnormal BP readings immediately after birth.
- Nurses Oxman, Heffernan, and O'Brien (the nursing supervisor) were placed on two-years probation and required to attend classes because they had failed to recognize the seriousness of the patient's condition.

The state board of medical examiners investigated the obstetrician.

Case Commentary

Undesirable Patient Outcome

Assessment Not one of the nurses caring for Terri did a full assessment of: (a) predisposing factors, (b) findings of the physical examination, (c) laboratory data, or (d) pain (sources and severity).

Diagnosis No nursing diagnoses were documented in the patient record.

Planning No nursing care plan was developed.

Implementation Since no plan of care was formulated, no nursing interventions were identified or implemented. When notifying the physician, the nurses reported only Terri's pain, nausea, and vomiting. The physician stated that he was *never* informed of the patient's elevated BP readings. Nurse Smith gave Terri Mylanta for epigastric pain without a physician's order or use of a collaborative protocol.

Evaluation The nurses failed to establish any outcome measures of nursing care to evaluate progress or lack of progress toward goals.

Desirable Patient Outcome

Assessment Nurses caring for Terri were not aware that: (a) PIH could develop postpartally in a woman without PIH ante- or intrapartally; (b) primigravidas are at risk for developing PIH; (c) complaints of epigastric pain, headache, and elevation of blood pressure are significant symptoms of developing PIH; and (d) the patient's condition was deteriorating.

No staff nurse, charge nurse, or nursing supervisor *ever* compared BP values with prenatal baseline readings (available in the patient's record). Nurse Oxman called the BPs "slightly elevated" and stated in her deposition that it was: (a) unimportant to check baseline BP values, and (b) blood pressures don't matter since all postpartum patients have either an elevated or decreased BP after delivery. Nurse Williams did not review baseline values since she did not think the BPs were high enough to warrant concern. Nurse Heffernan, the charge nurse from 1900-0700, took BPs at 1955 and 2025 of 220/120 and 170/110. She described a systolic BP > 30–40 mm Hg above baseline and a diastolic > 90 mm Hg as concerning. However, she *never* checked Terri's baseline BP values. In her deposition, Nurse Smith stated that elevated BP was not associated with PIH or HELLP syndrome.

Given Terri's elevated BP readings in the first two hours after delivery, BP values were not assessed sufficiently. The nurse should assess BP "every 1 to 4 hours; more frequently if indicated by medicine or other changes in the woman's status" (Olds, et al., 1996, p. 501) throughout postpartal care, especially when acute pain and life-threatening BP readings are discovered. At 0100 and 0115 (in the original note) and 0220 (in the altered note), when Terri was difficult to arouse, Nurse Smith did not assess her BP despite the previous BP readings that were seriously elevated. In her deposition, Nurse Smith testified that she hadn't taken a BP at these times "because she had left her stethoscope at the desk."

The nurses never assessed Terri for presence or absence of edema, urinary output, urinary protein, and specific gravity (Olds, et al., 1996). They also failed to assess integrity of the central nervous system, including: (a) deep tendon reflexes or clonus, (b) visual disturbances, (c) headaches, and (d) level of consciousness. If Terri's nurses had assessed these factors, they might have discovered and acted on the findings. Although Nurse Oxman stated in her deposition that she checked reflexes, she did not document her findings in the chart, a violation of the professional standards of care (ANA, 1991; NAACOG, 1991). Neither Nurse Williams, Smith, or Heffernan equated Terri's complaints of headache, stomach pain, and elevated BP with developing PIH and a deterioration of her condition. According to Terri's parents, she was not arousable after 2230, but Nurse Smith wrote (in the altered chart entry) that Terri was verbalizing and ambulating at that time. Not until 0100 (in the original chart entry) and 0220 (in the altered chart entry) did Nurse Smith document her assessment of changes in Terri's level of consciousness—2 1/2 to 4 hours *after* the family's assessment. The family's assessment of Terri's deteriorating status, including her escalating pain, unarousability, and "dying quiver," were not only unheeded but denigrated by the nursing staff.

Pain is "an unpleasant sensory and emotional experience associated with actual or potential tissue damage or described in terms of such damage" (International Association for the Study of Pain, 1979, p. 249). Thus, pain functions as a cue of potential tissue injury. Pain after childbirth may be a part of the postpartal process (e.g., hemorrhoidal or perineal pain, sore breasts, involution, etc.) or represent a pathologic condition. The objectives of pain assessment are to determine: (a) the presence of pain, (b) the impact of the pain, (c) pain-relieving interventions, and (d) effectiveness of interventions (Porter, 1993). Since pain is a subjective experience, the patient must self-report. Terri's repeated complaints of headache, escalating pain, and the lack of relief from analgesia went unheeded for hours by the nursing staff.

Objective criteria (e.g., behavioral, physiologic, endocrine/metabolic) assist the care provider in pain assessment. When they were assessing Terri's pain, her nurses did not consider the family's assessment of her escalating pain and their report of her "stoic" nature in the presence of pain. Not one of the nurses objectively assessed Terri's self-report of pain by assessing: (a) location, (b) quality, (c) duration, (d) quantity (on a scale of 0–10), and (e) precipitating and relieving factors. Moreover, complete vital signs were not taken prior to administration of narcotics at 1955, 2050, and 2325.

Nurses Oxman and Smith both stated in their separate depositions that epigastric pain, headache, and nausea and vomiting had nothing to do with elevated BP, PIH, or HELLP syndrome. Nurse Smith testified that the patient complained of stomach rather than epigastric pain. However, she never assessed the difference between the terms for the patient experiencing the pain. She also failed to assess the amount, frequency, force, precipitating or relieving factors, and character of Terri's nausea and vomiting.

Although Nurse Maroon was one of the three authors of the hospital's PIH policy, no nurse caring for Terri knew the criteria for PIH or HELLP syndrome. This lack of competence rendered them incapable of recognizing the significance of the information they had gathered in their assessments. This incompetence resulted in failures to (a) collect additional/pertinent data using appropriate assessment tools and techniques (ANA, 1983, 1991), (b) "detect subtle and significant changes in health . . . status" (ANA, 1983, p. 15), (c) "monitor at-risk individuals . . . for actual or potential . . . health problems" (ANA, 1983, p. 13), (d) collect data in a systematic, ongoing fashion (ANA, 1991), (e) involve "the client, significant others, and health care providers" (ANA, 1991, p. 9), and (f) document the data "in a retrievable form" (ANA, 1991, p. 9).

Comparison of the original chart entry and the altered chart entry in Table 8-1 illustrates significant discrepancies between the assessment data in the two records. Sworn information from the family disputes the kind and amount of assessment data charted in the altered chart entry. Despite the fact that Nurse Heffernan took the life-threatening BP readings, she did not document these values in the chart because "you never chart on a patient's chart if you're not taking care of that patient." This, of course, is untrue: a nurse must chart her nursing care of any patient and sign her entries. Since the assessment data (in the altered chart entry) were relied on by subsequent care providers, it appeared that Terri was well monitored by the nurse and coherent until the chart entry of 0220. Subsequent care providers did *not* have access to the assessment data in the original chart entry (at 0100) nor the information of the family that Terri was unresponsive from 2230.

Diagnosis In her deposition, Nurse Heffernan stated that she "thought about PIH when obtaining the two life-threatening blood pressures at 1955 and 2025." However, her "thought about PIH" was not formulated into a nursing diagnosis, nor used as the basis of a plan of care. Nurse Smith postulated medical diagnoses (e.g., food poisoning, gallbladder disease) for the patient's pain, nausea, and vomiting. Since Nurse Smith was *not* an advanced practice nurse, she was unqualified (by her state's nurse practice act) to formulate medical diagnoses. Within the scope of professional nursing practice, as mandated by the Nurse Practice Act, and the standards of professional practice and care (ANA, 1983, 1991; NAACOG, 1991), Nurse Smith failed to formulate appropriate nursing diagnoses:

Risk for Injury related to the possibility of convulsions secondary to cerebral vasospasm or edema (Olds, et al., 1996).

Risk for Injury related to hematologic and hepatic abnormalities secondary to the HELLP syndrome (Olds, et al., 1996).

Knowledge Deficit of patient, family (and nurses) related to lack of information about PIH and HELLP syndrome (Olds, et al., 1996).

Planning Because none of the nurses formulated appropriate nursing diagnoses, an individualized, collaborative, continuous, and documented plan of care was not developed (ANA, 1983, 1991; NAACOG, 1991). Additionally, no nurse planned to: (a) compare the patient's postpartum BP values with baseline values, (b) review the hospital's PIH/HELLP syndrome policy/protocol (NAACOG, 1991), or (c) inform the obstetrician of the elevated, life-threatening BPs and the patient's complaints of pain.

Not one of these nurses included the patient or her family as collaborators in her care as required by the Joint Commission on Accreditation of Health Care Organizations (JCAHO, 1995), standards of care and professional practice (ANA, 1983, 1991; NAACOG, 1991), and the code of ethics (ANA, 1985). In their behavior toward the patient and family, these nurses did not "provide services with respect to human dignity and the uniqueness of the client" (ANA, 1985, p. 2). They not only discounted and ignored the patient's complaints of pain and her family's assessment of her condition and their concerns about her welfare, but even berated, belittled, and denigrated Terri's family.

Within the patient's 20-hour postpartum course, five nurses provided care: (a) Nurse Maroon for two hours, ten minutes, (b) Nurse Oxman for seven hours (c) Nurse Williams for two hours, (d) Nurse Heffernan (took two BP readings), and (e) Nurse Smith for nine hours. This fragmented care was described by the family as "different nurses in and out all day." Nurse Oxman said her assignment was four to six patients and that she was busy, but not busy enough to ask for help. Nurse Smith, whose presence was

Signs and Symptoms of Worsening PIH

Increasing edema (especially hands and face)
Worsening headache*
Epigastric pain*
Visual disturbances
Decreasing urinary output
Nausea/vomiting*
Bleeding gums*
Disorientation*
Generalized complaints about not feeling well*

*Signs and symptoms (as documented in patient record) manifested by Terri Keaton

From: Olds, S., London, M., & Ladewig, P. (1996). *Maternal-newborn nursing,* 5th ed. Menlo

described as "sporadic" by the family, was also caring for two other postpartum patients. As Terri's condition deteriorated, the charge nurse, Nurse Heffernan, failed to: (a) alter Nurse Smith's assignment, (b) supervise Nurse Smith's care, (c) personally assume care of Terri, or (d) notify the nursing supervisor of the changes in Terri's condition. The changes in Terri's acuity (i.e., "the intensity of nursing resources required by the patient as an indirect measure of the severity of the illness" [NAACOG, 1989, p. 7]) required alterations in the plan of care, care delivery, and the allocation of competent nursing resources (ANA, 1983, 1991; NAACOG, 1991).

Implementation Neither the staff nurses nor the supervisory nurses were competent and clinically proficient in recognizing obstetrical complications (ANA, 1983, 1985, 1991; NAACOG, 1991). All failed to recognize the significance of: (a) elevated BPs, (b) life-threatening values, (c) the potential for CNS injury, and (d) manifestations of the HELLP syndrome. Having failed to appreciate the cardinal signs of PIH, the nurses then failed to: (a) recognize numerous signs and symptoms of worsening PIH, listed in the accompanying box, (b) review the protocol for PIH/HELLP syndrome, (c) review nursing and medical resource texts, and (d) notify a physician.

This hospital employed an in-house "deck doctor" who was asleep in the call room and who was *never* called by any nurse to emergently examine the patient as her condition deteriorated. As a patient advocate, the nurse must know the standard of medical care for treatment of PIH (see Table 8-2) and advocate that the patient receive the standard of care (ANA, 1985, 1994). Use of narcotics is *not* included in the standard of care for PIH. The goals of medical treatment for HELLP must include: (a) prompt diagnosis, (b) prevention of central nervous system, hematologic, renal, and hepatic sequelae and disease, and (c) prevention of fetal/neonatal complications (Olds, et al., 1996).

Essential nursing interventions in the presence of unstable PIH are outlined in the box on p. 124. In prescribing and administering medication (i.e.,

Table 8-2 Medical Treatment for PIH

Treatment	Rationale
1. Complete bedrest, preferably on left side.	Decreases environmental stimuli that could trigger a seizure. Increases glomerular filtration rate.
2. High-protein, moderate-sodium diet.	Adequate replacement of proteins that affect intra/extravascular fluid movement. Excessive sodium intake may worsen edema and blood pressure.
3. Anticonvulsants: Magnesium sulfate, diazepam (Valium), pentobarbital (Nembutal), Dilantin (phenytoin sodium).	CNS depressants that reduce the risk of seizure and promote complete bedrest.
4. Fluid and electrolyte replacement: oral and IV.	Balance between correcting hypovolemia and preventing fluid overload.
5. Antihypertensives: Aldomet (Methyldopal), Normodyne (labetalol), and nifedipine (Procardia).	Acute treatment of hypertension for a diastolic pressure of ≥ 100 mm Hg to maintain diastolic between 90 and 100 mm Hg.

Adapted from: Olds, S., London, M., & Ladewig, P. (1996). *Maternal-newborn nursing*, 5th ed. Menlo Park, CA: Addison-Wesley Nursing (pp. 497–500). Adapted with permission.

Mylanta) for Terri's "stomach pain," Nurse Smith violated: (a) the state's nurse practice act, (b) JCAHO standards (1995), (c) professional standards (ANA, 1985, 1991; NAACOG, 1991), and (d) the hospital's policy, which required a physician's order for medications to be administered to hospitalized patients.

Evaluation Every RN caring for Terri failed to detect: (a) the presence of symptoms indicating PIH, (b) the severity of her PIH symptoms, (c) the increasing severity of her PIH symptoms, and (d) the development of HELLP syndrome early in its course so that appropriate treatment measures could be initiated (Olds, et al., 1996). After administering medications (i.e., Percocet, Demerol, and Phenergan), the nurses all failed to evaluate their effectiveness or ineffectiveness. Lack of pain-relief with multiple doses of narcotics did not cause any nurse to revise assessments, nursing diagnoses, interventions, or the plan of care, as required by professional standards (ANA, 1983, 1991; NAACOG, 1991) and the state's nurse practice act. Neither the patient, her family, nor other health care providers were an integral part of evaluations of Terri's responses to interventions (ANA, 1983, 1991; NAACOG, 1991).

This institution's organized nursing services did not utilize the nursing process as "the framework for providing nursing care" (ANA, 1988, p. 5) as required by the nursing profession (ANA, 1983, 1991; NAACOG, 1991). Additionally, the *Standards for Organized Nursing Services* (ANA, 1988) requires nursing services to be "administered by qualified and competent nurse administrators" (p. 3). The director of nursing (DON) at this institution had only a baccalaureate degree and no management education. She was unqualified to fulfill her responsibilities as the nursing administrator of the organization and her actions resulted in negligence. The role of the DON is

Essential Nursing Interventions for Unstable PIH

The criteria for unstable PIH include:

- BP ≥ 160/110
- proteinuria of 5 grams
- urine output < 30 mL/hour
- edema of 3+ or 4+

Nursing interventions include:

- Take vital signs, including BP, every two hours.
- Record hourly I/O; specific-gravity and dipstick all urine.
- Monitor IV and/or Swan-Ganz.
- Administer IV Magnesium Sulfate at loading dose of 4–6 grams; continuous infusion of 1–2 grams/hour. Have Calcium Gluconate antidote available. Monitor reflexes, respirations, and urine output.
- Assess reflexes and clonus.
- Monitor fetus continuously.
- Auscultate lung sounds every four hours.
- Assess edema qid and weigh daily.
- Follow seizure precautions.
- Provide a quiet, low-stimulus environment.
- Interpret ordered lab tests, including CBC, platelets, Hct, creatinine, BUN, uric acid, clotting studies, liver enzymes, and electrolytes.

Adapted with permission from: Olds, S., London, M., & Ladewig, P. (1996). *Maternal-newborn nursing,* 5th ed. Menlo Park, CA: Addison-Wesley Nursing (pp. 490 and 505–507).

to provide "leadership and vision for nursing's development and advancement within the organization" (ANA, 1988, p. 9). Specifically, this nurse executive did not "ensure the establishment and implementation of standards of nursing practice consistent with standards of professional organizations and regulating agencies" (ANA, 1988, p. 10). Placing nurses in specialty practice (see Chapter 4) without documenting their educational and experiential competence violates regulatory agency standards (i.e., JCAHO and state health departments) as well as professional standards (ANA, 1983, 1985, 1988, 1991; NAACOG, 1990, 1991).

Two of the nurses caring for Terri, Nurses Maroon and Heffernan, were working without current nursing licensure as registered nurses. Nurse Oxman, whose last experience in obstetrical care was as a student (18 years earlier), was unqualified to care for Terri or any other obstetrical patient without appropriate supervision. This institution had: (a) *no* orientation for obstetrical care, (b) *no* obstetrical skills checklists or competency tests (these standards were initiated five months after Terri's death), (c) *no* inservice/continuing education documented in nursing personnel files (although the state required continuing education for relicensure), (d) *no* reference texts on the postpartum unit, and (e) *no* orientation to charge-nurse roles and responsibilities.

The hospital failed to conduct a formal evaluation, or to recommend disciplinary action or remediation for the nurses for their negligent nursing care and malpractice, yet an evaluation by the DON immediately after Terri's cardiopulmonary arrest resulted in alteration of patient records. The depositions of Nurses Smith, O'Brien (the shift supervisor), and Tower (the DON) reveal significant discrepancies in sworn versions of the events indicating that tampering with medical records had occurred. After Terri's cardiopulmonary arrest, Nurse O'Brien copied the original record, took a copy to the ICU, gave one to Dr. Dale at his request, and notified Nurse Tower, who arrived at 0330. Nurse Tower testified that she told Nurse O'Brien to instruct Nurse Smith to add a late entry at 2045 that the physician had been notified of the elevated BP. Nurse Smith testified that she wrote two versions of the patient record, at two separate times, and "threw away" the original version per Nurse O'Brien's instruction. Nurse O'Brien denied that she instructed Nurse Smith to destroy the original record. However, in discussing the record with Nurse Smith, Nurse O'Brien said she told her: (a) that the case would be reviewed by the DON and physicians, (b) that the chart needed to be as clear and accurate as possible, and (c) that she wanted her to write a note on a separate sheet of paper before she charted, so Nurse O'Brien could review the note. Nurse O'Brien said she assumed that entries would be added after the last nursing note, rather than from the beginning of the shift.

Nurse Smith gave Nurse O'Brien a rewritten, completed record, rather than a draft. Not agreeing with the content of the "rewritten" note, Nurse O'Brien asked Nurse Smith for the "old, original record" and was informed that it had been "thrown away." Neither nurse retrieved, reviewed, or compared the discarded note to the altered version that was entered into the permanent chart.

Two months after Terri's death and after the state health department's investigation, a copy of the original record surfaced (in the possession of Dr. Dale, whose privileges were under review). The discrepancies between the original and altered versions were apparent to both Dr. Dale and the hospital's administration. At that time, the DON made an undated, untimed, unsigned note and drew lines through blank spaces on a copy of the original note that was placed in the patient's chart (along with the altered version). Testifying that she altered/tampered with the original copy version on advice of counsel, the DON testified that notes could be rewritten if: (a) original notes were not entered into the permanent record, and (b) if the information had not been acted on. The DON's alterations of the patient record, whether she acted on her own or on advice of counsel (which should have been declined), violated federal and state statutes, the hospital's policy, and professional standards.

The content and completeness of patient records is governed by: (a) federal and state statutes, (b) municipal codes, and (c) hospital accreditation agencies (Mahoney, 1987). For hospitals participating in federally funded programs (i.e., Medicare, Medicaid), the federal government delineates specific patient record requirements. Within each state, hospital licensing statutes and/or hospital regulatory agencies such as state health departments promulgate rules and regulations for patient records in licensed hospitals. JCAHO's accreditation manual (1995) requires the maintenance of and specifies the content and completeness of patient records. State, federal, and accreditation agencies also require each hospital to have policies that govern patient records, storage, and retention. Professional standards of practice and care require adherence to the above legal statutes and preservation of patient records (ANA, 1983, 1985, 1988, 1991, 1994; NAACOG, 1990, 1991).

Nurse O'Brien's attempts to: (a) "edit" and "supervise" Nurse Smith's documentation, (b) instruct Nurse Smith to destroy the original document, and (c) conceal the alteration/destruction of patient records were illegal, unethical, and unprofessional. Whether she acted alone or was instructed by the supervisor and DON, Nurse Smith's alteration and destruction of the original record and failure to disclose the destruction violated state and federal statutes, the hospital policy, and professional standards. Alteration of patient records also enables plaintiff's attorneys to destroy the credibility of the entire record. In *Hiatt v. Grace* (1974), the court held that a clear discrepancy in the patient record justifies the jury's findings that if the record is erroneous in one area, it could be erroneous in other areas. Not only the record, but the professional authors of the record, lose credibility. In court, late entries are less credible if made "after a motive to falsify," such as regulatory-agency investigation or threatened litigation, has arisen (Mahoney, 1987, p. 5). Alterations made after litigation (either threatened or filed) subjects the entire record to suspicion that the revisions were made under a consciousness of negligence (*Pisel v. Stanford Hospital*, 1980).

Deliberate and intentional altering, falsifying, or tampering with patient records is a criminal offense and may subject the professionals and the institution to license revocation by regulating agencies. In this case, altered patient records resulted in: (a) allegations of a cover-up by the institution to attempt to avoid responsibility for actions of the nursing staff and administrators, (b) multiple investigations by federal and state agencies, (c) disciplinary action by the state board of nursing, and (d) a counter-lawsuit by the physician against the nurses and hospital for conspiracy and damages resulting from their attempt to place blame for Terri Keaton's death solely on the physician.

Case 2

Facts

On August 29 at 0350 Janet Donaldson, a 33-year-old G3 P2, arrived at the labor and delivery department of a rural level I hospital that delivered 700 births per year. Janet was at term and in active labor after a normal, low-risk prenatal course. One of Janet's previous children had been delivered by cesarean for breech presentation.

On Janet's arrival, Nurse Crown collected the admission data and the following events occurred.

0436: External fetal monitor (EFM) applied: FHR 130s.
0440: Cervix: 2 cm dilated, 50% effaced.
0500: Vital signs: T 36.4 C; P 56, R 22, BP 100/60. Height 5 feet 7 inches; weight 156 pounds, pregnancy weight gain of 25 pounds. Contractions: every 3 minutes, 40–95 seconds, firm. Membranes leaking clear fluid. FHR 120–140 beats per minute (bpm), baseline rate: long-term variability (LTV) present.
0530: EFM: occasional variable decelerations to 90–100 bpm over 20 seconds beginning at the peak of uterine contractions (UC) and then returning to baseline (130s). Patient on left side.
0600: EFM: variable decelerations continued, LTV present. Dr. Howard notified.
0620: Lactated Ringers (LR) IV started and butorphanol (Stadol) 1 mg slow IV push administered.
0640: EFM: continued to have late onset variables; decelerations to 110s over 30–40 seconds and return to baseline 10 seconds after contraction ends.
0655: Oxygen per face mask at 8 liters/minute. LR infused wide open after late onset variable to 80 bpm lasting 60 seconds.
0700: Nurse Bowls assumed care of Janet. Cervix: 2 cm dilated, 50% effaced, –3 station, bulging bag of waters. FHR 130–140s.
0710: Janet turned more on left side with wedge; oxygen per mask; IV wide open.
0725: BP 130/80. Dr. Howard called and given report about moderate variables with consistent late onset and interventions.
0730: No repeat of late decelerations in last 20-minute strip. FHR 140s with LTV present. Oxygen discontinued.
0735: Dr. Howard on the way to the hospital. Only mild, occasional variable decelerations. FHR 120s.
0750: EFM: mild variable decelerations during and after contractions. FHR decreased to 100s with good return to baseline: LTV present, BP 102/70.
0828: Dr. Howard arrived. Cervix: 2–3 cm dilated. Dr. Howard artificially ruptured membranes. Meconium-stained amniotic fluid was noted to be "light" amount (by physician) and "moderate" amount (by nurse). An internal fetal monitor (IFM) was placed: FHR 120–130s with short- and long-term variabilities.
0845: Cervix: 3–4 cm dilated. FHR 130s with mild variable decelerations.
0855: Stadol 0.50 mg × 2 administered slow IV push, BP 106/60, P 68.
0920: Cervix: 4–6 cm dilated, BP 120/78, P 87. FHR 130s with STV and LTV. IFM: late-onset decelerations with slow rebound followed by two more over next contraction.
0922: FHR 130–140s.
0943: Epidural anesthesia administered in sitting position, BP 95/57, P 64. FHR not documented.
0945: BP 85/57, P 66. FHR 120s with STV and LTV.

0948: Cervix: 5–6 cm dilated, BP 101/76, P 80. FHR 120s with STV and LTV.
0955: Cervix 75% effaced; 2–3 cm dilated; high station, BP 98/62.
1000: Dr. Howard observed fetal monitor strip and decided to perform cesarean delivery for fetal distress (i.e., consistent late-onset decelerations and no progress in dilation). BP 88/45, P 70.
1007: BP 97/58, P 75.
1010: Cervix: 5–6 cm, T 36.1 C, P 76, BP 92/50. FHR 130s with STV and LTV.
1030: Electronic fetal monitoring discontinued and patient taken to operating room.
1115: An 8 lb. 14 oz. (4026 grams) male infant with nuchal cord × 1 was delivered. APGARS 5, 8(5), 8(10). The infant required suction for meconium at the cords, FiO_2 100%, and bag and mask ventilation.
1120: On admission to the nursery, the infant was flaccid with intermittent respirations and CPAP ventilation. He was placed in an oxyhood with FiO_2 30% and pulse oximetry in the 80% range.
1130: Initial cord blood pH 7.02.
1145: Naloxone (Narcan) 1 cc given IM.
1150: Arterial blood gas repeated: pH 6.98.
1150–2255: The infant's respiratory distress worsened with increasing FiO_2 to 100% (by 2015), numerous apneic episodes, and seizure activity at 1245 requiring phenobarbital (Luminal) administration.
2330: Baby was transported to a level III neonatal intensive care unit.

Outcome

Severe perinatal asphyxia required a 9-day hospitalization. Severe bilateral hearing loss also occurred. At 9 months, the baby was diagnosed with growth retardation and cerebral palsy with profound neurologic handicaps.

Legal

This case is currently under litigation.

Case Commentary

Undesirable Patient Outcome

Assessment From admission to birth of the baby (i.e., 7 hours and 20 minutes), a complete set of Janet's vital signs were taken only once, on admission. A temperature was taken on admission (0500), and six hours later (1010), with leaking amniotic fluid. Janet's nurses took her pulse on admission, at 0855 with the second Stadol administration, at 0920, 23 minutes before the epidural, and after the epidural (7×) respiratory rate was taken on admission only. The nurses measured Janet's blood pressure on admission, after oxygen was started, with the second Stadol dose, and after epidural insertion (7×).

The nurses' assessments of fetal well-being also were deficient. They did not assess FHR often enough even for a low-risk patient, nor did they increase frequency when the fetus was clearly at risk. They also failed to assess FHR before and after artificial rupture of membranes, and during epidural anesthesia. External or internal EFM was not assessed often enough even for a low-risk patient, nor was frequency increased when the fetus was at risk. Janet's nurses did not assess FHR during transport or while waiting for operative delivery. They administered oxygen from 0655 to 0730. No assessment of need for supplemental oxygen was made during the mother's hypotension after the epidural.

Diagnosis No nursing diagnoses were made.

Planning No nursing plan was formulated to guide nursing interventions and evaluations.

Implementation The nurses failed to notify Janet's physician of "occasional variable decelerations" at 0600. They started oxygen at 0655 and discontinued it at 0730. Oxygen was *not* restarted during the mother's hypotension after epidural administration, nor were measures to correct hypotension initiated.

Evaluation These nurses did not recognize or act upon the ominous FHR patterns, indicative of fetal distress, in a timely manner.

Desirable Patient Outcome

Assessment The obstetrical nurse caring for the laboring woman must assess two patients (i.e., the mother and the fetus) using various methods (e.g., palpation, auscultation, external and internal EFM, ultrasound, and laboratory data) (Olds, et al., 1996). Data collection and interpretation are systematic, ongoing, and collaborative with the patient, family, and other health care providers (ANA, 1983, 1991; NAACOG, 1991). Nursing assessment of maternal and neonatal parameters and frequency of assessments during labor and birth are outlined in Table 8-3. During significant labor events, FHR auscultation, assessment, and documentation did not occur at or after: (a) initiation of labor-enhancing procedures (e.g., artificial rupture of membranes), (b) administration or initiation of analgesia/anesthesia, (c) rupture of membranes, (d) administration of medication (i.e., at peak action), (e) vaginal exams, and (f) evaluation of analgesia/anesthesia (NAACOG, 1990, p. 5). Discontinuation of the fetal monitor did not result in continued auscultation assessments by the obstetrical nurses. Throughout Janet's labor, these nurses failed to interpret correctly findings in the FM strips and failed to recognize and document FHR as follows:

0451: In early labor, first late deceleration with no acceleration noted after late deceleration (Figure 8-1, p. 131).
0510: Decrease in long term variability (LTV); an almost flat pattern for 4 minutes with late decelerations and no accelerations (Figure 8-2, p. 131).
0532: A sinusoidal FHR pattern is noted and persists for 13 minutes (Figure 8-3, p. 132).
0547: Late decelerations continue.
0610: Repetitive variable decelerations continue with a decrease in LTV.
0626: Decreased long-term variability.
0632: Long (i.e., 45 seconds) late deceleration to 100 bpm with no accelerations noted.

Table 8-3 Nursing Assessments During Labor and Birth

Stage/Phase	Mother	Fetus
First Stage		
Latent Phase	*Vital signs:* T q 4 hrs; T q 1 hr if > 37.5 C or membranes ruptured, BP and R q 1 hr if in normal range *Uterine contractions:* q 30 min	*Low risk:* FHR q 1 hr* *High risk:* FHR q 30 min*; note fetal activity If EFM assess reactive NST
Active Phase	*Vital signs:* T, P, R, and BP q 1 hr if in normal range *Uterine contractions:* q 30 min With epidural: baseline T, P, R, BP before medication administration, BP q 1–2 min for 10 min; q 5–15 min after medication administration, monitor P, R	*Low risk:* FHR q 30 min* EFM tracing q 15–30 min† *High risk:* FHR q 15 min* EFM tracing q 15 min† Note FHR/EFM tracing before/after epidural
Transition	*Vital signs:* P, R, BP q 30 min *Uterine contractions:* time frames vary according to individual patient condition	*Low risk:* FHR q 30 min* *High risk:* FHR q 15 min*
Second Stage	*Vital signs:* P, R, BP q 5–15 min *Uterine contractions:* palpated continuously	*Low risk:* FHR q 15 min EFM tracing q 5–15 min† *High risk:* FHR q 5 min EFM tracing q 5 min†
Third Stage	*Vital signs* and *Uterine contractions:* time frame for both vary with individual patient condition	Apgar score one and five minutes

*If normal (i.e., average variability; baseline 120–160 bpm; no late or variable decelerations)
†As long as FHR pattern is reassuring. If *any* nonreassuring characteristics or patterns appear, the time interval for nursing assessment should be shortened.

Adapted from: Olds, S., London, M. & Ladewig, P. (1996). *Maternal-newborn nursing,* 5th Ed. Menlo Park, CA: Addison-Wesley Nursing (pp. 613, 614, 652, 655).

0715: Decreased variability continues.
0759: Late decelerations to 90 bpm, lasting 60 seconds, followed by repeated late decelerations.
0835: Variability better but late decelerations persist.
0900: Late decelerations to 100 bpm lasting 70 seconds (Figure 8-4, p. 132).
0930: Late decelerations (FHR 140s down to 120s) without acceleration.
0935: FHR 120s with decelerations to 70s.
0950: Late decelerations continue, are repetitive without accelerations, decreased variability (Figure 8-5, p. 133).

Janet's nurses assessed these decelerations as variable; however, they were not variable decelerations because in the FM strips: (a) the shape was not variable, (b) the timing was not variable, and (c) they were not variable in depth. Despite a stable baseline FHR, these decelerations were late, not variable, because they were: (a) uniform in shape, (b) occurred after the peak of the contraction, and (c) did not return to baseline immediately after the contraction ceased (Adelsperger, Carr, Davis, Feinstein, & Schmidt, 1993). "Late-onset variable" is dated terminology; decelerations should be labeled either

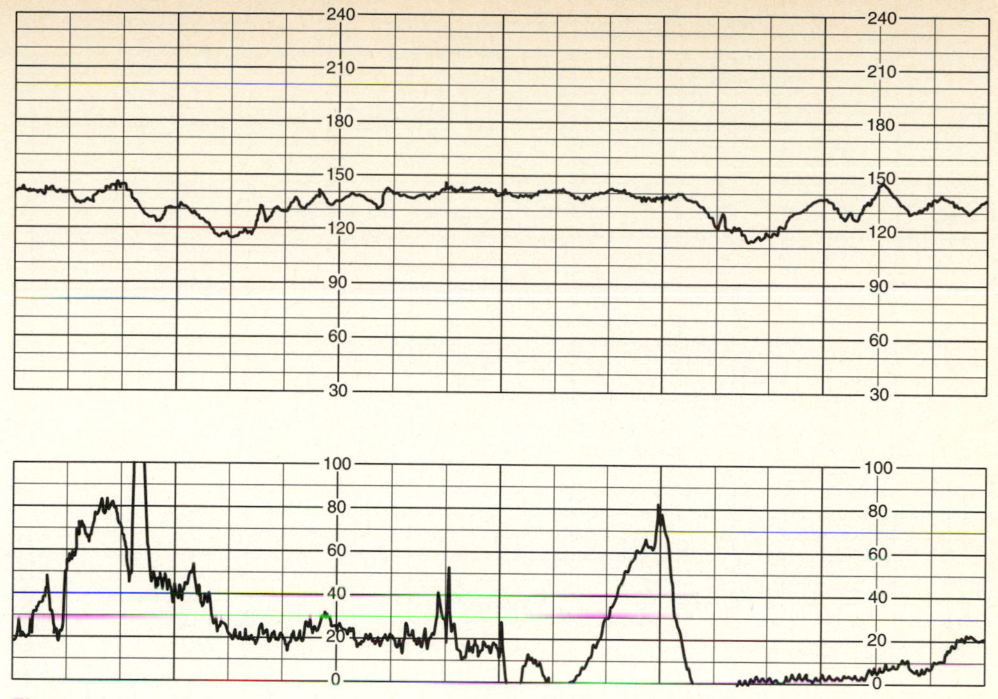

Figure 8-1 0451—External fetal monitor shows first late deceleration with no acceleration noted on EFM tracing.

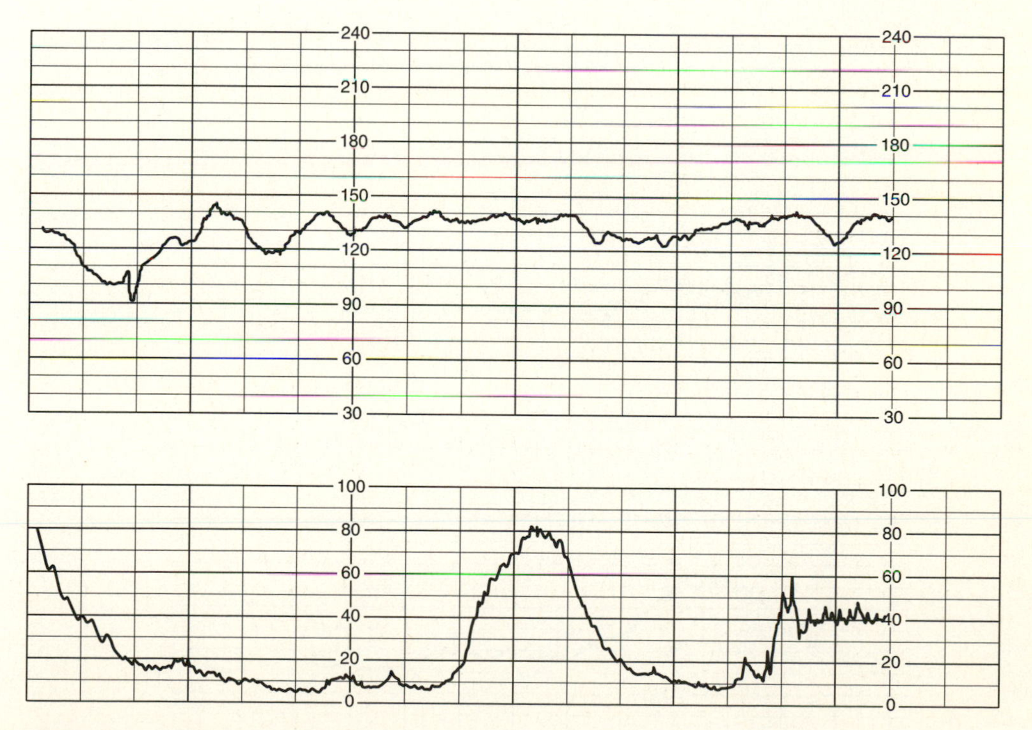

Figure 8-2 0510—External fetal monitor shows decreased LTV; an almost flat pattern for 4 minutes with late decelerations and no accelerations.

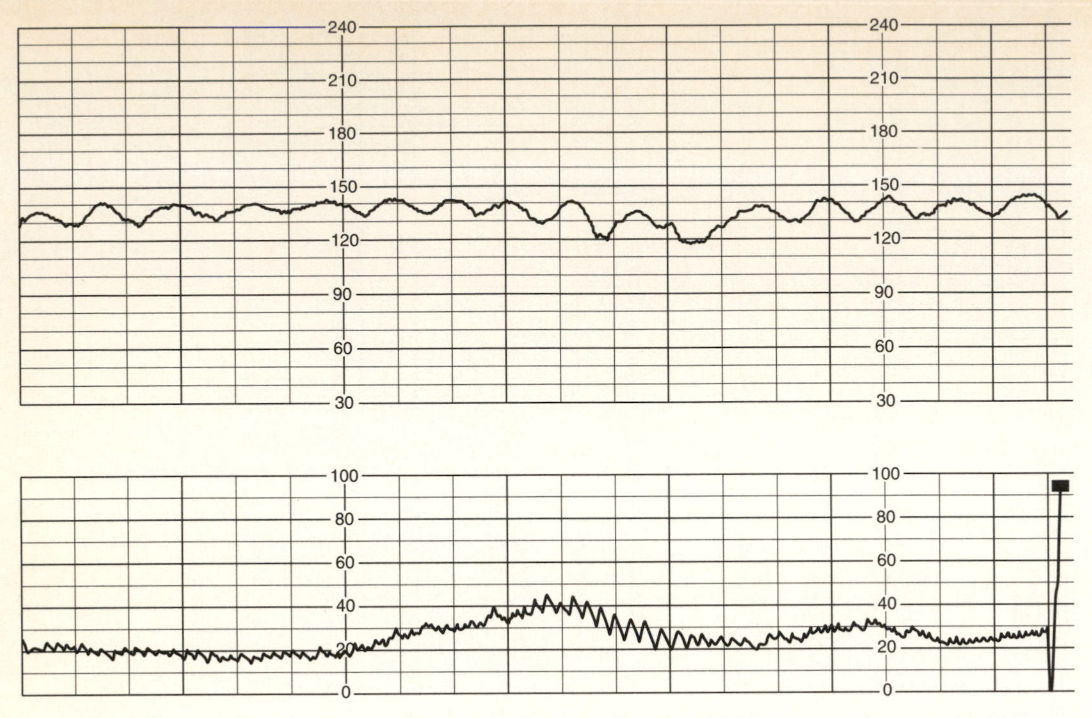

Figure 8-3 0532—External fetal monitor shows a sinusoidal FHR pattern that persists for 13 minutes.

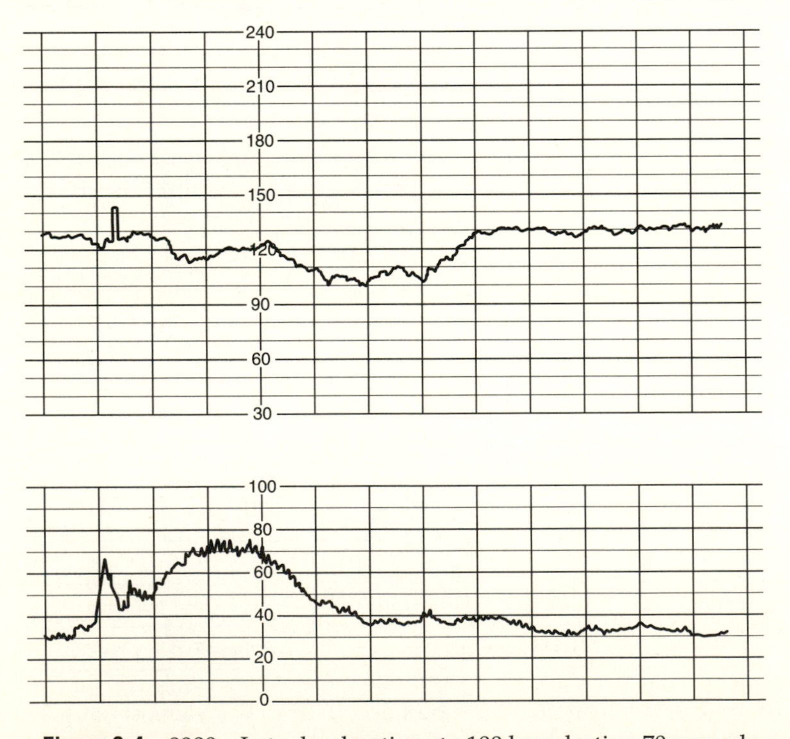

Figure 8-4 0900—Late decelerations to 100 bpm lasting 70 seconds.

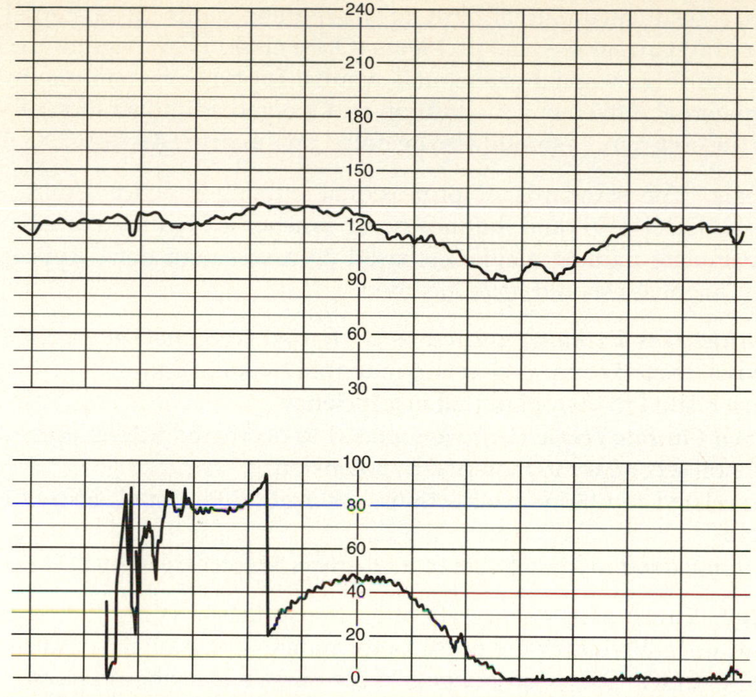

Figure 8-5 0950—Internal fetal monitor shows a late deceleration with the FHR returning to baseline after the contraction is over; no FHR accelerations. Decreased short- and long-term variability.

variable or late decelerations. No accelerations, a reassuring sign, were ever documented, and a sinusoidal pattern, suggestive of severe asphyxia, was missed. Late decelerations are "due to uteroplacental insufficiency as a result of decreased blood flow and oxygen transfer to the fetus through intervillous space during uterine contractions causing hypoxemia" and are "always an ominous sign" (Olds, et al., 1996, pp. 623–624). Repetitive and worsening decelerations, tachycardia, or a decrease in variability may require other assessment techniques (e.g., fetal blood sampling) to evaluate fetal acid-base status (Olds, et al., 1996).

Skill and competence *must* be maintained by nurses assessing and evaluating fetal monitor strips (ANA, 1985, 1991; NAACOG, 1991). Through inservice and continuing education programs, competence in FM interpretation and appropriate interventions for nonreassuring patterns can be maintained (AWHONN, 1993; Chez & Harvey, 1994; McRae, 1993; NAACOG, 1991). Nurses must record assessment data on the narrative nurses' notes and the fetal monitor tracing (Olds, et al., 1996). Missing fetal monitor tracings containing the only documentation of care preclude adequate nursing defense in malpractice litigation. Basic information on the monitor strip should include: (a) date/time, (b) patient's name, (c) hospital number, (d) age, (e) para and gravida, (f) estimated date of birth, (g) membrane status, (h) maternal vital signs, and (i) current medical problems (Olds, et al., 1996). Significant labor occurrences (e.g., vaginal exams and results; rupture of membranes; vital signs; maternal movement; medication and oxygen administration) and the time of the occurrences should also be noted on the strip (AAP-ACOG, 1992).

Diagnosis The standards of professional nursing practice (ANA, 1983, 1991; NAACOG, 1991) and the state nurse practice act required Janet's nurses to formulate nursing diagnoses based on assessment data. Appropriate nursing diagnoses should have included:

Impaired Gas Exchange related to decreased oxygenation secondary to possible cord compression and maternal hypotension
Injury related to uteroplacental insufficiency
Altered Cardiac Tissue Perfusion related to decreased uteroplacental perfusion secondary to maternal hypotension
Pain related to uterine contractions, cervical dilation and descent of the fetus
Anxiety related to knowledge of fetal stress and cesarean birth

Planning Given assessment data and appropriate nursing diagnoses, the standard of care requires the nurse to formulate a plan of care (ANA, 1983, 1991; NAACOG, 1991). Components of the nurse's plan should have included: (a) review institutional policy / protocol regarding fetal distress and nursing management during and after epidural anesthesia, (b) consult physician in a timely manner about EFM strips indicative of significant fetal distress, and (c) consult nursing colleagues and / or supervisor.

Implementation Nonreassuring FHR patterns, meconium-stained amniotic fluid, and repetitive late decelerations with decreased variability required timely nursing interventions (Table 8-4). Timely consultation with the physician for interpretation of FM strips early (0451) and throughout labor, and interventions when FM strips indicated significant fetal distress, did not occur (ANA, 1983, 1985, 1991; NAACOG, 1991). Janet's nurses also failed to consult with colleagues such as other obstetrical nurses to verify nursing assessments, diagnoses, plan, and interventions. Nurse Bowls did not notify the nursing supervisor regarding her patients (i.e., the mother and fetus) and their change to high-risk status in a timely manner. Nurse Bowls also delayed initiation of oxygen and interventions for maternal hypotension after epidural administration. The nurses failed to perform an adequate nursing assessment of maternal and fetal status prior to the administration of Stadol or after the insertion of the epidural for pain relief.

Evaluation Continued deterioration in this fetus' condition (i.e., late decelerations, decreasing variability, meconium-stained amniotic fluid, and lack of accelerations) with the interventions utilized should have resulted in a reevaluation and revision in the plan of care. Since Janet's care providers failed to establish outcomes, the effectiveness of their interventions could not be evaluated (ANA, 1991). As the patient's advocate, Nurse Bowls failed to

Table 8-4 Nursing Interventions for Signs of Fetal Distress

Assessment	Interventions
Late decelerations	• Oxygen 7–10 L/min by face mask. • Explain and reassure patient and family. • Continuously monitor for FHR pattern changes. • Position on left side. • Increase IV fluids (NS or LR) for hydration and treatment of hypotension. • Discontinue oxytocin. • Monitor maternal BP, P for hypotension; treat hypotension per protocol/MD orders. • Assess labor progress. • Notify MD/CNM immediately. • Assist with fetal blood sampling: pH > 7.25—continue monitoring and resample; pH 7.20-7.25 or <7.20—prepare for birth.
Late decelerations with decreasing variability	• All of the above. • Prepare for immediate cesarean birth.
Meconium-stained amniotic fluid	• Continuously monitor FHR. • Evaluate cervical dilatation (assess for umbilical cord prolapse). • Evaluate presentation (vertex/breech). • Position on left side. • Notify MD/CNM immediately.
Maternal hypotension (i.e., < 100 mm Hg systolic pressure)	• Position: left lateral; elevate foot of bed (10–20 degrees). • Increase IV rate. • Oxygen 7–10 L/min by face mask. • Vasopressors: Ephedrine 5–15 mg IV (if BP does not increase within 1–2 min). • Manually displace uterus laterally to the left.

Adapted from: Olds, S., London, M., Ladewig, P. (1996). *Maternal-newborn nursing,* 5th Ed. Menlo Park, CA: Addison-Wesley Nursing (pp. 631, 654, 682, 689). Adapted with permission.

ensure patient safety, avoid poor birth outcome, and provide competent care that meets the standard of care (ANA, 1983, 1985, 1991; NAACOG, 1991).

Case 3

Group B streptococcal (GBS) infection is the leading cause of sepsis in the immediate newborn period. Although 5–35% of pregnant women are colonized with GBS, only about 1% of infants born to colonized women (i.e., 1–5 cases/1000 live births) develop early onset disease (AAP, 1992; AAP-ACOG, 1992). Overall mortality for early (i.e., within hours through the first week of life) and late (i.e., 7 days to 3 months) onset neonatal and infant infection is 10–15% respectively. A higher mortality rate exists for preterm (25–30%) compared to term infants (2–8%) (AAP, 1992). Perinatal morbidity includes: (a) maternal endometritis, amnionitis, and urinary tract infections, and (b) neonatal/infant sepsis, pneumonia, meningitis, permanent neurologic sequelae, and death.

Perinatal (i.e., antepartal or intrapartal) maternal antibiotic treatment appears to prevent GBS disease in the neonate and decreases maternal postpartal endometritis (Boyer & Gotoff, 1986). Neonatal sepsis has been reported with: (a) fewer than 4 hours of maternal antibiotics at term, and (b) up to 48 hours in preterms (Weisman, Stoll, Cruess, Hall, Merenstein, Hemming, & Fisher, 1992). In order to prevent GBS, the American Academy of Pediatrics (AAP, 1992) issued practice guidelines and the American College of Obstetricians and Gynecologists (ACOG, 1992) issued a technical bulletin concerning screening and chemoprophylaxis. The AAP guidelines (1992) recommend: (a) vaginal/rectal cultures of all pregnant women at 28 weeks gestation, and (b) intrapartum antibiotic prophylaxis to women with positive GBS cultures in the presence of perinatal risk factors.

Although ACOG's educational aid discusses several treatment and management options, including selective treatment of women with GBS-positive cultures and perinatal risk factors, universal screening of pregnant women is not recommended (ACOG, 1992). Even though there is a lack of consensus between these two professional organizations, according to one study most obstetricians who did not agree with universal screening would treat positive culture results with antibiotics without regard for other risk factors (Gigante, Hickson, Entman, & O'Quist, 1995). AAP and ACOG's *Guidelines for Perinatal Care* (1992) requires that exposure to GBS be among other pertinent information transmitted to the physician (and other health care providers) caring for the infant after delivery.

Facts

On December 17, at 1600, Lauren Kastle, a 17-year-old, G1, P0 unmarried high school student entered the local hospital in active labor. Her contractions began at 0800, and she was now having contractions every 3–4 minutes, increasing to every 2–3 minutes with intact membranes. According to her prenatal records, Lauren began receiving care on 9/27, at 28 weeks gestation. Her initial screen showed: (a) blood type/Rh: O+, (b) Hct 32.8/Hgb 11.7, (c) nonreactive serology, (d) rubella immune, (e) hepatitis B/HIV nonreactive. On 9/29 an obstetrical ultrasound estimated a gestational age of 26.9 to 29.9 weeks. Cervical cultures taken on 10/3 showed: (a) gonorrhea—negative, (b) chlamydia—negative, (c) candida—positive, and (d) group B streptococcus (GBS)—positive. From 10/18 through 12/15, the fetus remained active and the mother had a normal prenatal course.

Admission data assessed by Nurse Tinker included:

December 17:
1700: FHR baseline 142–160, STV+, IV of LR started.
1730: Vital signs: T 37.3, P 120, R 20, BP 118/74, cervix 2 cm dilated, –1 station, 90% effaced. Dr. Lavin, Lauren's obstetrician, artificially ruptured membranes with clear fluid obtained, and FHR accelerations.
1735: Complete blood count: WBC 19,700, RBC 4,190, Hgb 13.5 gm/dL, Hct 38.4 gm/dL, Segs 78%, Bands 6%, Lymphocytes 12%, Monocytes 4%. The

family practice resident's admission note included the vital signs (taken by Nurse Tinker), FHR, dilatation, and artificial rupture of membranes (AROM) performed by Dr. Lavin. A note in the left margin cited + for GBS.
1800: FHR 140, +STV, + accelerations.
1815: FHR 140, +STV, + accelerations.
1835: Cervix 3 cm, –1 station, 90% effaced/Dr. Lavin. BP 123/54, Nubain (Nalbuphine) 10 mg IV, Phenergan (Promethazine) 12.5 mg IV, FHR 140, + accelerations.
1900: Cervix 4 cm, –1 station, 90% effaced/Nurse Jackson. FHR 145, FHR shows decrease to 120/110, supine.
1930: FHR 134–140, + accelerations, BP 136/82.
2000: Cervix 5 cm, –1 station, 90% effaced/Nurse Jackson.
FHR 125–130 with decelerations, pt. crying and complaining of backache, placed on left side, BP 127/72.
2015: BP 144/90, FHR 125–130 with decelerations.
2030: BP 127/12, FHR 125–130 with Nubain 10 mg, Phenergan 12.5 mg IVP.
2045: BP 123/81, FHR 125–135 with + accelerations.
2100: Cervix 8 cm, +1 station, 100% effaced/Nurse Jackson.
Pt. crying with contractions, FHR 130–140, + accelerations.
2105: Pt. thrashing about in bed, instructed to breathe with contractions.
2145: Completely dilated, Dr. Lavin notified. Pt. instructed to push.
2229: Delivery with vacuum extraction of a male infant with Apgars of 6 and 8 (5 minutes), and birth weight of 7 lbs. 10 oz. (3459 grams).
2240: On admission to the nursery the baby's vital signs were: T 37.2, P 172, R 56, pulse oximetry 96% in room air.
2300: Lauren's temp 37.3.

December 18:
0820: Physical examination by pediatrician within normal limits. Pediatrician checked "No risk factors noted" section of charting. Lauren's temperature decreased during day after delivery. Baby was active, vigorous, nippled well and had vital signs WNL.

December 19:
0750: Discharge physical of baby charted as WNL.
2255: Discharged to mother with follow-up in two weeks with pediatrician.

December 25:
Parents and family noticed baby was irritable, vomiting, with poor feeding, listless with a weak cry and not moving correctly. Baby was taken to hospital emergency room. Vital signs were: T 34.6, infant pale, lethargic, listless, no suck reflex, seizure activity noted. After cultures were done, intravenous antibiotics were administered. Infant was transferred to a university medical center for confirmation of sepsis, meningitis, life support. Life support was withdrawn with subsequent survival.

Outcome

Group B streptococcal sepsis and meningitis led to cerebral vascular infarction, hydrocephalus, developmental delays and significant neurologic sequelae.

Legal

This case is currently under litigation.

Case Commentary

Undesirable Patient Outcome

Assessment Lauren's temperature was taken only on admission (1730), and thirty minutes after delivery (2300) despite the fact that her membranes were artificially ruptured by the physician on admission (1730). There was no evidence of Nurses Tinker or Jackson interpreting the 1735 laboratory results. Lauren's prenatal records accompanied her to the hospital and were available to both nurses.

Diagnosis No nursing diagnoses were formulated or documented during the labor process for this patient.

Planning No nursing plan based on assessment data and nursing diagnoses was formulated to guide nursing interventions and evaluations.

Implementation No nursing actions based on assessment data, nursing diagnoses, and plan were implemented related to this patient's positive GBS culture, ruptured membranes, and elevated WBC.

Evaluation No evaluation criteria were established that could be used to evaluate the effectiveness of interventions. No nursing interventions related to positive Group B streptococcus occurred that could be evaluated. No revisions in the plan of care (e.g., use of intrapartum antibiotic prophylaxis) occurred.

Desirable Patient Outcome

Assessment Data collection and interpretation were not systematic, ongoing, or collaborative (ANA, 1983, 1991; NAACOG, 1991). Lauren's prenatal records clearly showed a positive GBS culture at 28 weeks and no treatment (i.e., antibiotics) prenatally. In the left margin of the admitting family-practice resident's note, + GBS is documented. The obstetrical nurses: (a) did not review the mother's history, and/or (b) did not understand the significance of + GBS cultures.

Although the maternal temperatures documented at 1730 and 2300 were lowgrade (i.e., 37.3) in elevation, more frequent assessment was warranted (see Table 8-3). Inadequate assessment by the nurses resulted in insufficient data to determine if this mother had a fever during labor. If the mother is a GBS carrier (i.e., + GBS culture), determination of one or more risk factors should result in intrapartum intravenous antibiotic therapy that significantly decreases neonatal infection (AAP, 1992; ACOG, 1992; Boyer & Gotoff, 1986; Pylipow, Gaddis, & Kinney, 1994). Risk factors in maternal GBS carriers are listed in the box on page 139.

In addition to collecting the blood for CBC, the nurse is responsible for interpreting test results (ANA, 1983; NAACOG, 1991). There is no indication

Risk Factors in Maternal GBS Carriers*

- Preterm labor at 37 weeks gestation
- Premature rupture of membranes at 37 weeks gestation
- Fever during labor
- Multiple births
- Rupture of membranes beyond 18 hours at any gestation

*If maternal colonization is unknown, presence of one or more risk factors may warrant antibiotic prophylaxis.

From: AAP (1992). Guidelines for prevention of group B streptococcal (GBS) infection by chemoprophylaxis, *Pediatrics, 90*(5), p. 777. Reprinted with permission.

that Nurses Tinker or Jackson interpreted the elevated WBC count or communicated the data to either the resident or the obstetrician. Failure to: (a) review perinatal history, (b) understand the significance of pertinent information, (c) collect adequate and timely data, (d) understand the risk factors in GBS carriers, and (e) interpret laboratory data violates the nurse's duty to practice competently (ANA, 1983, 1985, 1991, 1994; NAACOG, 1991).

Diagnosis Formulating appropriate nursing diagnoses is required by the state nurse practice act and professional standards of practice (ANA, 1983, 1985, 1988, 1991; NAACOG, 1991). Appropriate nursing diagnoses should have included:

Infection: Maternal related to AROM and + GBS culture
Injury: Neonatal related to GBS infection
Maternal Hyperthermia related to AROM

Planning The standard of care requires the nurse to formulate a plan of care for each patient (ANA, 1983, 1991; NAACOG, 1991). Components of the nurse's plan should have included: (a) review of institutional policy/protocol for GBS, (b) review of nursing/medical resource texts and/or national technical bulletins and practice guidelines, (c) advocate for intrapartum antibiotic prophylaxis and timely consultation with physicians regarding low-grade temperatures, (d) consult with nursing colleagues and/or supervisor, and (e) communicate GBS maternal colonization to all neonatal care providers.

Implementation During labor, Nurse Jackson failed to advocate for this mother and baby so they would receive the standard of medical/nursing care for GBS (ANA, 1983, 1985, 1991; NAACOG, 1991). Nurses must know the standard of medical care as well as nursing care. Nurse Jackson failed to advocate for the standards of medical care (i.e., intrapartum antibiotic prophylaxis) by: (a) reviewing the perinatal history and recognizing the significance of + GBS cultures, (b) ongoing assessment of temperature, especially after AROM, to evaluate presence/absence of this significant risk factor, (c) questioning and confronting the physicians about Lauren's GBS status and elevated WBC. Nurse Jackson could not advocate for Lauren, since she lacked knowledge of what the standard of medical care required. Both the nursing *Code of Ethics* and the standards for professional practice/care require the nurse to be competent in rendering nursing care (this includes patient advocacy) (ANA, 1983, 1985, 1991; NAACOG, 1991).

After delivery, Nurse Jackson failed to advocate for the continued health care of Lauren's infant. She did not communicate either verbally or in writing to any neonatal health care provider (i.e., nursery nurses or pediatrician) that Lauren was + GBS prenatally and had not received intrapartum antibiotic prophylaxis. The *Guidelines for Perinatal Care* (AAP, 1992; ACOG, 1992) state that "information to be transmitted to the physician caring for the infant after delivery includes . . . exposure to group B streptococci" (p. 83). If Lauren had demonstrated no fever during labor (with appropriate intervals of assessment) and a medical decision to forego antibiotic therapy had been made, Nurse Jackson still would have had an obligation to report GBS exposure to the neonatal careproviders to alert them to the probability of ascending infection secondary to 5 hours of ruptured membranes in the absence of a vaginal birth. Maternal, prenatal records and maternal progress notes did not accompany the infant to the nursery; the neonatal care providers relied on the labor/delivery summary sheet and the verbal report of the obstetrical nurses. The presence of a + GBS culture was never communicated to neonatal care providers by any of the obstetrical care providers (i.e., nurses or physicians). This communication was a shared responsibility of nurses and physicians. The nurses had 100% responsibility for nursing actions (ANA, 1985) and the physicians had 100% responsibility for medical actions.

Evaluation After delivery, the patient's temperature was the same as the admitting temperature, but lack of hourly evaluations did not preclude a fever during labor. No nurse evaluated the elevated WBC or AROM as a source of infection. Postpartally, Lauren's temperature decreased from 37.3 C and she was discharged with "no signs of infection" at 48 hours postpartum. An "early" discharge with no maternal complications resulted in the nurses evaluating this mother as being in "stable condition" at discharge.

Failure of the obstetrical nurses to alert all neonatal care providers of the + GBS culture and the lack of intrapartum antibiotic prophylaxis resulted in: (a) lack of higher suspicion of infection , (b) inadequate assessments of the infant, (c) a decision not to culture the infant, (d) no opportunity to treat the infant with prophylactic antibiotics, (e) no opportunity to delay discharge, (f) no opportunity to decide on early follow-up, including early clinic visit after discharge (sooner than 2 weeks) and home visits, and (g) no opportunity to decide on instructing parents regarding signs and symptoms of sepsis.

References

Adelsperger, D., Carr, J., Davis, D., Feinstein, N., & Schmidt, J. (1993). *Fetal heart monitoring: Principles and practice.* Washington, D.C.: AWHONN.

American Academy of Pediatrics. (1992). Guidelines for prevention of group B streptococcal (GBS) infection by chemoprophylaxis, *Pediatrics, 90*(5), pp. 775–778.

American Academy of Pediatrics-American College of Obstetricians and Gynecologists. (1992). *Guidelines for perinatal care,* 3rd ed. Washington, D.C.: Author.

American College of Obstetricians and Gynecologists. (1992). Group B streptococcal infections in pregnancy. *ACOG Technical Bulletin #170.* Washington, D.C.: Author.

American Nurses Association. (1983). *Standards for maternal child health nursing practice.* Washington, D.C.: Author.

American Nurses Association. (1985). *Code for nurses.* Washington, D.C.: Author.

American Nurses Association. (1988). *Standards for organized nursing services.* Washington, D.C.: Author.

American Nurses Association. (1991). *Standards of clinical nursing practice.* Washington, D.C.: Author.

American Nurses Association. (1994). *Guidelines on reporting incompetent, unethical, or illegal practices.* Washington, D.C.: Author.

Association of Women's Health, Obstetrics, and Neonatal Nurses. (1993). *Didactic content and clinical skills verification for professional nurse providers of basic, high-risk, and critical-care intrapartum nursing.* Washington, D.C.: Author.

Aumann, G. & Baird, M. (1993). Risk assessment in pregnant women. In R. Knuppel & J. Drukker (Eds.), *High-risk pregnancy: A team approach,* 2nd ed. Philadelphia: Saunders.

Boyer, S. & Gotoff, S. (1986). Prevention of early-onset group B streptococcal disease with selective intrapartum chemoprophylaxis. *New England Journal of Medicine, 314,* pp. 1665–1669.

Chez, B. & Harvey, C. (1994). *Essentials of electronic fetal monitoring.* Washington, D.C.: AWHONN.

Committee on Perinatal Health (1993). *Toward Improving the Outcome of Pregnancy II.* White Plains, N.Y.: March of Dimes Birth Defects Foundation.

Gigante, J., Hickson, G., Entman, S., & O'Quist, N. (1995). Universal screening for group B streptococcus: Recommendations and obstetricians' practice decisions. *Obstetrics and Gynecology, 85,* pp. 440–443.

Hiatt v. Grace, 215 Kan. 14, 523 P. 2d 320 (1974).

International Association for the Study of Pain, Subcommittee on Taxonomy. (1979). Pain terms: A list with definitions and notes on usage. *Pain, 6,* pp. 249–252.

Joint Commission on Accreditation of Healthcare Organizations. (1995). *The Joint Commission accreditation manual for hospitals.* Oakbrook Terrace, IL: Author.

Mahoney, D. (1987). The chart as a legal document. Paper presented at St. Francis Hospital, Colorado Springs, CO.

McRae, M. (1993). Litigation, EFM, and the OB nurse. *Journal of Obstetrics, Gynecologic, and Neonatal Nursing, 22*(5), pp. 410–419.

Nurses' Association of the American College of Obstetricians and Gynecologists. (1989). *Mother-baby care.* Washington, D.C.: Author.

Nurses' Association of the American College of Obstetricians and Gynecologists. (1990). *Fetal heart rate auscultation.* Washington, D.C.: Author.

Nurses' Association of the American College of Obstetricians and Gynecologists. (1991). *Nursing practice, competencies, and educational guidelines: Antepartum fetal surveillance and intrapartum heart monitoring.* Washington, D.C.: Author.

Olds, S., London, M., & Ladewig, P. (1996). *Maternal-newborn nursing,* 5th ed. Menlo Park, CA: Addison-Wesley Nursing.

Pisel v. Stanford Hospital, 41 C.L.J. 43 (1980).

Porter, F. (1993). Pain assessment in children and infants. In N. Schecter, C. Berde, & M. Yaster (Eds.)., *Pain in infants, children, and adolescents.* Baltimore, MD: Williams & Wilkins.

Pylipow, M., Gaddis, M., & Kinney, J. (1994). Selective intrapartum prophylaxis for group B streptococcus colonization: Management and outcome of newborns. *Pediatrics, 93*(4), pp. 631–635.

Weisman, L., Stoll, B., Cruess, D., Hall, R., Merenstein, G., Hemming, V., & Fisher, G. (1992). Early-onset group B streptococcal sepsis: A current assessment. *Journal of Pediatrics, 121,* pp. 428–433.

9

Low-Risk Neonatal Care: Level I Nursery

Toni M. Vezeau, RNC, PhD
Sandra L. Gardner, RN, MS, CNS, PNP
Mary I. Enzman Hagedorn, RN, PhD, CNS, CPNP

Risk management is unique in the level I nursery because the environment in which the registered nurse manages care is very different from most other areas in perinatal nursing. Ninety-five percent of all births in the United States are the result of healthy term pregnancies (Bobak & Jenson, 1993) with positive outcomes for infant, mother, and family. The newborn nursery, a wellness area, provides "low-tech" care aimed at health maintenance, health promotion, and illness prevention. The philosophy of care in the newborn nursery is that infants are considered well until proven otherwise. Focusing newborn care on wellness, the nurse may attribute questionable infant signs as variations of normal rather than signs that require further investigation. Determination and maintenance of a newborn's health status is only the starting place of level I nursing care.

Birth is a normal process rather than a disease, or medical phenomenon. The arrival of a newborn is a socio-cultural event that, in our present family-centered care environment, is determined and planned by the family with assistance from the nursing and medical team. Families have the final say in the style of the birth and the care of newborns. After assuring physiologic stability of the newborn, parent advocacy becomes the nurse's most important priority. The ethical principle of advocacy—protection of family autonomy in this instance—is supported by the American Nurses Association (ANA), the Association of Women's Health, Obstetrics, and Neonatal Nurses (AWHONN) (formerly NAACOG), and the Joint Commission on Accreditation of Health Care Organizations (JCAHO) standards of nursing care (ANA, 1985; NAACOG, 1991; JCAHO, 1992).

Essential to advocacy that is aimed at supporting parental autonomy is the effective teaching of families in the care of their newborns. However, the current care situation involves many barriers to effective teaching, including: a 30% no-care rate in urban areas (Mattson & Smith, 1992), high percentages of non-English-speaking families, and a decrease in indigent families' participation in prenatal preparatory classes. In addition, hospital stays commonly last 24 hours or less, so that care is discharge-focused. Brief-encounter nursing diminishes the nurse's ability to establish nurse-family relationships that support comprehensive teaching and evaluation of learning. Nursing care of newborns is quintessentially proactive: there is no possibility of retroactively addressing nursing concerns of the well newborn.

To overcome some of these barriers, nurses are relying increasingly on home visitation by community health nurses shortly after discharge. Implementation of appropriate referrals to the community is often the only safety net in the care of newborns.

The first two cases presented in this chapter explore the medico-legal uniqueness of level I care. The first case emphasizes the need for evaluation of family teaching, home assessment, and referral. The second case illustrates the fact that advocacy by nurses must proceed with extreme care so that everyone's rights—infant, family, and nurse—are protected. The third case explores nursing's failure to screen an at-risk infant for hypoglycemia and the disastrous outcome.

Case 1

Facts

In August, three-week-old Jose was brought by his father, mother, and uncle to a small rural hospital for emergency treatment. Jose was febrile (38 degrees C), lethargic, and pale with circumoral cyanosis. Other physical signs included sunken fontanelle, dry buccal mucosa, redness and drainage at the umbilicus, and skin wasting. The mother, through an interpreter, reported that the infant had been vomiting and having frequent watery stools. He had not eaten in a day and a half. Jose was airlifted to the regional care center for a neonatal intensive care unit (NICU) admission. Despite efforts to treat him for sepsis and dehydration, he died two days later.

Investigation by police and local health authorities noted that the home lacked refrigeration, running water, and kitchen facilities; had dirt floors; was infested with insects and was not ventilated in severe summer heat. Six adults and fourteen children, migrant farm workers from Mexico, lived in the one-room shack.

On interviewing the family, the community health nurse noted that the family seemed generally unaware of the need to refrigerate milk, of signs of illness in infants, and of where to obtain medical and health advice and care. The mother applied bourbon to the umbilical cord, under a tight belly band. The nurse also noted that this was the couple's first child, and they had no family nearby except for an uncle. They also were not enmeshed in the social community of the migrant camp. The uncle encouraged the couple to sue since they were "never taught" how to care for their infant.

Outcome

The outcome in this case was infant death secondary to sepsis.

Legal Status This case is currently under litigation.

Case Commentary

Undesirable Patient Outcome

Assessment Jose was born at a tertiary care center which often takes care of migrant workers for whom English is not the primary language. Prior assessment was unavailable in the record since the family did not receive prenatal care. The care plans for both the mother and infant on the mother-baby unit did not reflect adequate assessment of the family. Their nurse noted only that the family did not speak English.

There was no documentation of the use of an interpreter for family assessment or for teaching of newborn and self-care. There was no documentation of how the mother performed care for the infant. Despite one nurse's notation that questioned whether the family had material resources to care for the infant, no social service referral was made. The infant was discharged twenty hours after delivery. Although a referral was made to an agency for a postpartum home visit, the address written by the discharge RN was not correct and the agency did not locate the family.

Diagnosis On the infant care plan, Jose's nurses noted some common nursing diagnoses:

Altered Family Process
Knowledge Deficit
Risk for Infection (umbilicus)
Ineffective Thermoregulation

Planning The standard care plan for the newborn was placed in the chart. This care plan was never individualized to this child/family.

Implementation The plan of care on the infant's record did not identify the specific needs of this family.

Evaluation Jose's nurses failed to document any evaluation of learning or of the safety of this discharge. Effective evaluation could only have been accomplished through an interpreter, and no interpreter was present at discharge.

Desirable Patient Outcome

Communication Establishment of a communication venue is primary in any nursing situation, but it is critical in a brief nursing care encounter such as early discharge of a newborn infant (Bobak & Jenson, 1993; Sherwen, Scoloveno, & Weingarten, 1991). In these situations, communication concerns precede the nursing process. When the family does not speak the language of the dominant culture, an appropriate translator is necessary. Some helpful guidelines are:

- A translator speaking the same language may not be sufficient. This is especially true when a family member is used for translation. Rules in the culture often determine what may be said to another in terms of bodily function (Galanti, 1991). Bilingual care providers as well as in-house facility employees *with special training* are better choices. In perinatal areas, female translators may have less proscription on communication.

- Clients and translators often appear to understand when they do not. The reasons that may account for this include: true misunderstanding of complicated information; respect for authority figures; the need of the family and/or translator to "save face" when misunderstanding occurs; and the desire of the family to avoid causing the care provider to "lose face" when a misunderstanding occurs (Galanti, 1991). The perinatal nurse needs to be careful not to assume that a yes, a nod, or a smile indicates comprehension. Verbal responses and return demonstration on all essential elements of learning can help ensure that the family understands normal newborn care. Avoid questions that are answered with a yes or no. This is time-consuming, but ultimately, it is the only safe and prudent approach to patient teaching.
- Nurses should instruct translators to translate what the patient says word for word if possible. While some interpretation is inevitable due to differences in words available, it is important that translators understand their role.
- Care providers need to make the use of a translator part of the plan of care. The use and name of the translator should be documented in the care plan. All signed documents should be signed by the RN (or other care provider), the translator, and the appropriate family member.
- Nurses should not assume that written, audio, or video education materials in the family's primary language eliminate the need for verbal response and return demonstration. It is rarely feasible for nurses to assess the literacy of clients using another language.
- Nurses should not assume that multiparas already understand the basics of newborn care. As with any client, knowledge must still be assessed and documented.

Assessment In care situations involving patients who do not speak the language of the dominant culture, it is imperative that the nurse assess patient/family learning and the family's living situation. The preceding section addresses the issue of assessment of learning by verbal response and return demonstration through the use of a translator. Areas of teaching to emphasize are: signs of illness, safety, feeding (breast or formula preparation/storage), follow-up visits, and phone numbers for questions and emergencies.

In addition, the discharge RN needs to know the cultural variations within the population served. When suspecting a lack of material resources or family support, the nurse must initially assume there is more to know about the family. In agricultural states, non-English-speaking families returning to a rural, farm environment may be migrant workers. This often means that the living conditions of these families are uncertain. Nurses caring for these populations should request a full assessment of the family by a social worker, as well as home visits by a community health RN who monitors migrant health issues in that area.

Diagnosis The nursing diagnoses listed in the medical record were appropriate for this family. However, they should have been tailored to the family's needs. With migrant workers, appropriate disposal of formula, use of isopropyl alcohol for cord care, limited use of "belly bands" for the umbilicus, recognition of infections, and temperature regulation for an infant would have been important expansions to the standard care plan. Again, the nurse must know the variants within the population served to make appropriate expansions to the nursing diagnoses. Two additional nursing diagnoses are often indicated in similar care situations:

Impaired verbal communication
Knowledge Deficit (infant care) related to the lack of material resources and lack of nursing education of the family

Planning The nursing care plan should have reflected the need for a translator, how one was obtained, and the specific one involved with this family. The plan should have included the need for a social-services referral and the need to initiate special home visit follow-up by the community health RN working with migrant workers in that area. These referrals should have been completed *prior to discharge of the family.*

Implementation The discharge RN should have checked the accuracy of the family's address and phone number, as well as message numbers, if any, to assist in the community health nurse follow-up. Discharge information for families should have been written down by the translator in the primary language of the family. Since no prenatal care was obtained, Jose's nurses should have noted on the referral form that the community health nurse must assist the family in obtaining a care provider for follow-up. Phone numbers for questions or emergencies should have been written down for the parents as well. Educational material written in the family's primary language could also have been offered to the family, but only as a supplement to verbal instruction and evaluation of learning.

Evaluation Ongoing evaluation of the parents' knowledge level concerning infant care and access to follow-up care would have alerted the nurse to question the early discharge of a family lacking resources. The nurses did not use an interpreter for discharge instructions; therefore, it would be difficult to evaluate the parents' understanding or knowledge base concerning the information given.

Case 2

Facts

In June, twelve-week-old Crystal was brought by her father to the emergency room to treat a four-day history of vomiting and watery stools, irritability, and skin rash. The ER record noted that Crystal's temperature was below normal (35.2° C) despite adequate clothing. Also, Crystal had a musty odor, and her reflexes were hyperactive. Crystal's father reported that his wife breastfed the infant exclusively, and that during the initial hospitalization, she had refused all medication and blood draws on her baby.

Crystal's newborn chart noted one entry by the admission RN that her parents "refused all formula supplement, medication (e.g., eye prophylaxis and Aquamephyton [vitamin K]), blood draws, and stays in the nursery." The same was noted on the parents' prenatal birth plan. No medical personnel charted any counseling related to the refusal of genetic screening. The parents did not sign any statements of refusals. No one noted these refusals on the referral form for visiting nurse services.

Outcome

The infant was stabilized in the NICU and dehydration was reversed. Crystal's parents gave permission for blood draws. She was found to have phenylketonuria (PKU). Further testing noted developmental lags in the infant, prompting further assessment of neurological impairment.

Legal

Upon learning the medical diagnosis, Crystal's parents sued the hospital where she was born, since the risks of refusing testing were "not explained well." This case is presently under litigation.

Case Commentary

Undesirable Patient Outcome

Assessment Crystal's birth chart did not note assessment of the parents' understanding of the risks involved with their refusals of medication and blood draws. No assessment of parental risk assumption was documented on either the mother's prenatal or her postpartum record.

Diagnosis While it may have been difficult to determine which NANDA-approved nursing diagnoses would have been appropriate in this situation, no part of the infant care plan addressed this aspect of the infant's care. The most obvious nursing diagnosis was:

Parental Knowledge Deficit regarding newborn screening

Planning No plan of care was developed for this infant.

Implementation Neither nursing, nor medical personnel documented any intervention related to the parents' refusal of newborn screening, medications, and care.

Evaluation None of Crystal's care providers documented an evaluation of risk assumption either in the hospital or in the home visit. No opportunity was made for the visiting health nurse to evaluate risk assumption since no notation of this issue was made on the referral form.

Desirable Patient Outcome

Assessment The nurse has a legal responsibility to ensure that informed refusal of care follows the same guidelines as an informed consent: assessment of the family's competence, parental understanding of the explanation of risk, documentation of the parents' comprehension, and an explanation of the family's right to alter their decisions. The following questions may help the nurse assess parental knowledge and competence in a refusal situation:

- Is the family *competent* to make an informed choice? If refusals are made during painful or stressful events, the clients should be reassessed on their decision.
- Has the care team, including the nursing and medical personnel, *explained the risks involved in the refusal of care*? All possible risks, however unlikely, need to be explained to the family.
- How well does the family *comprehend* the risks they are assuming in the refusal of care? This assessment should use open-ended questions. A "yes" response to the question "Do you understand?" is insufficient.
- Has the nurse *documented* that the risks of refusal have been explained and parental comprehension assessed? Consultation with the facility's legal department can be made during the negotiation of this situation. Forms can be drawn up by the legal department for the refusal of eye prophylaxis, Aquamephyton (vitamin K), blood draws, and genetic screening. These forms should specify in clear, nonmedical terms the medical risks for the parents.
- Do the parents understand that they can *change their minds* at any time?
- Is there an *increased risk of harm to the infant* by this refusal? For example, if the mother or father had PKU, there would be an increased genetic predisposition toward PKU, and refusal in this situation involves much greater risk to the infant.

Diagnosis The infant's care plan should have included the following diagnoses:

Caregiver Role Strain related to conflict over advocacy for the family and infant

Decisional Conflict related to refusal of standard of care for newborns

Parental Knowledge Deficit regarding newborn screening

Planning The care plan should indicate the notification of medical staff or primary care provider, related educational needs, and follow-up by the visiting health nurse. The referral to the visiting health nurse should reflect the same plan of care. Case record charting should reflect that the care plan was fully carried out.

Implementation As stated earlier in this chapter, it is a nursing responsibility to advocate for family autonomy in the care of their infant (ANA, 1985; Kelly, 1991). The nurse advocate assists the family in self-determining the infant's care, but also explains the rights and responsibilities implicit in informed choice (Sherwen, et al., 1991).

The nurse involved in the infant's care must carefully document the notification of parental wishes to the medical staff and, as the family's advocate, assist in obtaining informed choice from the family. While the nurse does not need to duplicate documentation on the signed refusal form, it is her shared obligation to assess the family's continued comprehension. If questions arise related to this issue, immediate notification of the medical staff is indicated.

If the family refuses standard care for their infant, *even if such care is mandated by the state,* nurses may not perform such care without the backing of a court order (Legal Office, University Hospital, Denver, 1994, personal communication). To do otherwise could, in most states, result in a charge of battery and/or assault. Certainly, in this situation a nurse performing a blood draw for PKU on this infant would be found unethical and probably out of the bounds of the law. Likewise, giving medications (e.g., Aquamephyton [vitamin K], or eye prophylaxis) without parental consent would place the nurse in a similar situation.

Evaluation Although proactive nursing response to the refusal of care would not have prevented Crystal's poor outcome, it is prudent for nurses to take on a proactive style of addressing such decisional conflicts to ensure documented informed choice for their own protection. In this society, parents have the right to assume risks for poor outcome and even refuse standard testing and treatment.

Case 3

Facts

At 1902 on March 31 Jeannie Choi was born at Denver General Hospital. Her G1 P0 Korean mother had an unremarkable prenatal course and was in labor for 17 hours. The baby weighed 3810 grams (8 lbs. 6 1/2 oz.), was 40 weeks by dates and estimation of gestational age, and had APGARS of 9 and 9.

At 1925, on admission to the newborn nursery, Jeannie's nurse noted the following findings: axillary T 36.6° C ; P 168; R 60; BP no entry; Dextrostix: light 90. At 2100 the infant took 30 ccs. formula. On April 1, her formula feedings included:

2400–0100: 40 ccs. formula nippled slowly.
0500–0600: 30 ccs. formula nippled; active; loud cry; feeding fair, out to mom, feeding slowly.
0900: 30 ccs. formula nippled slowly.
1200: 45 ccs. formula nippled slowly.
1500–2330: still active; loud cry; feeding good; mom encouraged to feed more.
1700–1800: 60 ccs. formula nippled slowly.
2100: 45 ccs. formula nippled slowly.

No Dextrostix was documented in the nursery flow sheet.

On April 2 at 0430 (at 33 hours of age), Jeannie was found face down in her crib with no heartbeat or respirations. There was no vomitus in her mouth or nares. (Her last feeding was 30 ccs. formula at 2400–0100.) Cardiopulmonary resuscitation (CPR) was begun with an initial IV infusion of 4 ccs. D50W.

Laboratory data after the resuscitation indicated severe metabolic acidosis; and negative blood and cerebral spinal fluid cultures. Her CT scan showed blood/fluid level in left occipital horn (ventricle) without obvious source. A chest X ray showed no infiltrate initially, but left upper lobe infiltrate by April 3rd. Her EEG showed seizures with observed clinical signs.

Outcome

The short-term outcome was a hypoglycemic episode with apnea and/or seizure that resulted in cardiopulmonary arrest at 33 hours of age. Jeannie was discharged at 18 days of age on phenobarbital (Luminal) 10 mg BID with gavage feedings. The long term outcome was that, by 1988, when the lawsuit was filed, this 6-year-old child was profoundly developmentally delayed with profound cerebral palsy.

Legal

The jury awarded the family $2,000,000 (*Choi v. City and County of Denver*, 1988).

Case Commentary

Undesirable Patient Outcome

Assessment The nurses assessed this infant as appropriate for gestational age (AGA) although the physician assessed and documented the infant as borderline LGA. After his assessment, the physician ordered the routine hypoglycemia protocol. An initial Dextrostix assessment at 23 minutes of age was a "light 90." No further assessment was documented over the next 33 hours of life despite poor feeding behavior. The only documentation indicating an assessment of the infant's feeding pattern was "feeding fair; feeding slowly; mom encouraged to feed more." The physician's orders were not timed. The nurse signed off the orders at 0300, 7 1/2 hours after admission. Admission vital signs (without blood pressure) were the only vital signs assessed except for one axillary temperature in the first 33 hours of life.

Diagnosis Nursing diagnoses for this LGA newborn were developed from a standard care plan as:

> ***Altered Nutrition: Less than Body Requirements*** related to poor feeding secondary to risk for hypoglycemia

Planning The level I nursery's "Standard Nursing Care Plan for Well Newborns" required the nurses to do an initial physical assessment and estimated gestational age, follow procedures for infants at risk for hypoglycemia (e.g., SGA, AGA, LGA), and continue assessment of physical state at least twice a shift. The specific care for an LGA was: Dextrostix every hour for 3 hours, then every 3 hours before feeding for a total of 12 hours. In addition, nurses were to begin feedings immediately and follow a feeding schedule of every 3 hours for 24 hours, then every 4 hours unless otherwise ordered.

Implementation Nurses did not implement the unit's policy for "Standard Nursing Care Plan for Well Newborns" or its "Procedure for LGA Infant

Admission." Nurses did not clarify the discrepancy of gestational age between RN and physician at 0300 when orders were transcribed. The nursing care for this infant was carried out primarily by unlicensed assistive personnel under the supervision of an RN.

Evaluation No evaluation of the glucose status was performed beyond the initial Dextrostix. In addition, no ongoing evaluation of the feeding patterns of this infant were done. Although a documentation on the nursery flowsheet indicated that the mother was encouraged to "feed more," there was no documentation on how she was instructed (the mother spoke only Korean) or if this goal was attained.

Desirable Patient Outcome

Assessment Since the late 1960s when newborn classification was introduced, it has been recognized that certain classifications of infants are at increased risk for the development of certain morbidities (Battaglia and Lubchenco, 1967; Lubchenco, 1976). Correct nursing assessment of this neonate would have initiated the nursery procedure for admission and screening of LGA infants. Having recognized Jeannie as an at-risk infant, the admission nurse should *not* have been reassured by a Dextrostix at 23 minutes of age, since this reflects maternal, *not* neonatal glucose status. She should have assessed the infant according to a standard protocol (ANA, 1983, 1991; NAACOG, 1990, 1991). The erroneous nursing assessment could have been corrected and the protocol initiated at 0300 when the nurse cosigned the physician's orders for "LGA protocol." Documentations of poor and slow feedings were not followed by further assessments of vital signs, Dextrostix, specific gravity, or intake (ANA, 1983, 1991; NAACOG, 1990, 1991).

Diagnosis Appropriate nursing diagnosis for this infant should have included:

Altered Nutrition: Less than Body Requirements related to poor feeding secondary to risk for hypoglycemia
Risk for Injury
Risk for Hypothermia
Impaired Verbal Communication related to Korean-speaking family

Planning Accurate nursing assessment and diagnoses should have resulted in a plan of care with specific, measurable interventions, outcomes, and evaluation criteria (ANA, 1983, 1991; NAACOG, 1990, 1991). An example of a care plan for an infant at risk for developing hypoglycemia is contained in Table 9-1.

Implementation Implementation should have included a standard procedure for care of the LGA infant at risk for developing hypoglycemia (Figure 9-1, p. 154).

Evaluation No ongoing evaluation was performed for Jeannie's feeding patterns, glucose homeostasis per LGA classification, thermoregulation, or the parents' knowledge of infant care. When nurses took the original order

Table 9-1 Nursing Care Plan

Patient Needs/ Nursing Diagnosis	Patient Outcomes	Nursing Intervention/ Collaborative Actions	Evaluation
Altered Nutrition: Less than Body Requirements related to poor feeding and LGA classification.	Normoglycemic. Maintain/preserve neurologic integrity: • no seizure activity • no apnea/bradycardia • no respiratory distress.	Follow algorithm in Figure 9-1.	Glucose levels 40–45 mg/dl. Feeding behavior: • demands feedings • awakens easily to feed • intake: 50–80 kcal/kg in first 24 hrs. 110–120 kcal/kg by 3rd day of life • no vomiting • no symptoms of hypoglycemia: neurologic • poor feeding • abnormal cry • hypothermia • tremors • jittery • hypotonia • irritability • lethargy • seizures cardiorespiratory • cyanosis • pallor • tachypnea • periodic breathing • apnea • cardiorespiratory distress

Adapted from: McGowan, J., Hagedorn, M., Price, W., & Hay, W. (1993). Glucose homeostasis. In G. Merenstein & S. Gardner (Eds.), *Handbook of neonatal intensive care,* 3rd ed. St. Louis: Mosby-Yearbook (p. 179). Adapted with permission, Mosby-Yearbook, 1993.

off at 0300, they failed to detect the discrepancy between their assessment of gestational age and the physician's assessment and subsequent orders.

Care was provided in this level I nursery by unlicensed assistive personnel (UAPs). This alone does not present problems; however, in this infant's situation, the only ongoing assessments documented on the flowsheet were made by the UAP. The ANA defines UAPs as "individuals who are trained to function in an assistive role to the registered professional nurse in the provision of patient/client care activities as delegated by and under the supervision of the registered professional nurse" (ANA, 1994a, p. 2). UAPs are not licensed to practice nursing, have no legal scope of practice, and therefore have no legal authority to practice nursing (ANA, 1994a).

Professional nurses may delegate *tasks* of care, but may not delegate their responsibility and accountability for that care. Nursing activities that include the core of the nursing process and/or require specialized knowledge, judgment, and/or skill should *not* be delegated (Table 9-2). The Colorado Nurse Practice Act prohibits "unauthorized practice"; that is, "the practice

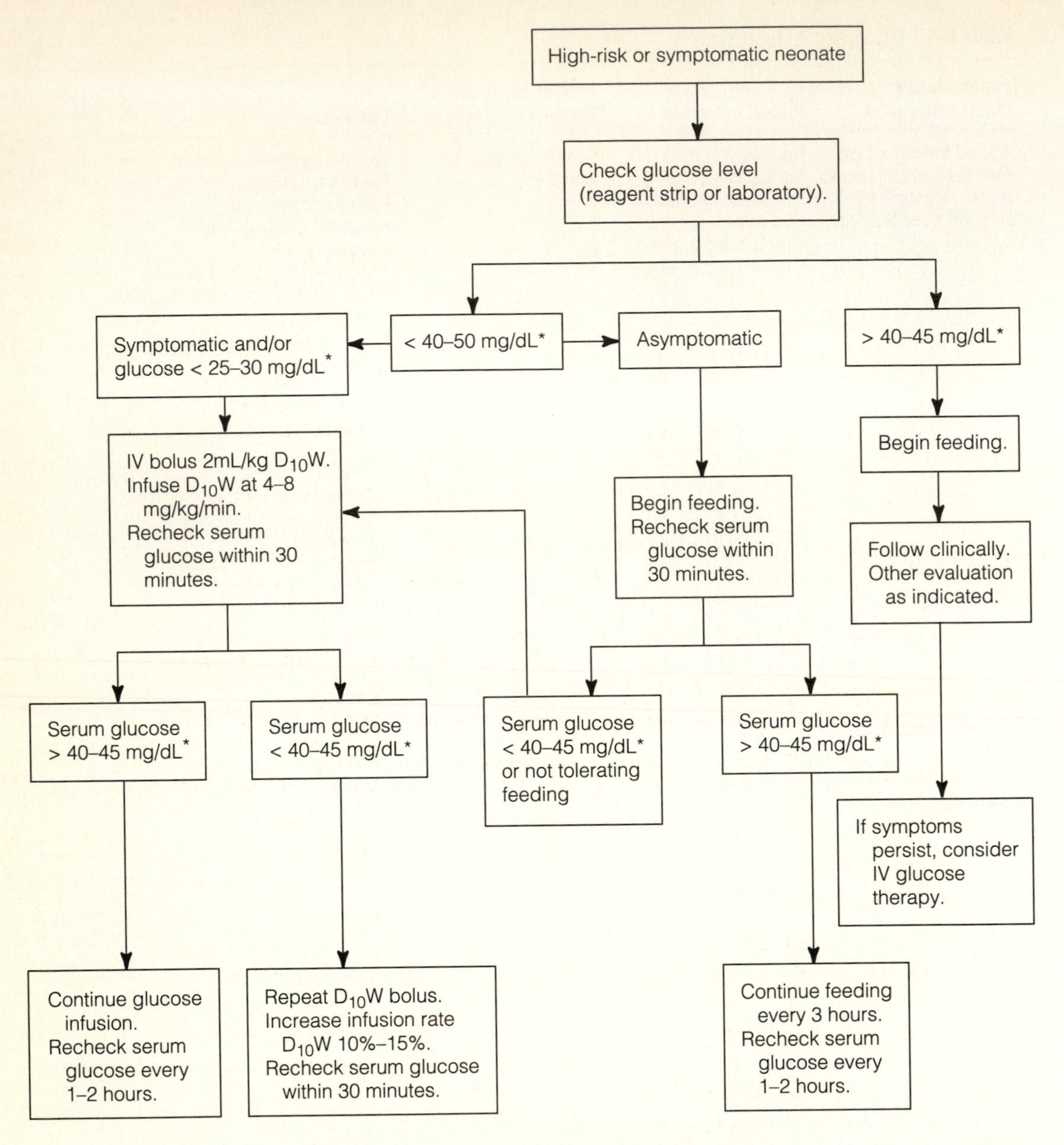

Figure 9-1 Decision tree for management of neonate with hypoglycemia.

SOURCE: McGowan, J., Hagedorn, M., Price, W., and Hay, W. (1993). Glucose homeostasis. In G. Merenstein and S. Gardner (Eds.), *Handbook of neonatal intensive care*, 3rd ed. St. Louis: Mosby-Yearbook. (p. 179). Reprinted with permission.

Table 9-2 Do Not Delegate

Nursing Process	Comments
Assessment	Initial and any subsequent assessment that requires professional nursing knowledge, judgment* and skill
Diagnosis	Nursing diagnosis and delineation of nursing goals
Planning	Development of nursing plan of care
Implementation	An intervention that requires professional nursing knowledge, judgment*, and skill
Evaluation	Of the patient's progress/lack of progress in relation to the nursing care plan

*Nursing judgment is the intellectual process that a licensed professional nurse (RN) utilizes in forming an opinion and reaching a conclusion by analyzing the data.

Adapted from American Nurses Association. (1994). *Registered professional nurses and unlicensed assistive personnel.* Washington, D.C.: Author (p. 12). Adapted with permission, ANA, 1994.

of practical or professional nursing by any person who has not been issued a license under the provisions of the nurse practice act" (Colorado Nurse Practice Act, C.R.S., 1991, p. 3). In its annual report, the Colorado State Board of Nursing (1990–91) listed tasks *not* within the LPN scope of practice: these include total body physical assessment. The annual report continues with a list of tasks *not* within the RN's scope of practice: supervision of nonlicensed personnel performing tasks for which a license is required (Colorado State Board of Nursing, 1990–91). If an LPN with a 9–11-month curriculum is unqualified to perform a total body physical assessment, a nurse's aide (i.e., UAP) certainly is unqualified. Neither the individual nurse *nor* the hospital can authorize actions beyond the scope of practice mandated in the state nurse practice act (ANA, 1994b). Such practice constitutes illegal practice (ANA, 1994b).

In 1991, Colorado joined several other states with a delegatory clause to their nurse practice act. Delegation, "the transfer of responsibility for the performance of a task from one person to another" (ANA, 1994a, p. 10), does not transfer accountability or task outcome. Since accountability and responsibility for the nursing process remain with the licensed professional nurse, delegating the entire assessment and care planning process is inappropriate and violates the state nurse practice act and national practice standards (ANA, 1994a). Table 9-3 represents a composite of violations of the standards of care in each level in the nursing process surrounding the care of Jeannie Choi.

Although UAPs provided direct care to newborns in the level I nursery and were deposed in this case, they were not defendants in the lawsuit. The physicians were excluded from the lawsuit by the judge in a pretrial hearing. The professional nurses who were legally liable for breach of duty (i.e., failure to properly assess, make accurate nursing diagnoses, plan care, intervene, and evaluate the neonate's ongoing condition) became the sole defendants in the lawsuit.

Table 9-3 Nursing Care and Standard of Care Violations

Nursing Process	Violations in Standards of Care
Assessment: • Nursing assessed infant as AGA. • MD assessed as borderline LGA (wrote order to do routine LGA care). • Initial (and only) Dextrostix assessment at 23 minutes of age. • Documentations during first 33 hours of life: "feeding fair; feeding slowly; mom encouraged to feed more." • No documentation of any Dextrostix assessment of poor feeding behavior (a sign/symptom of hypoglycemia). • MD orders not timed; RN signature at 0300 (7 1/2 hours after admission when discrepancy between nursing/medical assessment apparent). • Admission vital signs (without blood pressure) *only* vital signs (except one axillary temperature) assessed in first 33 hours of life.	*Standard of Clinical Nursing Practice (ANA, 1991):* *Standard I:* The nurse collects client health data. • Pertinent data are collected using appropriate assessment techniques. • The data collection process is systematic and ongoing. • Relevant data are documented in a retrievable form. *Code of Ethics (ANA, 1985):* • The nurse acts to safeguard the client . . . when health care and safety are affected by the incompetent, unethical, or illegal practice of any person. • The nurse assumes responsibility and accountability for individual nursing judgments and actions. • The nurse maintains competence in nursing. • The nurse exercises informed judgment and uses individual competence and qualifications as criteria for seeking consultation, accepting responsibilities, and delegating nursing activities. *Standards of Maternal and Child Health Nursing Practice (ANA, 1983):* *Standard I:* The nurse helps children and parents attain and maintain optimal health. • Takes a health history and does a physical assessment using appropriate screening and assessment tools. *Standard III:* The nurse intervenes with vulnerable clients and families at risk to prevent potential developmental and health problems. • Collects data about individual/family using appropriate assessment and screening tools. • Uses knowledge of risk factors to identify individual families at risk. • Monitors at-risk individuals/families for actual and potential developmental and health problems. *Standard V:* The nurse detects changes in health status and deviations from optimum development. • Collects baseline data about health/developmental status. • Detects subtle and significant changes in health and developmental status. *Nurse Providers of Neonatal Care (NAACOG, 1990):* • Obtain perinatal history. • Perform physical assessment (which includes determining gestational age and interpreting diagnostic data). • Distinguish, report, and record normal and abnormal conditions. • Identify life-threatening or emergency situations. *Standards for the Nursing Care of Women and Newborns (NAACOG, 1991):* *Standard I:* Comprehensive neonatal nursing care focuses on helping newborns, families, and communities achieve their optimum health potential. This is best achieved within the framework of the nursing process.

Low-Risk/Healthy Newborn Nursing Practice: Transitional care practices include a complete history and assessment. Initial assessment . . . may include: (a) identification of the at-risk newborn, (b) physical assessment, (c) gestational age assessment, (d) routine laboratory assessment, (e) initiation/facilitation of feedings.

Standard IV: Comprehensive nursing for women and children is provided by nurses who are clinically competent and accountable for professional actions and legal responsibilities inherent in the nursing role.

Nursing Diagnosis:

Newborn classification of LGA places this infant in an at-risk category for:

Altered Nutrition: Less than Body Requirements related to increased risk for hypoglycemia

Standard of Clinical Nursing Practice (ANA, 1991):

Standard II: The nurse analyzes the assessment data in determining diagnoses.

- Diagnoses are derived from assessment data.
- Diagnoses are validated with . . . health care providers when possible.
- Diagnoses are documented in a manner that facilitates the determination of expected outcomes and plan of care.

Standards of Maternal and Child Health Nursing Practice (ANA, 1983):

Standard I: The nurse helps children and parents attain and maintain optimum health.

- Identifies immediate, interim, and long-term health needs of client.
- Identifies human responses and reactions to actual and potential health problems.

Standard V: The nurse detects changes in health status and deviations from optimum development.

- Diagnoses physical and psychological responses to changes in health status and developmental status.

Standard VI: The nurse carries out appropriate interventions and treatment to facilitate survival and recovery from illness.

- Uses data collected about physiologic and psychologic responses of clients to illness to make nursing diagnoses.
- Identifies nursing problems related to illness in the interdependent domain.

Nurse Providers of Neonatal Care (NAACOG, 1990):

- Formulates conclusions; makes diagnoses.

Standards for Nursing Care of Women and Newborns (NAACOG, 1991):

Standard I: The nurse formulates and makes diagnoses.

Planning

Standard Nursing Care Plan for Well Newborns:

- Do nursing physical assessment.
- Follow procedures for SGA, AGA, and LGA
- Continue assessment of physical state at least twice a shift.

Institutional standard of care violated: hospital policy, procedures, and *Standard Nursing Care Plan for Hypoglycemia* not implemented.

(Continued)

Table 9-3 Nursing Care and Standard of Care Violations (*Continued*)

Nursing Process	Violations in Standards of Care
Procedures for LGA Infant Admissions: • Defined as infants of diabetic mothers and infants in LGA range on gestation weight chart (Lubchenco & Bard, 1971). • Dextrostix q hr. x 3 hrs., then q 3 hrs. a.c. for a total of 12 hrs. • Begin feeding immediately. • Feed q 3 hrs. for 24 hrs. then q 4 hrs. unless otherwise ordered.	*Standards of Clinical Nursing Practice (ANA, 1991):* *Standard III:* The nurse identifies expected outcomes individualized to the client. • Outcomes are derived from the diagnoses. • Outcomes are documented as measurable goals. • Outcomes are mutually formulated . . . with health care providers. • Outcomes include a time estimate for attainment. • Outcomes provide direction for continuity of care. *Standard IV:* The nurse develops a plan of care that prescribes interventions to attain expected outcomes. • The plan is individualized to the client's condition or needs. • The plan is developed . . . with health care providers. • The plan reflects current nursing practice. • The plan is documented. • The plan provides for continuity of care. *Standards of Maternal and Child Health Nursing Practice (ANA, 1983):* *Standard I:* The nurse helps children and parents attain and maintain optimum health. • Formulates a plan of care in consultation with client and/or family and with nurse experts and other professionals as needed. *Standard III:* The nurse intervenes with vulnerable clients and families at risk to prevent potential developmental and health problems. • Formulates a plan of care for at-risk management of vulnerable clients and families. *Nurse Providers of Neonatal Care (NAACOG, 1990):* B. Planning (develop a nursing plan of care based on appropriate data base and rationale that identifies short and long term goals, and expected outcomes . . .).
Implementation: • Nurse did not implement Standard Nursing Care Plan for Well Newborn or Procedure for LGA Infant Admission. • Nurse did not clarify discrepancy of gestational age between RN/MD assessments at 0300 and begin LGA protocol as ordered by MD.	Institutional standard of care violated: hospital policy, procedures, and *Standard Nursing Care Plan* not implemented; written physician order not carried out by RNs. *Standards for the Nursing Care of Women and Newborns (NAACOG,1991):* *Standard III:* Written policies, procedures, and protocols clarify the scope of nursing practice and delineate the qualifications of personnel authorized to provide care to women and newborns within the health care setting. *Standards of Clinical Nursing Practice (ANA, 1991):* *Standard V:* The nurse implements the interventions identified in the plan of care. • Interventions are consistent with the established plan of care. • Interventions are implemented in a safe and appropriate manner. • Interventions are documented. *Standards of Maternal-Child Health Nursing Practice (ANA, 1983):* *Standard I:* The nurse helps children and parents attain and maintain optimum health. • Refers health problems requiring other services to appropriate professionals. • Carries out physical interventions when indicated . . . *Standard III:* The nurse intervenes with vulnerable clients and families at risk to prevent potential developmental and health problems.

Nursing aides provide direct care in the newborn nursery.

Evaluation:

- No Dextrostix done to evaluate glucose status.
- No evaluation of poor feeding (a sign of hypoglycemia):
  - caloric intake
  - specific gravity
  - Dextrostix
  - vital signs
- "Mom encouraged to feed more"—no documentation on how (since mom did not speak English) and no evaluation of whether she understood directions.

- Intervenes therapeutically with high-risk individuals . . .
- Collaborates with other disciplines in treatment and referral of at-risk clients and families.
- Monitors clients' and families' reactions to at-risk status involved.

Standard V: The nurse detects changes in health status and deviations from optimum development.

- Intervenes to treat physical and psychological responses to changes in health status and developmental deviations.
- Initiates treatment in collaboration with other health professionals to improve health/developmental status.
- Monitors health and developmental status following changes or provides for monitoring by others.
- Coordinates delivery of care when other health professionals are involved.

Standard IV: The nurse promotes an environment free of hazards . . .

- Consults with nursing specialists and other professionals as needed.
- Carries out therapeutic interventions to facilitate physical and psychological recovery from illness and prevent complications.
- Provides for the client's basic physical needs as indicated by health status.

Nurse Providers of Neonatal Care (NAACOG, 1990):

C. Intervention which includes monitor, performs physical care, performs technical procedures, uses interventional strategies that maintain current standards of nursing practice.

Practice Guidelines: Professional nurses are the preferred neonatal caregivers. Aspects of infant care, however, may occasionally be delegated. All neonatal care must be provided by, or under the direct supervision of, a professional nurse.

Standards for the Nursing Care of Women and Newborns (NAACOG, 1991):

Standard I: The nurse helps children and parents attain and maintain optimum health.

- Ongoing assessment to provide data for planning newborn's care includes: (a) performs vital signs (temperature, heart rate, respiratory rate, and blood pressure), (b) performs and interprets indicated diagnostic tests, (c) collects laboratory specimens, (d) coordinates, facilitates, and evaluates nutritional status and feeding patterns, (e) assesses the physical, neurological, behavioral, and developmental status of the newborn.

Standards of Clinical Nursing Practice (ANA, 1991):

Standard VI: The nurse carries out appropriate interventions and treatments to facilitate survival and recovery from illness.

- Evaluation is systematic and ongoing.
- The client's responses to interventions are documented.
- The effectiveness of interventions is evaluated in relation to outcomes.
- Ongoing assessment data are used to revise diagnoses, outcomes, and the plan of care, as needed.
- Revisions in diagnoses, outcomes, and the plan of care are documented.

Standards of Maternal-Child Health Nursing Practice (ANA, 1983):

Standard I: The nurse helps children and parents attain and maintain optimum health.

- Evaluates nursing interventions with the client and/or family on the basis of specific goal-oriented client outcomes.
- Reassesses and reorders priorities with the client and/or family including setting new goals and revising care plans.

(Continued)

Table 9-3 Nursing Care and Standard of Care Violations (*Continued*)

Nursing Process	Violations in Standards of Care
	Standards of Maternal-Child Health Nursing Practice (ANA, 1983):(Continued) *Standard III:* The nurse intervenes with vulnerable clients and families at risk to prevent potential developmental and health problems. • Evaluates nursing interventions on the basis of specific goal-oriented client outcomes. • Reassesses at-risk status of clients and/or families and sets new goals and priorities. *Standard V:* The nurse detects changes in health status and deviations from optimum development. • Alters the plan of management collaboratively with the client and family, nurse experts, and other professionals as needed. *Standard VI:* The nurse carries out appropriate interventions and treatment to facilitate survival and recovery from illness. • Evaluates nursing interventions on the basis of specific goal-oriented client outcomes. • Reassesses and reorders priorities, including setting new goals and revising plans of care. *Nurse Providers of Neonatal Care (NAACOG, 1990):* D. Evaluation—determine effectiveness of interventions in relation to expected outcomes on an ongoing basis. *Standards for the Nursing Care of Women and Newborns (NAACOG, 1991):* *Standard VII:* Nurses caring for women and newborns . . . evaluate nursing practice to improve the outcomes of care.

Adapted from: American Nurses Association. (1983). *Standards of maternal-child health nursing practice.* Washington, D.C.: Author. American Nurses Association. (1985). *Code for nurses, with interpretative statements.* Washington, D.C.: Author. American Nurses Association. (1991). *Standards of clinical nursing practice.* Washington, D.C.: Author. Nurses' Association of the American College of Obstetricians and Gynecologists. (1990). *Nurse providers of neonatal care.* Washington, D.C.: Author. Nurses' Association of the American College of Obstetricians and Gynecologists. (1991). *NAACOG Standards for the nursing care of women and newborns,* 4th ed. Washington, D.C.: Author. Association of Women's Health, Obstetric and Neonatal Nurses. Adapted with permission.

References

American Nurses Association. (1983). *Standards of maternal-child health nursing practice.* Washington, D.C.: Author.

American Nurses Association. (1985). *Code for nurses.* Washington, D.C.: Author.

American Nurses Association. (1991). *Standards of clinical nursing practice.* Washington, D.C.: Author.

American Nurses Association. (1994a). *Registered professional nurses and unlicensed assistive personnel.* Washington, D.C.: Author.

American Nurses Association. (1994b). *Guidelines on reporting incompetent, unethical, or illegal practices.* Washington, D.C.: Author.

Battaglia, F. & Lubchenco, L. (1967). A practical classification of newborn infants by birth weight and gestational age. *Journal of Pediatrics, 71,* 159–163.

Bobak, I. & Jenson, M. (1993). *Maternity and gynecologic care: The nurse and family,* 5th ed. St. Louis: Mosby-Yearbook.

Choi v. City and County of Denver, No. 84 C.V. 8868 Colorado (1988).

Colorado Nurse Practice Act, C.R.S. Section 12-38-103(s).

Colorado State Board of Nursing. (1990–91). *Annual report.* Denver, CO: Author.

Galanti, G. (1991). *Caring for patients from different cultures.* Philadelphia: University of Pennsylvania Press.

Joint Commission on Accreditation of Healthcare Organizations. (1992). *Standards of nursing practice.* Oakbrook Terrace, IL: Author.

Kelly, L. (1991). *Dimensions of professional nursing,* 6th ed. New York: Pergamon Press.

Lubchenco, L. (1976). *The high-risk infant.* Philadelphia: Saunders.

Mattson, S. & Smith, J. (1992). *Core curriculum for maternal-newborn nursing.* Philadelphia: Saunders.

McGowan, J., Hagedorn, M., Price, W., & Hay, W. (1993). Glucose homeostasis. In G. Merenstein & S. Gardner (Eds.), *Handbook of neonatal intensive care,* 3rd ed. St. Louis: Mosby-Yearbook.

Nurses' Association of the American College of Obstetricians and Gynecologists. (1990). *Nurse providers of neonatal care.* Washington, D.C.: Author.

Nurses' Association of the American College of Obstetricians and Gynecologists. (1991). *Standards for the nursing care of women and newborns,* 4th ed. Washington, D.C.: Author.

Sherwen, L., Scoloveno, M., & Weingarten, C. (1991). *Nursing care of the childbearing family.* Norwalk, CT: Appleton & Lange.

Resource Material

American Nurses Association. (1994). *Every patient deserves a nurse.* Washington, D.C.: Author.

10

Medium-Risk Neonatal Care: Level II Nursery

Sandra L. Gardner, RN, MS, CNS, PNP
Mary I. Enzman Hagedorn, RN, PhD, CNS, CPNP

In addition to providing level I neonatal care services, level II nurseries provide care for moderately low birth-weight infants (1500–2500 grams, 32–36 weeks gestation) and management of infants with a moderate degree of illness that are admitted or transferred from a level I nursery (AAP-ACOG, 1992). Level II nurseries are located in either community or teaching hospitals with or without intensive care (level III) facilities. The nursing staff in level II nurseries must be able to perform emergency resuscitation, monitor and stabilize cardiopulmonary status and thermal and metabolic functions, and assist with special procedures (e.g., exchange transfusions, endotracheal intubation, and umbilical catheterization) (AAP-ACOG, 1992). Guided by protocols, nursery nurses must be educated in neonatal care and be "able to initiate, modify, or stop treatment when appropriate even if a physician or neonatal nurse practitioner is not present" (AAP-ACOG, 1992, pp. 8–9).

This chapter presents three cases occurring in level II neonatal centers. In the first case, both the health care providers and administration failed to establish practice guidelines consistent with the standard of care. In order to contain costs, the supervising institution did not have neonatal nurse practitioners or neonatologists within the community nursery at all times. The second case illustrates mismanagement of a neonate with seizures, and failure of the neonatal nurse to advocate for the infant to receive the standard of care. The last case illustrates that the reliance on physician actions does not obviate nurses from responsibility and accountability for their own practice.

Case 1

Facts

On the weekday afternoon of July 3rd at 1448, baby girl Baker was born in a community hospital whose level II nursery was staffed and administered by the local children's hospital. The primiparous mother's expected date of confinement (EDC) was June 27th. On July 2nd, she had a spontaneous rupture of membranes at 1700 and was admitted to the hospital at 2100. Her blood pressure was 130/90 (>20 mm Hg over her prenatal value), with 2+ reflexes. At 0450 (on July 3rd) she had three late decelerations with baseline return after 20–30 seconds; another late deceleration at 0510 resulted in physician notification. At 0530 the physician placed an internal fetal monitor and noted meconium in the amniotic fluid. At 1112–1117, 2 doses of Nisentyl 20 mg were given subcutaneously to the mother. She was completely dilated at 1330 and delivered at 1448 with 2+ meconium.

The baby was given APGARS of 8 and 9 and was Delee suctioned on the perineum. She was dusky at birth on 40% oxygen blowby. Resuscitation consisted of bag and mask ventilation and naloxone (Narcan).

Significant documentation on admission to the level II nursery included:

1449: Very dusky.
1459: Neonatologist called.
1505: Infant continued to be dusky in 40% blowby.
1510: First vital signs: T 36 Ax, P 146, R 40, BP 32/D.
1515: Obstetrician placed 3.0 ET tube, bagging with 100% oxygen, continued cyanosis. ABG (radial): pH 7.07, $paCO_2$ 43, pO_2 21, O_2 saturation 21%, BE –18.
1518: Obstetrician placed umbilical venous catheter (UVC).
1522: $NaHCO_3$ 4 meq/UVC.
1529: Infant bagged, BP 32/D, UVC removed by obstetrician and reinserted.
1533: Infant placed on ventilator.
1546: Neonatologist arrived. Reintubated infant with a 3.5 ET tube for air leak. Vital signs: T 35.7 skin/36.3 Ax, ABG (radial): pH 7.26, $paCO_2$ 30, paO_2 29, O_2 sat 46%, BE –12.
1600: T 35.5, UVC/umbilical artery catheter (UAC) reinserted.
1624: Chest X ray showed bilateral pulmonary infiltrates.
1626: 40 ccs. 5% albumin given. Bagging with 100% oxygen. Infant still cyanotic.
1634: Phenobarbital 70 mg; Pancuronium (Pavulon) .25 cc; vital signs: T 35.2, BP (postductal) 54/P, $NaHCO_3$ 10 meq IV push, bagging continued. ABG (UAC): pH 7.24, $paCO_2$ 62, paO_2 19, O_2 sat 29%, BE –3.
1640: BP 80/P (preductal).
1700: Dopamine 10 mcg/kg/min at 2 ccs./hr; 3 ccs given before UVC lost. ABG (UAC): pH 7.01, $paCO_2$55, paO_2 12, BE –19. CBC: Hct 41, WBC 19,000, platelets 435,000.
1715: Several attempts to get peripheral intravenous (PIV) in—unsuccessful.
1730: T 35.6. Bagging with 100% oxygen. ABG (UAC): pH 7.11, $paCO_2$ 14, paO_2 52, O_2 sat 80%, BE –24.
1740: Transport team arrived.
1745: Bradycardia—80/min, still bagging. MD attempted UVC again. ABG (UAC): pH 6.97, $paCO_2$ 38, paO_2 30, O_2 sat 39; BE –24. Infant placed on portable warmer for low temperature (35.8 Ax). Infant servocontrol (ISC) increased by transport nurse.
1810: Four attempts to start PIV—not successful.

1830: PIV started.
1835: $NaHCO_3$ 15 meq IV push.
1845: T 35.9 Ax/37.4 skin. Ventilator settings: Rate 162; FiO_2 100%, PIP 44, PEEP 8, poor peripheral perfusion (4–5 sec. cap refill), dopamine restarted at 10 mcg/kg/min.
1855: T 36 Ax.
1915: ABG (UAC): pH 7.35, $paCO_2$ 4, paO_2 272, BE –19.
1920: Suctioned blood from ET tube.
1930: ABG (UAC) ph 7.28; $paCO_2$ 4; paO_2 356; BE –21.
1950: $NaHCO_3$ 10 meq given.
2000: T 36 Ax/35.4 skin. Discontinued temperature per neonatologist (transport nurse's note). Suctioned large amounts of blood from ET tube.

Outcome

The short-term outcome for this infant was birth asphyxia. The sequelae of birth asphyxia for this infant included meconium aspiration pneumonia, persistent pulmonary hypertension, intracranial bleeding, acute tubular necrosis, and necrotizing enterocolitis. The long term outcome for this infant was severe cerebral palsy with severe developmental delays, cortical blindness, and spastic quadriplegia.

Legal

This case was settled out of court for hundreds of thousands of dollars.

Case Commentary

Undesirable Patient Outcome

Assessment Intrapartally this mother exhibited factors (e.g. late decelerations, 1+ meconium, and maternal hypertension with 2+ reflexes) that increased the neonate's risk of requiring a skilled resuscitation at birth (Golden & Peters, 1993; AAP, 1988; AAP, 1992).

At birth, the nursery nurse assigned APGARS of 8 and 9. No pulse oximetry assessment of duskiness or continued cyanosis was ever done.

Diagnosis No nursing diagnoses were developed to direct care. In anticipation of this infant's birth, appropriate nursing diagnoses should have included:

Ineffective Airway Clearance
Risk for Aspiration
Ineffective Breathing Pattern

Planning Given the perinatal history and potential nursing diagnoses for this neonate, the nurse should have planned for a skilled resuscitation team to be present at the delivery. At this institution, staff nurses were not educated or skilled in the practice of endotracheal intubation.

Implementation This baby's condition was poor enough that the nursery nurse took the infant immediately to the level II nursery (where both

APGARS were assigned). According to the transport nurse's notes, this infant's condition was too poor to weigh or measure on admission (at 8 days of life, the infant weighed 3.5 kg).

Because this infant was dusky and continued to be cyanotic with little movement, the nurse started oxygen by blowby at 40%, and at 22 minutes of life, oxygen was increased to 100% in an oxyhood. Positive pressure ventilation (e.g., CPAP, bag and mask) was not begun until 27 minutes of life, when the obstetrician intubated the baby. At 45 minutes of life, the infant was placed on pressure ventilation. At 58 minutes of life, the neonatologist arrived.

Evaluation The first arterial blood gas, at 27 minutes of life, reflected birth asphyxia: severe acidosis, severe hypoxia, metabolic acidosis, and respiratory acidosis (the infant was intubated and bagged, and the respiratory component of acidosis decreased with bagging). The nurse failed to perform pulse oximetry to evaluate the level of hypoxia and the effectiveness of oxygen administration. Despite the persistence of duskiness in 40% oxygen blowby, the nurse did not start 100% oxygen until 22 minutes of life. Despite obvious clinical signs of hypoxia, the nurse failed to initiate interventions immediately to improve oxygenation (e.g., CPAP and bag and mask ventilation).

Desirable Patient Outcome

Assessment "Nursing care of the newborn begins with anticipation and identification of high-risk newborns" (NAACOG, 1991, p. 65). Correct assessment of intrapartal risk factors should have resulted in anticipation of skilled resuscitation at delivery (AAP-ACOG, 1988, 1992; Golden & Peters, 1993). The professional nurse has responsibility and accountability for her actions and inactions. She must maintain clinical competence and use her knowledge of risk factors to identify those at risk (ANA, 1983, 1985; NAACOG, 1991). In addition to national standards, hospital policies, procedures, and protocols she must delineate risk factors requiring skilled resuscitation teams (NAACOG, 1991; AAP-ACOG, 1992).

Theoretically, the APGAR scoring system provides an objective quantitative measure of an infant's condition at one and five minutes of life. The APGAR score is both an indicator of the need for and an assessment of the infant's response to resuscitation (Golden & Peters, 1993). Degrees of asphyxia are qualitatively associated with APGAR scores (Table 10-1), so that a low score requires initiation of resuscitation (AAP-ACOG, 1992; Golden & Peters, 1993). Assignment of appropriate APGAR scores by the nurse fulfills the standards of care related to initial assessment and identification of at-risk newborns and life-threatening or emergency situations (NAACOG, 1990, 1991). Assigned APGARS of 8 and 9 do not correctly reflect this infant's condition. Despite these APGARS and a time lapse of 3 1/2 hours since the last dose of maternal analgesia, this infant was given Narcan at birth. Did the care providers assess this as a narcotized baby and thus give Narcan? Why was the Narcan given if this was a "non-asphyxiated" neonate? Utilizing documentation in the medical record, Table 10-2 represents "corrected"

Table 10-1 Association between APGAR Score and Degree of Asphyxia

APGAR Score	Degree of Asphyxia
8–10	No asphyxia
5–7	Mild asphyxia
3–4	Moderate asphyxia
0–2	Severe asphyxia

Adapted from Golden, S. & Peters, D. (1993). Delivery room care. In G. Merenstein & S. Gardner (Eds.), *Handbook of neonatal intensive care,* 3rd ed. (pp. 62–63). St. Louis: Mosby-Yearbook. Adapted with permission.

Table 10-2 "Corrected" APGARS Based on Documentation in the Medical Record

Medical Record Entry	"Corrected" APGARS
1448: Time of birth—bag and mask ventilation, Narcan, dusky	
1449: Assigned APGAR—8	*1449*
Very dusky	
0—color	0
2—heart rate	2
2—reflex	1–2
2—tone	1–2
2—respiration	1–2
	5–8 APGAR
1453: Assigned APGAR—9	
1510: (22 minutes) continues cyanotic—color	0
146/minute—heart rate	2
little movement—reflex and tone	1
40/minute; 100% oxygen—respiration	1–2
	5–6 APGAR
1515: (27 minutes)	
continues cyanotic; severe hypoxia (paO_2 21; O_2 sat 21%)—color	0
(no documentation)—heart rate	0–1
severe hypoxia; acidosis (pH 7.07; BE –18)—reflex and tone	0–1
bagging with 100% oxygen/ET tube—respirations	0–1
	2–5 APGAR

APGARS at 1, 22, and 27 minutes of life that illustrate this baby's poor and deteriorating condition.

Diagnosis Of the potential nursing diagnoses (see p. 165), this infant actually experienced:

Ineffective Airway Clearance
Risk for Aspiration
Impaired Gas Exchange
Inability to Sustain Spontaneous Ventilation

Failure to make appropriate nursing diagnoses violates national standards of nursing care (ANA, 1983, 1991; NAACOG, 1990, 1991) as well as the state standard of care (i.e., state nurse practice act).

Planning The first intrapartal documentation of late decelerations and meconium occurred hours before delivery. Level II nursery nurses had sufficient time to formulate a plan for skilled resuscitation at this infant's birth. Meconium-stained amniotic fluid requires specialized resuscitation techniques, including intubation, suction beyond the cords, and assisted ventilation with 100% oxygen for apnea, bradycardia, and poor respiratory effort (Golden & Peters, 1993). Since staff nurses were not skilled in airway management (e.g., laryngoscopy, endotracheal intubation, or suctioning of the airway), more qualified personnel were required for this resuscitation (AAP-ACOG, 1992).

Implementation As a patient advocate, the level II nurse has the obligation to anticipate and prepare for a complicated resuscitation by notifying more qualified care providers (e.g., pediatrician, neonatologist, or neonatal nurse practitioner) to be present at the birth (ANA, 1985; AAP-ACOG, 1992; Golden & Peters, 1993). Severe asphyxia (APGARS of 0–2) requires "at least three trained people working together as a swift, efficient team (Golden & Peters, 1993, p. 63). Corrected APGARS in Table 10-2 are as low as 2.

By failing to refer, collaborate, and/or consult with more skilled practitioners or to gather an adequate resuscitation team, the nurse violated the standard of nursing care (ANA, 1983, 1985, 1991; NAACOG, 1990, 1991) and is responsible and accountable for her actions (ANA, 1985; NAACOG, 1991). To provide the standard of care for this infant, other nursing actions should have occurred: (a) interventions for hypothermia (the first documented intervention for hypothermia was at 1745, a full 5 hours after birth, by the transport nurse), (b) initiation of CPAP (using bag and mask) to improve oxygenation in an obviously hypoxic infant, and (c) initiation of pulse oximetry to titrate oxygen administration.

Evaluation Evaluation of nursing interventions directs reassessment, formulation of new diagnoses and alterations in the plan and execution of care. If nursing interventions are not enhancing patient outcomes, evaluation directs a change in nursing practice for positive results (ANA 1983, 1985, 1991; NAACOG, 1990, 1991). Evaluation of this infant's continuing cyanosis and little movement (i.e., hypotonia) in 40% oxygen should have resulted in immediate attempts to improve oxygenation. Pulse oximetry monitors oxygen saturations and gives immediate data to evaluate the effect (or lack of effect) of interventions to improve oxygenation. The first arterial blood gas, at 27 minutes of age, showed severe hypoxia and acidosis, and required reassessment and alterations in interventions.

Despite the fact that there was no organized plan (e.g., collaborative practice guidelines), the nurse had the professional duty to be proactive in initiating the process of gathering a skilled resuscitation team. By maintaining a proactive approach, the nurse not only advocates for the patient but is able to maintain her own professional standards.

Case 2

Facts

In a community hospital with a level II nursery, baby boy Jensen was born on May 5, at 1957 hours, weighing 9 lbs. 7 oz. (4300 grams). He was 42 weeks by dates. APGARS of 5 and 9 were assigned. He was admitted to the nursery at 2035 with an axillary temperature of 35.2 C, respirations of 36 with nasal flaring, audible grunting, mild retractions, and blood pressure of 40/P. He was pink with slight circumoral cyanosis and his right arm was held in extension position.

The physician examined the baby at 2045 and ordered blowby oxygen at 100%. This "pinked up" the baby by 2105 and he had fewer retractions. By 2200 the baby warmed to 36.9 C Ax with a 36.8 radiant warmer temperature. A transcutaneous monitor (TCM) was attached, a "mid 60's" reading obtained, and the TCM discontinued. Initial reagent strip for glucose was 35 mg%. The infant breastfed and nippled formula after feeding. The following series of events then occurred.

May 6:

0700: Breastfed in A.M. Infant back in nursery. "Had a dusky spell and a little spitty."

1000: Out to mom—another episode of duskiness/spitting.

1700: Out to mom—having trouble breathing. Infant was described as extremely dusky with poor muscle tone. Rushed back to nursery while stimulating; given 100% oxygen. Infant pinked up but began seizure activity: arm twitching slightly, rhythmically, eyes deviating to left side, alternating staring and blinking; continued for 2 minutes. Physician called to evaluate.

1715: Drs. Jones and Smith examined infant and witnessed several dusky spells with tonic/clonic movements, hypertonicity, and abnormal Moro reflex.

1720: Another dusky spell with shallow, slow respirations. Labs drawn: CBC and differential showed normal results; platelets were normal; electrolytes were normal; glucose was normal; blood culture showed no growth.

1740: Physician orders included:
IV of D10W at 10 ccs./hr (started); IV phenobarbital 40 mg (10 mg/kg) to run over 20 minutes (changed order to IM); monitor; warmer; NPO.

1800 (May 6) to 1130 (May 7) (17 1/2 hours): 64 documentations of: color changes (dusky, pale, cyanotic [very]), tonic/clonic movements of extremities, shallow respirations/apnea, fixed dilated pupils, staring gaze, eye deviations, mouthing movements, completely unresponsive during episodes, TCM values dropped into the 20's with episodes which increased in length from 10–15 seconds to 60–90 seconds and occurred with increasing frequency from every 15–20 minutes to every 3–5 minutes).

Nursing interventions for these 17 1/2 hours included: physical stimulation, 100% oxygen by face mask, occasional bagging with oxygen.

1810: Phenobarbital 40 mg given IM; quiet, inactive; almost unresponsive to IV start.

1900: Both Drs. Jones and Smith saw the baby's seizure activity again.
1905: Lumbar puncture done—results normal. Dr. Jones' progress note: Loading dose of phenobarbital at 10 mg/kg; would give another 10 mg/kg at 12 hours if still seizing.
2020: Seizure witnessed by physician (1 hr 10 min after phenobarbital given IM).
2300: Nurse called Dr. Smith regarding 5 seizures in the last 2 hours. Orders given: TCM, O_2 via hood at 30% if needed.

May 7:
0200: Dr. Jones in and given progress report by RN: 26 episodes of seizure activity since he saw infant at 2000. MD progress note: Will continue to watch closely. Ordered: phenobarbital 40 mg IV slowly over 30 minutes at 0500.
0500: Phenobarbital given.
0700: Nurse called Dr. Smith and gave progress of baby. IV rate increased to 15 ccs./hr.
0800: Dr. Smith in. Progress note: Has received loading dose of phenobarbital of 20 mg/kg over last 12 hours and still seizing. Pyridoxine IV to rule out deficiency. CT scan this A.M.
0800: Neurology consult. Infant still experiencing frequent seizures with and without apneic spells and cyanosis. Often needs bagging with cyanotic episodes. Very bad prognosis. CT scan this A.M.
0830: CT scan showed bleeding in head.
0900: Dr. Jones in. Called transport team.
0950: Pyridoxine (vitamin B_6) 50 mg IV push.
1000: Phenytoin sodium (Dilantin) 60 mg IV.
1130: Transport team from level III nursery arrived.

Outcome

This child's outcome was mild to moderate retardation with developmental quotient of 65.

Legal

This case was settled out of court in advance of trial for multiple thousands of dollars.

Case Commentary

Undesirable Patient Outcome

Assessment Nursing assessments clearly timed and documented this infant's "dusky spells" and obvious (rather than subtle) seizure behaviors.

Diagnosis No nursing diagnoses were formulated from assessment data.

Planning This infant was admitted to a level II nursery and cared for in the first 19 hours of life by RNs. At 21 hours of life, he began obvious seizure activity while being cared for by a graduate nurse (GN). While this infant seized for the next 17 1/2 hours, he was cared for by the GN and two RNs. No RN, either as a direct care provider or as supervisor of the GN, planned this neonate's care based on assessment, nursing diagnosis, or the standard of care for a seizing neonate.

Implementation Nurses acted on the dependent aspects (i.e., physicians' orders) of patient care but did not carry out independent nursing actions (i.e., patient advocacy and affirmative action). Appropriate nursing interventions to support ventilation were utilized during the 17 1/2 hours of active seizures; however, appropriate medical intervention (i.e., administration of anti-epileptics to stop seizures and timely diagnosis of cause of seizures) was not done.

Evaluation Despite the fact that the nurses intervened to support ventilation during seizures and carried out physician orders, this infant continued to seize actively for a protracted time because of insufficient evaluation and treatment.

Desirable Patient Outcome

Assessment Although nurses appropriately assessed and documented this infant's seizure episodes, no arterial blood gas was done to calibrate TCM readings, and no pulse oximetry was used to assess inability to maintain adequate gaseous exchange during these episodes. No further evaluations of blood glucose status (with reagent strips) were done. These omissions clearly violate the nurses' duty to utilize collected data using appropriate assessment techniques on both an initial and ongoing basis (ANA, 1983, 1991; NAACOG, 1990, 1991).

Diagnosis Nursing diagnoses with appropriate plan of care are outlined in Tables 10-3 and 10-4.

Planning Since "all neonatal care must be provided by or be under the direct supervision of a professional nurse" (NAACOG, 1990, p. 4), the assignment of a GN to care for a seizing infant should have been re-evaluated by the supervising RN. If the supervising RN did not assume direct care for this infant, she certainly had the responsibility to "directly supervise" the GN and to plan appropriate nursing interventions (ANA, 1985; NAACOG, 1991).

Implementation Care of an at-risk infant requires nursing intervention by clinically competent professionals who are responsible and accountable for their judgments and actions (ANA, 1985; NAACOG, 1991). It is certainly doubtful that the GN in this case had enough clinical expertise to understand the implications of neonatal seizures and the standard of care in their management. However, the RNs in this case showed no more clinical competence than did the GN.

Through the duty of affirmative action, nurses must take positive, even forceful steps to ensure that the patient receives proper care. The *Code for Nurses* (ANA, 1985) requires that nurses advocate for the client's care and safety by "being alert to and taking appropriate action regarding incompetent, unethical, or illegal practices by any member of the health care team" (ANA, 1985, p. 6). In order to advocate that a patient receive proper care, the

Table 10-3 Plan of Care for Altered Tissue Perfusion: Cerebral

Patient Needs/ Nursing Diagnosis	Patient Outcomes	Nursing Interventions/ Collaborative Actions	Evaluation
Altered Tissue Perfusion: Cerebral related to hypoxia as evidenced by seizures	Seizure-free as a result of adequate pharmacologic management and stabilization of condition. Stable neurological status: No seizure activity, no apnea/ bradycardia.	1. Observe for and document all seizure activity. 2. Notify MD of all seizure activity. 3. Assist in diagnostic procedures related to seizure workup: blood draws, lumbar puncture, B mode, CAT/MRI scans, glucose monitoring. 4. Administer seizure medications and monitor for efficacy/adverse reactions (respiratory depression, hypotension blood dyscrasia). 5. Monitor blood levels of anti-seizure drugs. 6. C/R monitor with alarms set and emergency equipment (suction, bag and mask setup) available for resuscitation. 7. Daily OFC. 8. Maintain adequate oxygenation and ventilation using continuous pulse oximetry monitoring. 9. HOB up 30 degrees.	1. Lab results: • cultures negative • CAT/B mode negative for IVH, malformations • glucose (≥40 mg/dl) • calcium (>7 mg/dl) • magnesium (1.5–2.8 mg/dl) • blood gases: pH 7.35–7.45 paCO_2 35–45, paO_2 50–70 (altitude) 80–100 (sea level) O_2 sat 92–94% • electrolytes Na 133–146 K 4.6–6.7 Cl 100–117 CO_2 13.8–27.1. 2. Anti-seizure drugs cease seizure activity; if not, notify MD to obtain order for change/increase in drug. 3. Anti-seizure drug levels in therapeutic range: Phenobarbital: 20–25 mcg/cc Dilantin: 15–20 mcg/cc. 4. Pulse oximetry ≥92–94%.

Table 10-4 Plan of Care for Ineffective Breathing Pattern

Patient Needs/ Nursing Diagnosis	Patient Outcomes	Nursing Interventions/ Collaborative Actions	Evaluation
Ineffective Breathing Pattern related to inability to sustain spontaneous ventilation as evidenced by need for pressure ventilation, hypoxia	Infant will maintain adequate oxygenation/ ventilation: • apnea ceases, • R 30–60/min, • pulse oximetry 92–94%.	1. Apply continuous noninvasive monitoring for oxygenation (pulse ox; TCM). 2. Draw/monitor ABGs. 3. Administer FiO_2 to keep paO_2 ≥92–94%; use CPAP bag/ mask with 100% for apnea. 4. Cardiorespiratory monitor with alarms set. 5. Bag/mask, suction at bedside for resuscitation. 6. Endotracheal tray at bedside. 7. Ventilator changes to maintain ABG WNL and draw ABG within 15–30 minutes after ventilator change.	1. ABG within normal range: pH 7.35–7.45 paO_2 50–80 (altitude) 80–100 (sea level) paCO_2 35–45 O_2 sat 92–94% HCO_3 22–26 meq/l BE –4 to +4. 2. Color pink. 3. BP WNL for age/size. 4. R 30–60 BPM.

Acute Management of Neonatal Seizures

- Assess clinical situation—are the episodes seizures?
- Draw blood for glucose, calcium, magnesium, blood gas analysis, and electrolytes.
- Maintain adequate oxygenation and ventilation.
- Perform Dextrostix:
  If Dextrostix <25–45, give 100 mg/kg IV minibolus of glucose.
  If Dextrostix >25–45, give phenobarbital, 20 mg/kg IV.
- If seizures continue after 10–20 minutes, the following steps should be taken:
  Give additional doses of phenobarbital, 5 mg/kg each to a total of 40 mg/kg.
  Give Pyridoxine, 50–100 mg IV bolus.
- If seizures continue or recur after the above steps:
  Draw phenobarbital level.
  Correct calcium or magnesium if low.
  Give phenytoin, 20 mg/kg IV (no more rapidly than 10–20 mg/min.).
- If seizures persist or continue with the above treatment:
  Consider major intracranial etiology (malformation, bleed, etc.).
  Repeat metabolic studies (including NH_4) and blood levels of phenobarbital and phenytoin.
  Give diazepam, 0.3 mg/kg IV, or lorazepam, 0.05–0.1 mg/kg IV.
  Be prepared to intubate if drug-induced apnea occurs or to maintain ventilatory support.
  Consider diazepam or repeated doses of phenobarbital 5–10 mg/kg as necessary.
- Once seizures are under control, maintain phenobarbital levels at 20–30 mg/dl.
- Cultures (blood and CSF) should be considered as soon as the infant is stable.

From: Minarcik, C. & Beachy, P. (1993). Neurologic disorders. In G. Merenstein & S. Gardner (Eds.), *Handbook of neonatal intensive care*, 3rd ed. (p. 447). St. Louis: Mosby-Yearbook. Reprinted with permission.

nurse must be an expert in the management of specific health care conditions. Failure to follow accepted treatment modalities regarding management of neonatal seizures (see the accompanying box) resulted in 17 1/2 hours of compromised cerebral perfusion and ineffective spontaneous ventilation because of seizing.

Even though the nursing professionals caring for this infant carried out the physician's orders, "neither physicians' prescriptions nor the employing agencies' policies relieve the nurse of ethical or legal accountability for actions taken and judgments made" (ANA, 1985, p. 9). "Appropriate actions" by the nurses should have included: (a) referring to hospital policies, procedures, and protocols and/or neonatal textbooks regarding the management of neonatal seizures; (b) questioning, confronting, and/or challenging the attending physician regarding medications and necessity to transport; (c) operationalizing the chain-of-command (supervisory nurses and physicians); and (d) documenting each action taken.

Evaluation Evaluation criteria, outlined in the nursing care plans, validates the effect (or lack of effect) of interventions and directs reassessment and revision of interventions. Failure of this infant to cease seizing on 10 mg/kg of phenobarbital should have redirected nurses (and physicians) to other interventions (as shown in the box).

Nursing negligence (i.e., failure to know the standard of care) and nursing inaction (i.e., failure to advocate that this baby receive treatment to relieve seizures and a timely transport to a level III nursery) resulted in nurses being held legally accountable for violation of the standard of care.

Case 3

Facts

Rebecca Weeks was born on December 12th at 1317 in a community hospital by repeat cesarean section (due to fetal distress, maternal preeclampsia, thrombocytopenia, and possible HELLP syndrome) to a G3 P2–3 mother. Meconium was present at birth and APGARS were 8 and 9. Birth weight was 6 lbs. 4 oz. (2835 grams) and estimated gestational age was 38 weeks. In the level I nursery the following sequence of events occurred:

1355: Admitted with normal vital signs and an initial Dextrostix of <45 mg%.
1410: CBC: Hct 71; respiratory distress with sternal retractions.
1440: Dextrostix <45 mg%.
1443: STAT serum glucose: 30 mg%, no urine output.
1453: Private pediatrician called. Infant nippled 25 ccs. D5W slowly.
1550: Viscosity studies positive for hyperviscosity (central Hct 68).
1635: Dextrostix <45 mg%, STAT serum glucose 72 mg%.
1640: Pediatrician notified.
Transferred to level II nursery at 1715.
1900: Pediatrician arrived.
2000: Partial exchange transfusion started.
2025: Exchange completed with 45 ccs. sodium chloride. As UVC was removed, Rebecca became dusky. Heart rate stable; apneic; oxygen given and bagged with 100% oxygen. Repeated tongue thrusts; major motor convulsion noted.
2028: Phenobarbital 30 mg IV push. Respirations shallow, color dusky. Oxygen by CPAP.
2033: Phenobarbital 10 mg IV push. Color pale.
Transferred to level III nursery at 2036.
2036: Color pale. Oxygen by blowby.
2040: Phenobarbital 10 mg IV push.
2045: Pediatrician and neonatologist at bedside. CBC and lytes drawn.

2055: Dilantin 15 mg IV push.
2145: Cerebral ultrasound showed cerebral edema.
2215: Dexamethasone (Decadron) 1.5 mg IV.
2230: Lytes: Na 187 meq/L, Cl 167 meq/L. Pediatrician's note: After receiving report of initial electrolytes, the vials used in the exchange were dug out of the garbage can. Both vials were sodium chloride 120 meq (2.5 meq/cc). Received 112 meq Na in transfusion. Impression: Sodium intoxication secondary to accidental substitution of hypertonic for normal saline in exchange transfusion.
2235: No seizure activity.

December 13:
0115: More dusky, poorer peripheral perfusion, Na 184 meq/L.
0200: Na 174 meq/L, questionable seizure activity. Treated with 2.5 mg/kg of Dilantin.

December 14:
0025: Intubated to maintain patent airway during seizures and increasing apnea.
1915: Na 156 meq/L, less seizure activity. Cerebral ultrasound—no bleed, no ventricular dilation.

December 15:
0600: Na 151 meq/L; seizures × 2 overnight, controlled by Valium and early doses of phenobarbital.
2100: Na 147 meq/L; no seizures; phenobarbital level: 37.

December 14 through 18:
Baby intubated and ventilated because of increased phenobarbital levels and respiratory depression.

December 22:
Discharged to home.

Outcome

At age 9, Rebecca has mild motor delays and significant cognitive delays (IQ 70–75).

Legal

This case involved an out-of-court settlement with the pediatrician's insurance company for hundreds of thousands of dollars. In addition, there was a jury award of $139,400 for child; $88,020 for the plantiff's parents (*Weeks v. Memorial Hospital*, 1994).

Case Commentary

Undesirable Patient Outcome

Assessment Nurses in the level I nursery assessed Rebecca as small for gestational age (SGA). The Dextrostix at 1635 was <45 mg% (STAT serum glucose 72 mg%).

Diagnosis No nursing diagnoses were documented in the record.

Planning When the pediatrician talked to Nurse H. on the phone, he ordered the baby be transferred to the level II nursery, an IV started, and preparations made for a partial exchange transfusion with normal saline. Nurse H. wrote telephone orders for transfer and IV, but not for the exchange transfusion with normal saline.

In preparing for the exchange, Nurse H. questioned the pediatrician regarding the use of normal saline solution, since the hospital protocol states: 5% albumin or fresh frozen plasma. Nurse H. discussed use of normal saline with Nurse B. (evening charge nurse) since she was uncomfortable with using it. She then went to the level III nursery cabinet and removed two bottles of sodium chloride and two bottles of 5% albumin solution. Upon returning to the level II nursery she put the solutions on the baby's bed.

Implementation The pediatrician arrived and saw albumin on the baby's bed and stated he didn't want to use it because it was too expensive and increased the chance of AIDS. Nurse H. picked up the sodium chloride vials, held them up at about 18 inches from the doctor's face, and asked, "Is this the solution you want to use?" He said, "Yes, that's fine." Nurse B. witnessed this exchange but had not looked at the vials of sodium chloride. Nurse H. finished her charting and left the unit.

Since partial exchange transfusion was "new" to her, Nurse B. went to the level III nursery to discuss it with the charge nurse. They pulled out the procedure manual and the level III charge nurse talked to Nurse B. about gathering together the necessary equipment. From the vials, Nurse B. pulled up the sodium chloride solution into 10 cc syringes.

Evaluation As the transfusion was completed, the infant began to obviously seize. In searching for possible causes, a post-exchange workup was done. After serum electrolytes showed hypernatremia and hyperchloremia, the vials were retrieved and were obviously *not* normal, but hypertonic saline.

Desirable Patient Outcome

Assessment A 38-week, 2835-gram neonate is an appropriate for gestational age (AGA), not an SGA, infant. Although the second Dextrostix value was <45 mg% and correlated with a serum glucose level of 30, the next Dextrostix was also <45 mg% but did not correlate with the serum glucose level of 72 mg%. Such a discrepancy raises questions about technique of blood draw, freshness of Dextrostix supply, etc.

Diagnosis Appropriate nursing diagnoses based on assessment data should have included:

Altered Tissue Perfusion: cerebral, respiratory, renal, and gastrointestinal related to hyperviscosity syndrome, umbilical venous catheter placement, partial exchange transfusion, and sodium intoxication (use of hypertonic rather than isotonic saline)

Ineffective Breathing Pattern related to hyperviscosity syndrome during/after partial exchange transfusion as evidenced by tonic seizures

Impaired Gas Exchange related to tonic seizure activity and anti-seizure drugs necessary to stop seizures

Ineffective Infant Feeding Pattern related to CNS depression from use of anti-seizure medication

Fluid Volume Deficit related to NPO status

Planning In preparation for the transfusion, these nurses questioned the pediatrician, discussed among themselves, and consulted the written protocol regarding appropriate solutions. Since the protocol specified 5% albumin or fresh frozen plasma, the use of normal saline would violate the hospital's standard of care. The nurses did not consult any neonatal texts or reference materials. Although the medical director of the nursery was present in the level II nursery prior to the onset of the transfusion, no nurse planned to (or did) consult with this neonatologist regarding the use of a solution that deviated from the written policy. Not to consult with the neonatologist violates the standard of care, since the *Code of Ethics* (ANA, 1985) requires that the nurse exercise informed judgment and use individual competence and qualifications as criteria for seeking consultation. Certainly a neonatologist who has more training and expertise in care of the neonate should have been consulted about this proposed deviation from the protocol. The Standards of Maternal-Child Health Nursing Practice (ANA, 1983), The Standards of Clinical Nursing Practice (ANA, 1991), and the Standards for the Nursing Care of Women and Newborns (NAACOG, 1991) all require nurses to collaborate, coordinate, and consult with other professionals.

Implementation Even though Nurse H. phoned the pediatrician, took orders, and even questioned the use of normal saline, no medical orders for exchange with normal saline were ever written on the chart. In deposition she stated, "I normally don't write things to prepare for because he (the physician) could come in and write the order and write for specifically what he wants." However, in the interim she acted on the verbal orders, obtaining the vials of sodium chloride for the transfusion.

In deposition, Nurse H. stated that she "mistook hypertonic for normal saline; at the time I didn't know it wasn't normal saline." She further stated that she "saw sodium chloride on the label and didn't read the dilution; she assumed it was normal saline, was concerned about the content of the vial, not the concentration." When she showed the vial to the physician, she didn't know that it was concentrated, not normal saline.

Although Nurse B. saw Nurse H. hold up the vial for the physician to read, she admits she "didn't know how closely the physician examined it." In addition to being told by Nurse H., she also heard the pediatrician say that "he wanted normal saline." Nurse B. saw sodium chloride on the vials, didn't know the vial wasn't normal saline, didn't check the dilution, handled the vials, and aspirated the solution into syringes. She further conceded in her deposition that "If I had read the labels, I would have known the difference between normal and hypertonic saline since basic nursing training teaches the difference." Regarding the red warning labels, she said she "didn't recall reading that." She stated that she "relied on the physician reading the label"

The "Five Rights" of Drug Administration

- Right drug
- Right dose
- Right route
- Right time
- Right patient

From: Murphy, M. & Turner, B. (1993). Pharmacology in neonatal care. In G. Merenstein & S. Gardner (Eds.), *Handbook of neonatal intensive care,* 3rd ed. (p. 131). St. Louis: Mosby-Yearbook. Adapted with permission.

and didn't know until later that he didn't read the content on the label (in its entirety). In concluding the deposition, Nurse B. was asked if by showing the vial to the physician she was relieved of any obligation to assure that the ordered medication was the medication given. Her response was, "Yes, I feel he saw the bottle . . . I took it as an order."

In implementation, the nurse has a responsibility to interpret and carry out physician orders properly and safely (ANA, 1985, 1991; NAACOG, 1991; state nurse practice act). In addition, the nurse has the responsibility to implement independent nursing practice (e.g., those aspects of the nursing care plan that do not require physician's orders). The competent execution of the pediatrician's order for normal saline required both nurses to: (a) know that sodium chloride comes in various concentrations; (b) read the labels to determine the concentration in the vials; (c) recognize that the vials were hypertonic, not normal, saline; (d) heed the label's warning: "Caution: must be diluted"; and (e) not rely on the physician's reading of the labels. Failure to act in such a manner did not "promote, maintain, or restore health" (ANA, 1985, p. 8).

Clinical competence (ANA, 1985; NAACOG, 1990, 1991) in medication administration requires completing the "five rights" listed in the accompanying box. "Administering the correct dosage of a drug is a shared responsibility between the physician who orders the drug and the nurse who carries out that order" (Whaley and Wong, 1991, p. 1224). These nurses did not ensure that they had the right concentration of the drug (i.e., the solution of sodium chloride). Nurse H. had the opportunity to read the vial for the correct contents and concentration: (a) on removal from the cabinet, and (b) on holding the vials up for the doctor to see. Nurse B. had the opportunity to read and check the vials, (a) when she picked them up from the baby's bed, (b) before aspirating the solution into the syringes, and (c) after aspirating the solution into the syringes (Krug, 1963; Potter & Perry, 1991). The nurses' failures to demonstrate competence in performance of the technical procedures of fluids and medication administration were not ameliorated by the physician's reading of the vial.

The nurse must assume responsibility and accountability for individual nursing judgments and actions (ANA, 1985; NAACOG, 1991). As stated in the *Code for Nurses*, "the regulation and control of nursing practice by nurses demands that individual professional practitioners of nursing bear primary responsibility for the nursing care clients receive and be individually accountable for practice" (ANA, 1985, p. 8). This responsibility and accountability is not obviated by the physician's responsibility and accountability. Both nurses and physicians have a shared responsibility for the patient. The nurse has 100% accountability and responsibility for nursing actions and judgments while the physician has 100% accountability and responsibility for medical actions and judgments. The code further clarifies that "neither physician's prescriptions (i.e., orders) nor the employing agency's policies relieve the nurse of ethical or legal accountability for actions taken and judgments made" (ANA, 1985, p. 9). Nurse H.'s negligence in obtaining the wrong concentration of sodium chloride was compounded by her reliance on the physician's reading of the vial and Nurse B.'s drawing solution from an unread, unchecked container.

Evaluation Evaluation of nursing practice to improve goal-oriented patient outcomes is the last step of the nursing process (ANA, 1983, 1991; NAACOG, 1991). The ineffectiveness of these nursing interventions became very clear when the vials were retrieved and found to be hypertonic solution. "Having two nurses calculate and check the dosage decreases errors" (Murphy and Turner, 1993, p. 131). However, in this case two nurses handled the vials of solution but neither checked for the concentration of sodium chloride to assure normal versus hypertonic solution. In reconstructing the incident, normal and hypertonic saline were found next to each other in the cabinet (Cohen, 1994). Normal saline was available.

References

American Academy of Pediatrics and American College of Obstetricians and Gynecologists. (1988). Appendix C—Sample list of perinatal conditions that increase the risk for neonatal morbidity and mortality. In *Guidelines for perinatal care*, 2nd ed. (pp. 297–298). Washington, D.C.: Author.

American Academy of Pediatrics and American College of Obstetricians and Gynecologists. (1992). Perinatal care service. In *Guidelines for perinatal care*, 3rd ed. (pp. 1–33). Washington, D.C.: Author.

American Nurses Association. (1983). *Standards of maternal-child health nursing practice*. Washington, D.C.: Author.

American Nurses Association. (1985). *Code for nurses with interpretive statements*. Washington, D.C.: Author.

American Nurses Association. (1991). *Standards of clinical nursing practice*. Washington, D.C.: Author.

Cohen, M. (1994). Sodium chloride concentrate: No substitute allowed. *Nursing 94*, 15.

Golden, S. & Peters, D. (1993). Delivery room care. In G. Merenstein & S. Gardner (Eds.), *Handbook of neonatal intensive care,* 3rd ed. (pp. 55–75). St. Louis: Mosby-Yearbook.

Krug, E. (1963). Administration of medicines. In *Pharmacology in nursing* (pp. 93–124). St. Louis: Mosby-Yearbook.

Minarcik, C. & Beachy, P. (1993). Neurologic disorders. In G. Merenstein & S. Gardner (Eds.), *Handbook of neonatal intensive care,* 3rd ed. (p. 447). St. Louis: Mosby-Yearbook.

Murphy, M. & Turner, B. (1993). Pharmacology in neonatal care. In G. Merenstein & S. Gardner (Eds.), *Handbook of neonatal intensive care,* 3rd ed. (pp. 127–140). St. Louis: Mosby-Yearbook.

Nurses' Association of the American College of Obstetricians and Gynecologists. (1990). *Nurse providers of neonatal care.* Washington, D.C.: Author.

Nurses' Association of the American College of Obstetricians and Gynecologists. (1991). *Standards for the nursing care of women and newborns,* 4th ed. Washington, D.C.: Author.

Potter, R. & Perry, A. (1995). Administering medications. In *Basic nursing theory and practice,* 3rd ed. (p. 560). St. Louis: Mosby-Yearbook.

Weeks v. Memorial Hospital, No. 86 C.V. 2823, Division 3, County of El Paso, Civil Court, Colorado. (August 1, 1994).

Whaley, L. & Wong, D. (1995). *Nursing care of infants and children,* 5th ed. (pp. 1184–1246). St. Louis: Mosby-Yearbook.

11

High-Risk Neonatal Care: Level III Nursery

Sandra L. Gardner, RN, MS, CNS, PNP
Mary I. Enzman Hagedorn, RN, PhD, CNS, CPNP

Level III perinatal centers provide complete maternal and neonatal care in addition to high-risk intrapartal and neonatal care, consultation, transport, education, and data analysis (AAP-ACOG, 1992). The level III intensive care nursery provides comprehensive services to neonates with complicated medical and surgical problems and the highest risk (<1500 grams, <32 weeks gestation) (AAP-ACOG, 1992). Nursing staff in the level III nursery should have advanced training and experience in high-risk neonatal nursing to care for the family and unstable neonate with multisystem problems, requiring specialized technology (AAP-ACOG, 1992). *Guidelines for Perinatal Care* (AAP-ACOG, 1992, p. 9) also states that an "all professional registered nurse staff is preferable" when caring for the high-risk neonate. The NAACOG document *Nurse Providers of Neonatal Care* (NAACOG, 1990) states that "nursing care of infants should be provided by professional nurses" (p. 2) and "professional nurses are the preferred neonatal caregivers" (p. 4).

This chapter presents cases of nursing liability related to undertreatment of hypoglycemia, complications of umbilical catheters, and complications of endotracheal intubation and mechanical ventilation.

Case 1

Facts

On December 16 at 1725, baby girl Causteau was born at 40 weeks gestation weighing 8 lbs. 8 1/2 oz. (3870 grams). The G1 P0 mother had maternal hypertension (BP 130–152/108–110) with a 2+ urine protein. Spontaneous rupture of membranes had occurred at 1830 on December 15. When green meconium was noted in the amniotic fluid, labor was augmented with oxytocin (Pitocin) at 1155 (December 16). Fetal heart rate patterns showed "little variability" at 1330; "light greenish fluid" and "large amounts of meconium fluid" were noted at 1420. After a labor of 20 hours, including a second stage of 3 hours and 55 minutes, a primary cesarean section for cephalopelvic disproportion (CPD) was performed with very difficult extraction of the head through a large "criss-cross" incision.

Resuscitation consisted of bag and mask ventilation (for Apgar scores of 5 and 7). The baby was noted to have facial, head, shoulder, and chest contusions and was carried in the arms of Dr. Veslek to the level III nursery, where further care was initiated.

The following care occurred in sequence:

December 16:

1807: Dr. Rogers notified. Lab work (stat serum glucose and capillary gas) ordered.

1845: Lab technician arrived to draw blood. With FiO_2 at 36%, the following capillary blood gas was obtained: pH 7.24, PCO_2 54, PO_2 40, BE –5.

1915: Dr. Rogers was given the blood gas results.

1930: Lab technician redrew blood sugar.

2030: Color noted to be "ruddy" (Hct 62.5) and "dusky." FiO_2 was increased to 40%. Dr. Rogers called—no response. Dr. Black (neonatologist and director of unit) called.

2030–2100: Infant noted to have "dusky" color with a pulse oximeter below 70%. Infant was bagged with 100% oxygen for 1 minute, with an increase in the pulse oximetry reading. This process was repeated four times.

2115: IV was started and D10W initiated at 8 mL/hr; 6 mL IV dextrose given as IV bolus.

2130: Serum glucose 5 mg/dL.

2150: 6 mL of D10W given as IV bolus; IV increased to 10 mL/hr.

2230: Serum glucose 9 mg/dL.

2300: 6 mL D15W given IV bolus.

2330: Serum glucose 21 mg/dL.

2400: Vital signs: T 36.5 rectally (R), HR 128, R 72 (shallow with expiratory grunt). Warmer was turned up; FiO_2 increased to 48%.

December 17:

0020: 2330 serum glucose results phoned to Dr. Black.

0030: Serum glucose 8 mg/dL.

0100: T 36.6 (R); warmer turned up; blanket placed.

0140: Infant apneic; bagged for 1 minute with 100% oxygen.

0155: Serum glucose results of 0030 shown to Dr. Bates.

0207: Suspherine (Epinephrine) 0.03 mL ordered and given subcutaneously.

0210: 6 mL D15W IV bolus given.

0245: D10W discontinued; D15W started at 10 mL/hr.

0300: Vital signs: T 37.1 (Ax), R 80 and shallow; color slightly mottled; lips and nailbeds pink. FiO_2 of 48% with a pulse oximetry reading of 98%.

0320: Serum glucose 37 mg/dL.

0630: "Both hands in tight fists and toes curled up."

0655: Pulse ox: 63% in 32% FiO_2; color dusky; oxygen increased to 37%.

0810: Serum glucose 25 mg/dL.

0900: D15W discontinued; D20W started at 10 mL/hr. Infant described as fussy and gaggy; color dusky. O_2 per nasal cannula with improved color.

1000: Serum glucose 21 mg/dL.

1015: Color dusky, respiratory rate decreased and shallow; infant stimulated with color improvement.
1045: Dr. Bleacher arrived. Lab called for blood sugar results; results delayed.
1150: Infant noted to be "fussy"; glucagon given.
1300: Serum glucose drawn.
1310: Serum glucose 25 mg/dL.
1500: No further dusky episodes since A.M. Serum glucose 40 mg/dL.

December 21:
Phenobarbital and phenytoin (Dilantin) started to treat seizure activity.

Outcome

This child is multiply handicapped, with severe developmental delays and cerebral palsy.

Legal

This case was settled out of court for $1.7 million.

Case Commentary

Undesirable Outcome

Assessment On admission to the level III nursery, no vital signs, Dextrostix/Chemstrip, or estimation of gestational age were performed. The first set of documented vital signs occurred 6 hours and 30 minutes after birth. Although this neonate was on a radiant warmer, there is no documentation of her skin temperature or radiant-warmer control temperatures. Estimation of gestational age was done at 7 hours of age. No Dextrostix was obtained while waiting for the STAT lab work to be drawn and/or reported. At 1845, the STAT blood work was drawn, but since the lab did not believe the glucose value (0 mg%) this level was not reported and another specimen was drawn at 1930 (also 0 mg%). At 3 hours, 8 hours and 15 minutes, 9 hours and 35 minutes, 15 hours and 35 minutes, and 16 hours and 45 minutes of life this infant had respiratory distress requiring oxygen and bag and mask ventilation.

Diagnosis No nursing diagnoses were formulated from assessment data.

Planning On admission to the level III nursery, this infant was cared for by a graduate nurse (GN). Neither the GN nor the RN supervising her planned this neonate's care based on assessment data or nursing diagnoses.

Implementation An intravenous infusion of D10W at 8 mL/hr was begun at 3 hours and 50 minutes after birth, 2 1/2 hours after the first lab draw, 1 hour and 45 minutes after the second lab draw, and 45 minutes after the onset of "dusky spells" requiring bagging with 100% oxygen. "Increasing the temperature of the warmer and placing a blanket on the infant" was the only documented nursing intervention for hypothermia.

Evaluation Despite nursing interventions to support oxygenation and ventilation, this infant continued to have apnea and hypoxic episodes secondary to hypoglycemia and inadequate glucose administration. No pulse oximetry to evaluate the hypoxia and effectiveness of oxygen administration was performed during these periods of apnea and hypoxia.

Laboratory results were not obtained in a timely fashion. Care based on laboratory values was difficult; however, bedside reagent strips (Dextrostix or Chemstrip) were never used to quickly evaluate the infant's glucose status specifically when respiratory distress and seizure activity were noted. Use of these reagent strips could have resulted in more timely interventions on the nurse's part.

Desirable Patient Outcome

Assessment Since nursing care of the neonate "begins with anticipation and identification of high-risk newborns" (NAACOG, 1991), initial assessment must include: (a) review of perinatal history, (b) physical assessment, (c) vital signs (temperature, pulse, respiration, and blood pressure), (d) gestational age, and (e) interpretation of routine and indicated laboratory tests (NAACOG, 1990, 1991). A review of this infant's perinatal history reveals numerous factors that contributed to her increased risk for hypoglycemia: (a) prolonged labor, specifically second stage of labor, (b) fetal distress, (c) difficult extraction resulting in multiple contusions, (d) Apgar scores of 5 and 7, and (e) a maternal history of hypertension. A timely estimation of gestational age (i.e., within the first hour of life) would have alerted the nurse to the newborn's classification of full term, large for gestational age (FLGA) with a 4% incidence of hypoglycemia (Lubchenco & Bard, 1971; Olds, London, & Ladewig, 1996).

The standards of nursing practice also require the nurse to "identify life threatening and emergency situations" (NAACOG, 1990). An initial screening test (i.e., Dextrostix or Chemstrip) would have quickly determined the very low blood sugar. Certainly the return of the lab technician to redraw the specimen should have prompted the nurse to question why a redraw was necessary and to have elicited the information regarding the "unbelievable" blood sugar of 0 mg/dL! Intravenous glucose should have been initiated at 1930 instead of 1 hour and 45 minutes later; the initial hypoxic episodes could have been prevented.

Diagnosis Appropriate nursing diagnoses should have included:

Altered Nutrition: Less than Body Requirements related to LGA classification and increased risk for hypoglycemia.

Ineffective Breathing Pattern related to infant's inability to sustain spontaneous ventilation secondary to hypoglycemia.

Planning Obviously the GN caring for this infant was unable to accurately assess, diagnose, and formulate a plan of care (see Tables 9-1 and 9-2). If the supervising RN did not assume direct care, she had the responsibility to "directly supervise" the GN and plan appropriate and timely nursing interventions (ANA, 1985; NAACOG, 1990, 1991). Nursing management in the NICU violated the standard of care by not having written policies, procedures, and protocols readily accessible to clarify nursing's scope of practice (NAACOG, 1991).

Implementation Specific measurable interventions, outcomes, and evaluation criteria are delineated in Tables 9-1 and 9-2. The *Standards for nursing care of women and newborns* (NAACOG, 1991) require the nurse to: (a) provide and maintain neutral thermal environment; (b) establish and maintain cardiopulmonary function; (c) perform indicated lab tests; (d) establish parenteral therapy, providing and maintaining fluid and electrolyte balance; (e) assist with technical procedures as delineated by policies, procedures, and protocols; (f) utilize laboratory (and other) diagnostic data in providing care; (g) initiate and maintain oxygen and respiratory therapy; (h) monitor nutritional status and provide nutrition; and (i) intervene in emergency situations following written policies and procedures. These guidelines require the nurse to "use interventional strategies that maintain current standards of nursing practice" (NAACOG, 1990, p. 5).

Care of at-risk infants requires nursing intervention by clinically competent professionals who are responsible and accountable for their judgements and actions (ANA, 1985; NAACOG, 1991). If the GN primary caretaker did not have clinical expertise to understand the dynamics of hypoglycemia symptoms and management, the RN supervising her should have intervened. The *Code for Nurses* (ANA, 1985) requires nurses to advocate for the client's care and safety. In order to advocate for the neonate to receive appropriate care, the nurse must be an expert in accepted treatment modalities. Failure to follow the standard of care regarding medical management of hypoglycemia (McGowan, Hagedorn, Price, Hay, 1993) resulted in 21 1/2 hours of symptomatic hypoglycemia.

Even though the nurses carried out the physician's orders, "neither the physician's prescriptions nor the employing agency's policies relieve the nurse of ethical or legal accountability for actions taken and judgments made" (ANA, 1985, p. 9). The nurses should have: (a) referred to hospital protocols and/or neonatal textbooks regarding management of hypoglycemia; (b) calculated the amount of glucose this infant required to maintain a normal glucose level; (c) questioned, confronted, and/or challenged the physician; and (d) operationalized the chain of command.

Evaluation Continued serum glucose levels below 40 mg/dL and symptoms of hypoglycemia in the presence of undertreated hypoglycemia validate the ineffectiveness of interventions and require the nurse to redirect, reassess, and revise the interventions (i.e., provision of more glucose/kg). Failure of this infant's symptoms to subside and for the serum glucose level to be ≥40–45 mg % should have resulted in a reassessment and revision of the glucose therapy. Nursing's inaction resulted in 21 1/2 hours of symptomatic hypoglycemia and legal accountability for violation of the standards of care.

Case 2

Indwelling umbilical catheters (arterial or venous) are foreign bodies that promote fibrin deposition and thrombus formation around the catheter which is of clinical significance in <10% of neonates (Pierce & Turner, 1993). Compromised circulation most often results in ischemic disease due to emboli or spasms (Pierce & Turner, 1993). Catheter slippage and/or disconnection may result in significant blood loss. Bacterial contamination may result in clinical manifestations of sepsis that include generalized septicemia, localized omphalitis, osteoarthritis, and myelitis (Rao & Elhassani, 1980).

Optimal placement of an umbilical artery catheter (UAC) is in the lumbar 3–4 (L3–4) vertebrae for lower catheters and thoracic 8 (T8) vertebra for a high placement (Pierce and Turner, 1993). Although there are more complications with umbilical venous catheters (UVC), they are less severe than complications seen with UACs. Complications of high catheter placement (T8) are fewer but more severe than in low-placement (L3–4) catheters (Pierce and Turner, 1993).

Facts

On July 17 at 0811, baby boy Miller was born in an outlying community hospital by repeat cesarean section to a G2 P1 mother whose due date was July 27. Birth weight was 4 lbs. 2 oz. (1871 grams) at 34 weeks gestation. Apgar scores were 8 and 9 at 1 and 5 minutes. At 0950 the transport nurse found a flaccid, dusky infant in an oxyhood of 35% with the following vital signs: T 35.6 (R), P 160, and R 50. Grunting respirations and retractions ensued (hyaline membrane disease was diagnosed on chest X ray). At 4 hours of life, baby Miller was intubated and a UAC was placed. Stabilization of the infant occurred prior to transport to a level III regional NICU 40 minutes away. The following sequential care occurred:

July 17:
First arterial blood gas (ABG) revealed combined respiratory and metabolic acidosis and hypoxia.
Admission vital signs to NICU revealed hypothermia and tachycardia.
Infant was intubated and placed on a ventilator.
1630: CBC/WBC 7.7; platelet count 288,000.
All cultures were negative except a culture of the right eye, which was positive for *pseudomonas.* UAC was pulled back 2 cm, over T5 vertebra.

July 18:
0700: WBC 6.9; infant remained hypothermic, tachypneic, and tachycardic. ABGs revealed a combined metabolic/respiratory acidosis with hypoxia.

July 19:
Infant remained hypothermic and tachycardic with increasing sternal retractions. ABGs revealed an ongoing metabolic acidosis and hypoxia.

Chest X ray revealed the tip of the UAC at T10 vertebra.
Transducer was changed at the stopcock and tightened due to leakage (no amount of blood loss recorded).
UAC was flushed every hour from 1500 to 2200 (despite only one ABG draw). Blood pressure (through transducer reading) decreased from previous level.

July 20:
Infant remained hypothermic, tachycardic, tachypneic, and hypotensive; ABGs revealed an ongoing metabolic acidosis.
0800: Chest X ray showed correct tube placement, atelectatic changes in both lungs with decreasing aeration bilaterally.
1030: UAC removed and tip cultured; new UAC placed due to poor position on X ray (over T4).
1430: UAC was pulled back 3 cm.
2024: WBC of 3.1.
2200: Transducer blood pressure 38/18 (a 15–20 mm change from previous values).
Physician called, since order read: Call MD if systolic blood pressure is less than 40.

July 21:
Infant remained hypothermic (finally warming to skin temperature of 36.5 at 1200), tachycardic, and hypotensive. An X ray for placement of the UAC revealed the tip at T6.
1500: Nurse's notes read, "Not as active as yesterday at this time. Responds to stimuli most of the time. Nailbeds dusky."
1600: No spontaneous respiratory effort on ventilator; very little response to stimuli; no reaction to a heelstick for blood work.
2100: Very jaundiced, a little pinker on the cheeks than previously noted, moved arms and legs more spontaneously, had spontaneous opening and closing of eyes, but still no spontaneous respirations.
2200: Bradycardia × 2 with suctioning.
2230: "Red spots" on left leg which remained throughout the night; some spontaneous respirations.

July 22:
0400: "Red spots" on lower abdomen and legs spreading over buttocks to upper trunk; jaundice increased.
0800: "Red spots" continue on lower abdomen and left leg. Left foot slightly edematous. Irritable when disturbed. Pulling legs to body.
1030: Left leg continues to appear mottled; spreading over lower abdomen and buttocks; edema continues in left leg.
1145: Physician notified of rash and edema.
1200: UAC removed and the tip of the catheter sent for culture (report on July 24 was positive for *Staphylococcus Aureus*). Infant continued to hold left leg close to body; femoral and pedal pulses decreased in left leg.

July 23:
0600: Physician's orders read, "Keep left leg at the level of the body, apply warm packs, and keep down." Nurse's notes read, "Left leg wrapped in warm packs; to position leg lower than his body."
1600: Femoral pulses present; left leg remains mottled, left foot bruised; great toe and second toes are "very blue."
1630: First physician report regarding vascular insufficiency in left leg and foot with decreased pulses, and left foot and toes very dark and swollen. Cardiovascular consult: irreversible vascular changes in left foot and (?) lower leg; Doppler femoral and popliteal pulses present although weak.

July 24:
0130: Blood cultures obtained.
0200: Antibiotics started.
0500: Discoloration of the left foot increased since 2400.
0738: Lumbar puncture performed and documented as "normal."
0930: Platelet count of 19,000.

Outcome

Vascular insufficiency progressed. Eventually the neonate's left lower leg was amputated. At 9 years of age, the child was fitted with a lower-leg prosthesis.

Legal

The case was settled out of court for an undisclosed amount said to range in the "hundreds of thousands" of dollars.

Case Commentary

Undesirable Patient Outcome

Assessment Nursing assessments documented significant clinical data: (a) persistent hypothermia, (b) questionable placement and function of the UAC line, and (c) signs and symptoms of sepsis (on the fifth day) that went untreated for a long period of time. Prior to the obvious onset of lower-extremity circulatory compromise, nurses failed to assess and document the condition of the lower extremities and buttocks of an infant with a UAC. Descriptions of skin lesions as "red spots" fail to adequately assess and describe the change in skin and vascular perfusion (i.e., macules/papules; color; size; location; capillary refill; blanching with pressure; pattern of dispersement).

Diagnosis No nursing diagnoses were generated from assessment data.

Planning No plan of care based on assessment data and nursing diagnoses was established to direct nursing interventions.

Implementation The physician was finally notified of the "red spots" on the leg and abdomen 25 hours and 15 minutes after they first appeared; 6 hours and 45 minutes after the note about the rash spreading; 2 hours and 45 minutes after the note about edema of the left foot, and 1 hour and 15 minutes after the note about mottling and edema of the left foot spreading. Earlier physician notification of these significant findings, suggestive of infection, would have prompted earlier interventions (e.g., UAC removal, sepsis workup, and administration of antibiotics). These interventions would have prevented the undesirable outcome of amputation.

Evaluation No evaluation of nursing care was documented because no measurable outcomes were stated for this infant's hospitalization.

Desirable Patient Outcome

Assessment In gathering information about a patient's condition, the professional nurse is responsible not only for assessment of clinical conditions but also for interpretation of laboratory data (NAACOG, 1991). Complete nursing assessment of this preterm infant should have included: (a) clinical manifestations, (b) UAC placement, condition, removal, and replacement, and (c) laboratory data (i.e., decreasing WBC and platelet counts). Recognizing the significance of these data, the nurse should have been suspicious of infection and utilized the nursing process, "the structure for professional nursing practice and standards for practice" (NAACOG, 1990, p. 4), to formulate a plan of care. "Professional nurses are the preferred neonatal caregivers" (NAACOG, 1990, p. 4) because the nonverbal infant relies solely on the nurse's physical assessment and observational skills (Lepley, Gardner, and Lubchenco, 1993). Unfortunately, on July 21 this preterm infant was being cared for by a licensed practical nurse (LPN) and a graduate nurse (GN), *not* a professional registered nurse. Since neither the LPN nor the GN recognized the significance of the infant's clinical course or laboratory data, conclusions about the possibility of acquired infection were not formulated, nor was consultation sought with a supervising RN or the attending physician (ANA, 1983, 1985; NAACOG, 1991).

Diagnosis Even if aspects of the nursing process (e.g., assessment and implementation tasks) are delegated, the RN is legally (through state nurse practice acts) and professionally (through standards of practice) responsible for formulating nursing diagnoses and a plan of nursing care. Table 11-1 illustrates a proactive plan of care.

Planning Since "all nursing care must be provided by or under the direct supervision of a professional nurse" (NAACOG, 1990, p. 4), the assignment of an LPN or GN to care for this unstable ventilated preterm is in question. Nursing care must be delegated to a competent, knowledgeable, and qualified provider (Sullivan, 1994). Delegation of care by the RN must match the needs and acuity of the patient and the skill level of the caretaker. Certainly the supervising RN in this NICU bears the professional (ANA, 1985, 1991; NAACOG, 1991) and legal (state nurse practice act) responsibility for delegation of tasks after assessment of individual competence. As the charge or supervisory nurse, she also bears both professional and legal responsibility for direct supervision of those providing nursing care. Direct supervision of the LPN and GN by a competent RN would have provided earlier recognition and intervention for this infant's deteriorating condition.

Table 11-1 Proactive Nursing Care Plan

Patient Needs/ Nursing Diagnosis	Patient Outcomes	Nursing Interventions/ Collaborative Actions	Evaluation
Altered Tissue Perfusion: Peripheral related to placement of umbilical artery catheter (UAC)	Maintain/preserve tissue perfusion to lower extremities.	1. Verify catheter placement: Low placement: 3–4 High placement: 8.	Color in extremities remains pink.
		2. Assess lower extremities, upper legs, and buttocks q 1 hr for: color, perfusion, presence/absence of "catheter toes."	No blanching or blueness of extremities.
		3. Observe UAC and connections q 1 hr for patency.	No leakage of fluid or blood from UAC connections.
		4. Notify MD immediately for any change in color, pulses, notable changes in blood pressure.	
		5. If blanching occurs, remove UAC immediately; consider heparin therapy if blueness (mottling, cyanosis) present.	Circulation re-established and color returns to pink.
		6. If vasospasm occurs, apply warm wraps to opposite extremity, or to upper extremity if both legs are affected. Reheat wraps q 10–15 min until spasm resolves.	Reflex vasodilation re-establishes circulation and color of extremity is pink.
		7. Check peripheral pulses in lower extremities every shift by palpation or Doppler.	Pulses are easily palpated in extremities.
Risk for Infection related to: immature immune system; prematurity; presence of UAC	Infant remains free of infection.	1. Observe, document, and notify MD immediately of signs/symptoms of infection: • temperature instability (> or <) • respiratory distress (apnea, cyanosis, tachypnea) • lethargy/irritability • feeding difficulties (vomiting, increased residuals, abdominal distention) • increased jaundice • purpura/rashes/erythema • sclerema/pustules/omphalitis • pallor/cyanosis/mottling • hypotension • edema • tachycardia/dysrhythmias	No signs/symptoms of infection.
		2. Draw blood, assist with sepsis workup: • CBC, differential, platelet count • blood cultures • lumbar puncture: CSF glucose, protein, cell count, culture, gram stain • urinalysis, CIE or latex agglutination • urine culture	Cultures negative. CBC, WBC, differential WNL. Platelets 192–252,000. Lumbar puncture glucose 34–229 protein 20–170 gram stain negative.

Implementation Standards of nursing practice (ANA, 1983, 1991; NAACOG, 1990, 1991) require nurses to intervene, refer, collaborate, monitor, initiate, coordinate, supervise, consult, and carry out nursing care. The *Code for Nurses* (ANA, 1985) and NAACOG standards (NAACOG, 1991) require that nurses maintain competence, seek consultation, assume responsibility and accountability for individual nursing judgement and actions, and act as an advocate for the patient.

Competent nursing practice, requiring an understanding of the significance and ramifications of persistent hypothermia, demands not only documentation but also nursing interventions for low temperatures. Even though this neonate's central blood pressure values changed significantly (15–20 mm Hg) from previous levels, nursing corroboration of the validity of these values was not done. External measurements of extremity blood pressures, an evaluation of the blood pressure wave form (i.e., dampening related to transducer malfunction and / or thrombus formation) or a total change of the leaking transducer were interventions never documented (i.e., performed) or corroboration of true hypotension or equipment malfunction.

Nursing interventions include relaying all medically significant data to the physician in a timely fashion so as to prevent harm (Mandell, 1993). Less than 24 hours after the noninvestigated low WBC count, the nurses failed to recognize the clinical manifestations they documented as indicators of acquired infection. They did not report the skin lesions, edema, and discoloration of legs, abdomen, and buttocks to the physician in a timely fashion.

Patient advocacy requires the nurse to question, collaborate, and initiate action to safeguard the patient's care and safety (ANA, 1985). As advocates, this infant's nurses should have pointed out, questioned, confronted, challenged, initiated action, and consulted with the attending physician rather than resident physicians. Also, they should have invoked the chain of command at critical junctures in this infant's care: (a) If the significantly hypotensive values proved to be valid, why is this baby hypotensive? Is it hypovolemia due to hemorrhage, iatrogenic loss? Is the infant septic? (b) Is the WBC of 3.1 correct, or a lab error? What is the platelet count? Is this baby septic? Is a sepsis workup indicated? (c) Despite the presence of a low WBC count with signs and symptoms of infection, why was the removal of the UAC not accompanied by a sepsis workup and the initiation of antibiotic therapy? (d) What is the goal of wrapping the affected limb in warm compresses? Application of warm compresses to an extremity with circulatory compromise increases the basal metabolic rate and oxygen need and consumption, thus complicating cellular metabolism (Hodson & Belenky, 1975). If the goal is to increase circulation, the opposite lower extremity (provided that it is not affected) or the upper extremities should be warm-wrapped to obtain reflex vasodilation.

Evaluation Evaluation of nursing interventions directs reassessment, formulation of new diagnoses, and alterations in the plan and execution of nursing care. If nursing interventions are not enhancing patient outcomes, evaluation illuminates the needed changes in interventions for positive results (ANA, 1983, 1991; NAACOG, 1990, 1991). Evaluation criteria are outlined in Table 11-1.

Case 3

Respiratory diseases are the primary diagnosis found in infants admitted to level III nurseries. Many neonates suffering from respiratory illness are premature, but there is a population of post-term infants who suffer from other types of respiratory distress secondary to infection or meconium aspiration (Hagedorn, Gardner, & Abman, 1993).

Skilled placement of an endotracheal (ET) tube is key to the stabilization and ongoing management of infants with moderate to severe respiratory distress (Hagedorn, Gardner, & Abman, 1993). Optimal care of the infant with an ET tube requires that the nurse have expert skill in assessment and ongoing care (Hagedorn, Gardner, & Abman, 1993). Nurses must be able to determine that the tube is in appropriate position, and that with ongoing care it does not become displaced. If the tube should be dislodged or in incorrect placement without immediate intervention, long-term sequelae or death may occur (Hagedorn, Gardner, & Abman, 1993).

Facts

On December 19 at 0059, baby girl Bono was born in a community hospital with a level III nursery by emergency cesarean section to a G1 P0 mother whose due date was December 11. Birth weight was 7 lbs. 7 oz. (3370 grams) and the infant was 41 weeks AGA according to estimated gestational age scoring. Apgar scores were 2 at 1 minute and 3 at 5 minutes.

The pregnancy was described as uncomplicated and the mother was admitted on December 18 for prostaglandin induction. She was placed on oxytocin (Pitocin) and the labor was progressing. At 0020 on December 19, the mother received 10 mg of morphine sulfate for pain. Within minutes after morphine administration, significant variable decelerations to 50–60 beats were noted. The fetus developed persistent bradycardia for about 30–35 minutes (0025–0030) prior to the cesarean. The infant was delivered by emergency cesarean and noted to have no tone, respiratory effort, pale color, and a heart rate <100 beats per minute. The anesthesiologist, Dr. Kay, ordered 0.2 mg of naloxone (Narcan) to be given IM. The infant was bag and mask ventilated (with no manometer in place) by anesthesia and a family practice physician. When the infant's condition did not improve (Apgar 3 at 5 min), Dr. Kay orally intubated the infant with a 3.0 ET tube. The tube was suctioned for a moderate amount of fluid and bag ventilation was continued. Labor and Delivery (L&D) called a neonatologist, Dr. Door, to come immediately. Dr. Door ordered (over the telephone) chest X ray, capillary blood gas (CBG), and CBC with differential and asked the nurse to call back with information. A second call was made to Dr. Door to come immediately. Dr.

Door then called Dr. Rollo to come immediately. L&D made a third call to summon a neonatologist. The following sequencing of events then occurred:

December 19:

0115: Color poor, no tone, no respiratory effort, (+) grimace; Dr. Kay continued to bag ventilate infant.
0120: Color pale pink, minimal chest wall expansion, HR >120, (+) breath sounds on right; little movement on left (anesthesiologist told about these findings); few spontaneous breaths with retractions. Dr. Kay continued bagging ET tube; Narcan 0.2 mg IM repeated.
0125: Color mottled, HR >100, breath sounds unequal right greater than left; infant limp, (+) grimace (these findings reported to Dr. Kay). Dr. Kay repositioned ET tube and suctioned. Slight improvement noted on left side. Charge nurse of NICU came to L&D to tell Dr. Kay that infant needed to be brought to NICU immediately. After requesting ventilator settings, the nurse was told that they had no manometer on the bag. Dr. Kay ordered ventilator settings.
0130: RN picked up and carried infant to the NICU and placed her under radiant warmer. First vital signs: T 36.3, HR 170, R 60, BP 78/44, mean 57. Infant placed on ventilator with the following settings: 100% oxygen, PIP 20, PEEP 5, and Rate 60. Breath sounds decreased on auscultation; chest wall not expanding. Nurse requested extubation; Dr. Kay said no; gave 0.3 mg Narcan. Oxygen saturation 80–82.
0140: NICU nurses' notes: no respiratory effort, no tone, very pale, HR 152, (+) grimace, BP 69/58 (a decrease).
0145: The neonatologist, Dr. Rollo, arrived (46 minutes after the birth)! CBG results indicated a combined respiratory and metabolic acidosis: pH 6.96, Po_2 60, Pco_2 65, HCO_3 15, BE –17. Dr. Rollo documented a large air leak.
0150: Dr. Rollo extubated and attempted nasal reintubation × 2.
0200: Infant orally intubated with 3.5 ET tube.
0210: Umbilical artery catheter (UAC) placed.
0220: Umbilical venous catheter (UVC) placed.
0225: Infant moving about; over about a 30-minute period after reintubation, infant's Fio_2 was decreased from 100% to 54% with pulse oximetry readings >94%.
0230: Chest X ray ordered.
0235: Decreasing blood pressure 48/24; 37/LL.
0245: 35 mL albumin given over 40 minutes.
0310: T 37. UAC blood gas: pH 7.58, Po_2 65, Pco_2 16, BE –3.
0400: "Arms tightening"; Sao_2 <92%. Dr. Rollo notified; 50 mg phenobarbital IV; O_2 sat >97%.
0430: Seizure activity noted; 30 mg phenobarbital IV.
0455: Seizure activity continued; 1 mg dilantin (Phenytoin sodium) IV. ET tube suctioned for large amounts of pink secretions.
0500: Infant continued to seize; repeat chest X ray showed ET tube just above carina.
0505: Dilantin 50 mg given IV; ET tube pulled back.

0530: Infant continued to seize; 0.3 mg of Pavulon (pancuronium) given IV push.
0540: Infant continued to seize; 0.3 mg of Pavulon given IV push.
0600–0700: Oxygen adjusted from 97% to 94%.
0920: Seizure activity noted; Pavulon 0.3 mg given.
Throughout rest of the day when infant had seizure activity, Pavulon 0.3 mg was given (this occurred every 2–3 hours).

December 20:
0100–0800: Ventilator FiO_2 decreased to 32%; rate to 47; Pavulon 0.3 mg given × 2.
0830: Lorazepam (Ativan) given for seizure activity.
0900–1300: Pavulon given × 2. Albumin given × 1 over an hour.
1400: Head ultrasound done.
1505: Lorazepam given for seizure activity.
1530: Antibiotics started (Amcill [Ampicillin] and Gentamicin [Garamycin]).

Over the next several days, baby girl Bono's respiratory status gradually improved. She was extubated on the afternoon of December 27. An initial EEG performed on December 20 revealed extensive sharp activity bihemispherically. A second EEG performed on January 3 revealed activity within normal limits. Baby girl Bono remained on anticonvulsants and Pavulon until December 23, when Pavulon was discontinued. She remained on phenobarbital until December 28, when a level of 43 was noted, and the drug was not restarted. The infant's tone was hypotonic throughout the hospitalization, with a diminished suck/swallow which gradually improved over the hospitalization with intervention from speech therapy and occupational therapy; she was able to nipple feed by discharge on January 18.

Outcome

This child is multiply handicapped, with severe developmental delays and cerebral palsy.

Legal

Three years after the birth, the parents are still in litigation for long-term sequelae from perinatal asphyxia.

Case Commentary

Undesirable Patient Outcome

Assessment Nursing assessments documented significant clinical data: (a) persistent hypoxia, (b) questionable ET tube placement, (c) decreasing blood pressure indicating volume deficit, (d) seizure activity that continued for several hours into the next day. The fact that it took 46 minutes (in a level III nursery) for a neonatologist to arrive to care for the infant was obviously of great concern to the nurses who made several attempts to summon help from a neonatologist.

Diagnosis Several nursing diagnoses appeared in the chart and were frequently updated:

Impaired Gas Exchange related to asphyxia
Fluid Volume Deficit related to post dates
Risk for Infection related to invasive procedures
Altered Parenting related to NICU status and illness
Alteration in Neurological Function
Risk for Altered Nutrition related to poor suck

Planning Ongoing plan of care appeared in chart and was updated on a weekly basis. Interventions were documented shift by shift.

Implementation The lack of response by a neonatologist in the early resuscitation and stabilization period jeopardized the long-term outcome of this infant. The nurse questioned the placement of the tube and requested an extubation, but was denied by the anesthesiologist. No further intervention was attempted by nurses until the neonatologist arrived. The nurses made three attempts to summon a neonatologist to L&D. There was no further documented attempt to summon backup when these attempts were unsuccessful. After an unorganized attempt to resuscitate the infant for over 20 minutes in the delivery room, a nurse carried the infant to the NICU, exposing her to cold stress and further compounding the stress she was experiencing.

Once the infant arrived in the nursery, she was further stressed with two attempts at nasal intubation prior to a successful oral intubation. No IV line was in place for almost 3 hours after delivery.

Evaluation Despite nursing interventions to support oxygenation and ventilation, this infant continued to have hypoxia, decreased respiratory effort, poor tone, poor color, and a borderline heart rate. A skilled resuscitation team was not present for this high-risk delivery. Ongoing monitoring of the oxygenation of the infant did not occur in the delivery room. Pressures via bag resuscitation were not monitored because no manometer was in place.

Once the infant arrived in the NICU, stabilization and management began to occur, but several laboratory studies were delayed. The next three weeks were spent treating the sequelae of birth asphyxia.

Desirable Patient Outcome

Assessment Nursing care of the high-risk neonate starts with anticipation and identification of potential problems (NAACOG, 1991). Initial assessment must include: (a) a review of perinatal history, (b) physical assessment, (c) vital signs (temperature, pulse, respiration, and blood pressure), (d) estimation of gestational age, and (e) interpretation of routine and indicated laboratory tests (NAACOG, 1990, 1991). A review of the infant's perinatal history reveals several factors of concern that could have contributed to her increased risk for respiratory depression at birth: (a) induction of labor with Pitocin, (b) post gestational dates, (c) use of narcotics to control maternal labor pain, (d) signs of prolonged fetal distress, and (e) emergency delivery by cesarean (Olds, London, & Ladewig, 1996).

The standards of nursing practice require the nurse to identify life threatening events and emergency situations (NAACOG, 1990). The ongoing variable decelerations and persistent bradycardia required immediate intervention, certainly not monitoring for incidence of over 35 minutes. An emergency cesarean requires organization and the presence of a skilled resuscitation team (AAP-ACOG, 1992). Where was this skilled resuscitation team?

Diagnosis Appropriate nursing diagnoses were identified; however, the nursing diagnoses should reflect etiologies in which nurses can intervene. The first diagnosis, *Impaired Gas Exchange* related to asphyxia, is inappropriately written and combines a nursing and medical diagnosis. Asphyxia is a medical diagnosis and can only be confirmed with an arterial blood gas (ABG). Appropriate nursing diagnoses include:

Impaired Gas Exchange related to lack of spontaneous respirations secondary to aspiration
Fluid Volume Deficit related to NPO status and increased insensible water loss
Risk for Infection related to multiple invasive lines and invasive procedures
Altered Family Process related to unexpected NICU stay
Altered Tissue Perfusion: Cerebral related to decreased oxygenation secondary to birth asphyxia
Altered Nutrition: Less than Body Requirements related to ineffective nippling of formula

Planning Nursing management in the NICU violated the standard of care by not having written policies, procedures, and protocols readily accessible to clarify nursing's role in removing an ET tube when positioning or patency is questionable (NAACOG, 1991). The nurses should have followed a "chain of command" when summoning neonatal backup (in less than 46 minutes!) for a severely depressed infant. This infant required skilled resuscitation, stabilization, and management (AAP-ACOG, 1992; Golden & Peters, 1993). Skilled resuscitation also includes appropriate equipment (i.e., a bag with manometer to monitor pressures necessary to ventilate the infant).

Implementation Specific measurable interventions, outcomes, and evaluation criteria are delineated in the *Standards for the nursing care of women and newborns* (NAACOG, 1991) and require the nurse to: (a) provide and maintain neutral thermal environment; (b) establish and maintain cardiopulmonary function; (c) perform indicated lab tests; (d) establish parenteral therapy to provide and maintain fluid and electrolyte balance; (e) assist with technical procedures as delineated by policies, procedures, and protocols; (f) utilize laboratory (and other) diagnostic data in providing care; (g) initiate and maintain oxygen and respiratory therapy; (h) monitor nutritional status and provide nutrition; and (i) intervene in emergency situations following written policies and procedures. These guidelines require the nurse to "use interventional strategies that maintain current standards of nursing practice" (NAACOG, 1990, p. 5).

When the first two doses of Narcan failed to reverse the infant's respiratory depression, why was a third dose administered? The administration of morphine and the incidence of decelerations may seem to have some relationship, but when the infant did not revive after administration of Narcan, why were two more doses given?

A key nursing intervention in this case should have been the establishment and ongoing support of cardiopulmonary function. This infant had no spontaneous respirations and a probable misplaced tube that was further compromising respiratory status. A skilled nurse would have acted on the assessment of decreased breath sounds (on the left side) by summoning a physician, assisting with the repositioning of the tube, and/or extubation and reintubation of the infant if necessary (Table 11-2). Appropriate resuscitation equipment was not available in the delivery room for resuscitation of this infant. It took almost 3 hours to establish an intravenous line to provide

Table 11-2 Complications of Endotracheal Intubation

Complication	Comments
Immediate	
Malposition	
• Too low	Usually in right mainstem bronchus; no or diminished breath sounds in left chest or upper right lobe; asymetrical chest movement; atelectasis. (Withdraw tube until breath sounds are heard bilaterally and equally.)
• Too high	Inadequate ventilation bilaterally, especially at lung bases.
• Esophagus	Air movement auscultated in stomach with no or inadequate breath sounds.
Obstruction	
• Plug	Partial—no change or diminished breath sounds audible. Complete—distant or no breath sounds audible.
• Kinking of the tube	Flexion or extension of the head results in diminished or blocked air flow.
• Head position	
Perforation	
• Vocal cords	
• Trachea	
• Pharynx	
• Esophagus	
Infection	
Air leak	
Increased intracranial pressure	
Postextubation	
• Migratory lobar collapse	Prevent and treat with pulmonary hygiene.
• Diffuse microatelectasis	In very low birth weight infants, may be associated with apnea; treatable by pulmonary hygiene or nasal CPAP, or both.
Long Term	
General	Vocal cord inflammation, stenosis, and eventual dysfunction; tracheoesophageal fistula; subglottic stenosis; tracheal inflammation and stenosis; contributes to bronchopulmonary dysplasia.

Adapted from: Hagedorn, M., Gardner, S., & Abman, S. (1993). Respiratory diseases. In G. Merenstein & S. Gardner (Eds.), *Handbook of neonatal intensive care*, 3rd ed. (p. 328). St. Louis: Mosby-Yearbook. Adapted by permission.

fluids to her. The *Code of Ethics* (ANA, 1985) requires nurses to advocate for the client's safety and care. Nursing advocacy was absent during the crucial period of delivery which resulted in life-long sequelae for this patient.

Infants require thermoregulatory interventions to prevent cold stress (Blake & Murray, 1993). This infant was transported in the arms of a nurse to the NICU. She should have been transported in a warm isolette/transporter (Golden & Peters, 1993).

Nurses ultimately have legal and ethical accountability for actions taken and judgments made (ANA, 1985) regardless of the action or lack of action taken by physicians. The nurses in this case should have: (a) referred to hospital protocols relating to skilled resuscitation measures; (b) operationalized the chain of command when physician response did not occur; (c) questioned, confronted, and challenged the physician on ET tube placement; and (d) removed the ET tube and provided bag or mask ventilation until skilled personnel could reintubate (Hagedorn, Gardner, & Abman, 1993).

Evaluation Continued hypoxia and lack of spontaneous respirations validate the ineffectiveness of interventions and require the nurse to redirect, reassess, and revise interventions (questioning the placement of the ET tube). This infant's symptoms failed to subside; furthermore, she experienced ongoing stressors such as cold stress, fluid volume deficit, etc. These ongoing symptoms should have resulted in a reassessment and revision of the plan.

Nursing's inaction resulted in prolonged hypoxia in this infant and legal accountability for violation of the standards of care. The long-term sequelae may well have been avoided.

References

American Academy of Pediatrics-American College of Obstetrics and Gynecology. (1992). *Guidelines for perinatal care,* 3rd ed. Washington, D.C.: Author.

American Nurses Association. (1983). *Standards of maternal-child health nursing practice.* Washington, D.C.: Author.

American Nurses Association. (1985). *Code for nurses.* Washington, D.C.: Author.

American Nurses Association. (1991). *Standards of clinical nursing practice.* Washington, D.C.: Author.

Blake, W. & Murray, J. (1993). Heat balance. In G. Merenstein & S. Gardner (Eds.), *Handbook of neonatal intensive care,* 3rd ed. (pp. 100–115). St. Louis: Mosby-Yearbook.

Golden, S. & Peters, D. (1993). Delivery room care. In G. Merenstein & S. Gardner (Eds.), *Handbook of neonatal intensive care,* 3rd ed. (pp. 55–76). St. Louis: Mosby-Yearbook.

Hagedorn, M., Gardner, S., & Abman, S. (1993). Respiratory diseases. In G. Merenstein & S. Gardner (Eds.), *Handbook of neonatal intensive care,* 3rd ed. (pp. 311–364). St. Louis: Mosby-Yearbook.

Hodson, W. & Belenky, D. (1975). Management of respiratory problems. In G. Avery (Ed.), *Neonatology* (pp. 265–294). Philadelphia: Lippincott.

Lepley, C., Gardner, S., & Lubchenco, L. (1993). Initial nursing care. In G. Merenstein & S. Gardner (Eds.), *Handbook of neonatal intensive care* 3rd ed. (pp. 76–99). St. Louis: Mosby-Yearbook.

Lubchenco, L. & Bard, H. (1971). Incidence of hypoglycemia in newborn infants classified by birth weights and gestational age. *Pediatrics, 47,* 831–835.

Mandell, M. (1993). What you don't say can hurt you. *American Journal of Nursing, 93,* 15–16.

McGowan, J., Hagedorn, M., Price, W., and Hay, W. (1993). Glucose homeostasis. In G. Merenstein & S. Gardner (Eds.), *Handbook of neonatal intensive care,* 3rd ed. (pp. 127–140). St. Louis: Mosby-Yearbook.

Nurses' Association of the American College of Obstetricians and Gynecologists. (1990). *Nurse providers of neonatal care.* Washington, D.C.: Author.

Nurses' Association of the American College of Obstetricians and Gynecologists. (1991). *Standards for the nursing care of women and newborns,* 4th ed. Washington, D.C.: Author.

Olds, S., London, M., & Ladewig, P. (1996). *Maternal-newborn nursing,* 5th ed. Menlo Park, CA: Addison-Wesley Nursing.

Pierce, J. & Turner, B. (1993). Physiologic monitoring. In G. Merenstein & S. Gardner (Eds.), *Handbook of neonatal intensive care,* 3rd ed. (pp. 115–127). St. Louis: Mosby-Yearbook.

Rao, H. & Elhassani, S. (1980). Iatrogenic complications of procedures performed on the newborn, Part I: Intravascular procedures. *Perinatology - Neonatology, 4,* 25–31.

12

Outpatient Pediatric Care

Mary I. Enzman Hagedorn, RN, PhD, CNS, CPNP
Margaret M. Burns, RN, PhD
Sandra L. Gardner, RN, MS, CNS, PNP
Ellen Dore, RN, MS

Because of changes in the health care delivery systems that provide patient care, risk-management concerns are starting to shift to the outpatient care setting. Health care systems are integrating more clinics, ambulatory care centers, home care facilities, surgical centers, and outpatient operations (Japsen, 1994). The number of medical and nursing research studies conducted in pediatric ambulatory settings is increasing as well (Chamorro & Tarulli, 1990). Pediatric ambulatory care settings are becoming larger and serving a wider range of clients. To care for this ever increasing population, nurses are being asked to expand both their scope of practice and knowledge. A myriad of patient needs and complexities also accompany these changes. Institutions with ambulatory care systems are leaving themselves vulnerable to lawsuits by ignoring the uncharted areas of risk brought about by these changes (Japsen, 1994).

With these changes come the concern for the adequacy of these settings and the nursing skills required to provide this comprehensive care. Sound risk-management programs that include nursing standards, nursing protocols, and active quality-improvement/outcome studies are not routinely established in these sites. Nursing orientation and training programs are another deficiency found in the ambulatory care setting. Many new hirees are inexperienced in outpatient care (Chamorro & Tarulli, 1990).

Nurses in these settings must assume greater legal accountability for their actions as they emerge from the protective legal shadow of the physician and the health care facility. Sound risk-management practices must be established to minimize adverse effects from care provided to the patient. These are listed in the box on p. 202. Risk-management strategies are significant not only for the facility but also for the individual physician, nurse practitioner, or nurse who is concerned with personal protection from incidents and liability that lead to litigation (Chamorro & Tarulli, 1990). Anticipation of some of the more sensitive areas, increased awareness, and appropriate strategies may help the individual nurse clinician in limiting liability in the pediatric ambulatory care setting (Table 12-1).

Risk-Management Strategies for Enhancing Professional Accountability in the Pediatric Ambulatory Care Setting

Employment Parameters

- Evaluation of skills competency within the interview process
- Role descriptions/performance standards reflect actual practice
- Comprehensive orientation program including competency-training
- Individual records of competency-training/mandatory inservice-training as well as continuing education
- Training in medical devices and easy access to manuals containing standards of practice/procedures/protocols

Patient Care

- More interface with public; therefore the need to be courteous and attentive to patient concerns
- Protocols directing status/triaging of patient in the ambulatory care setting
- Patient care protocols for common diagnosis/illness treatment
- Patient admission and discharge criteria well-defined
- Sharp patient assessment and history-taking skills that integrate clinical pertinence (e.g., allergies, immunization status, medication list)
- Assurance that patients properly informed before treatment
- Prompt attention to diverse levels of care
- Request/authorization for medical records
- Assessment of cumulative effects of drugs in individuals
- Follow protocols/standards for medication administration
- Impeccable attention to universal precautions
- Monitoring and evaluation of patient status, reporting any change in patient status and performing appropriate and timely nursing assessments, interventions, and education
- Intervene if improper order or care, using chain of command
- Efficient/effective documentation system and accurate charting
- Guidelines for effective communication to evaluate patient-care status with physician
- Concise instructions for patient-administered treatments, medications, and equipment (i.e., written home care sheets directing the above patient-administered care)
- Protocols in place for telephone advice, triage, medical management, and follow-up care
- Guidelines for patients leaving without being seen or missed appointments
- Clear guidelines for follow-up care
- Guidelines for ongoing care and discharge of patients receiving medications that alter consciousness, and advice for performance of normal activities
- Guidelines for patient transfer to a different care setting

Professional Issues

- Open lines of communication and regard for patient/family input
- Foster excellent public relations
- Keep apprised of ever-changing pediatric care modalities in nursing literature
- Ongoing self- and peer-evaluation regarding provision of care, professional competency, and job performance
- Ongoing quality-improvement activities

Table 12-1 Common Litigation Situations in Pediatric Outpatient Nursing

Frequent Allegations	Prevention Tips for Nurses	Prevention Tips for Setting
Failure to ensure patient safety (toys, play, equipment)	1. Monitor patient in a timely manner. 2. Provide assistance for those patients who require it (use of toilet/bathtub). 3. Assess family capabilities to care for child. 4. Keep side rails raised for patients who are medicated or need supervision for ambulation. 5. Evaluate environmental risks. 6. Use appropriate restraint devices. 7. Provide age-appropriate toys.	1. Maintain adequate ratio and competency of staff. 2. Educate staff in age-appropriate techniques for performance of interventions.
Improper treatment or performance of treatment	1. Question interventions deemed improper. 2. Use proper techniques when performing treatments. 3. Follow outpatient guidelines when performing treatments. 4. Seek consultation for treatments beyond your scope of practice. 5. Update professional skills through continuing education.	1. Design a clear procedure for nurses to follow if medical treatment is inappropriate. 2. Provide resources for nurses to consult regarding treatments. 3. Provide appropriate procedures for nursing treatments. 4. Ensure a competency-based program to evaluate nursing skills. 5. Ensure consistency of performance standards of interventions across clinical areas.
Failure to monitor and report	1. Follow prescribed orders regarding monitoring of patients. 2. Report any requested information or significant changes in a patient's condition. 3. Perform appropriate and timely nursing assessments.	1. Verify nursing assessment skills. 2. Maintain an adequate nurse-patient ratio. 3. Establish a system to ensure prompt documentation of physician orders. 4. Provide for delegation of skills to appropriately trained staff.
Medication errors and reactions	1. Verify any questionable patient care orders. 2. Verify 5 R's of medication administration and allergy status. 3. Obtain history of patient's present medications and allergies. 4. Use references/resources to validate dosage, adverse effects, and usage.	1. Provide a clear policy on verbal and written medication orders. 2. Provide reference materials for medication administration. 3. Provide inservice education on medications and clear protocols regarding their administration.
Failure to follow outpatient procedure	1. Develop and revise policies and procedures in the outpatient setting. 2. Know your outpatient procedures. 3. If you must deviate from a procedure, discuss the incident with your supervisor and decide on the appropriate actions.	1. Provide necessary policies and procedures that are clear and concise. 2. Conduct ongoing quality-assurance programs that ensure compliance with outpatient policies and. procedures. 3. Conduct ongoing risk-management programs to evaluate outpatient programs.
Faulty equipment use	1. Know how to operate equipment in a safe and appropriate manner. 2. In teaching patients to use equipment, follow predetermined procedures with patient return-demonstration. 3. Provide patients with names of resource agencies where they can obtain medical durable equipment. 4. Coordinate referrals with home care agency if necessary. 5. Conduct routine equipment inventory and checks to evaluate proper functioning.	1. Provide competency-based learning for all equipment. 2. Have a system in place for documentation of ongoing education for equipment usage. 3. Verify that agency employees and personnel know equipment before assigning them to a particular patient or area.

(Continued)

Table 12-1 Common Litigation Situations in Pediatric Outpatient Nursing *(Continued)*

Frequent Allegations	Prevention Tips for Nurses	Prevention Tips for Setting
Inappropriate or insufficient documentation	1. Document significant information about your patients objectively and factually. 2. Be time-specific about the information, documenting when you performed actions, observations, or performed patient made assessments. 3. Document legibly, spell correctly, and only use organization-approved abbreviations. 4. Provide ongoing documentation of phone triage. 5. Provide documentation on discharge planning and follow-up care.	1. Provide effective methods of charting such as flow charts or computerized charting. 2. Develop critical care pathways and treatment protocols that can be customized to individual patient situations. 3. Utilize quality-improvement programs to evaluate and enhance patient care.

Potential liability in independent settings where nurses practice (e.g., clinics, emergency or after-hours centers, homes) are derived from: (a) employment parameters, (b) patient care, and (c) professional issues. An increasing number of litigations against home health agencies are focusing on the agency's responsibility to hire, train, and monitor employees appropriately (Hogue, 1992). Outpatient health care agencies need to design a system of checks and balances with a pre-employment screening and probationary period to evaluate the skills and knowledge of new employees. In home care and freestanding outpatient care models, most employees are away from the agency or alone, leaving providers in an extremely vulnerable position regarding acts of omission or incomplete decision-making or documentation (Sussman & Siegel, 1991). An organized, comprehensive orientation program that ensures competency of personnel in the provision of patient care, appropriate use of equipment, and the safe administration of medications and treatments must be provided. Ongoing evaluation must occur and a system devised to update skills and educate staff on new treatments and equipment as they are introduced.

All nurses practicing in the same specialty area are responsible for standards of care established for that specialty area regardless of the size of or services provided for the patient population (Allen, 1991). Adherence to accepted standards of nursing practice is a legal and professional responsibility (ANA, 1991). Failure to meet established standards places the nurse in a position of litigation and the patient in extreme danger (Allen, 1991). The nurse is ultimately responsible for the provision of care for patients with a variety of complex health care needs. Risk-management strategies include the comprehensive use of the nursing process from introduction of the patient to the system, as well as ongoing provision of patient education and care. Consistency is enhanced in these patient populations through the use of standards, protocols, and guidelines that guide the care and its documentation (Chamorro & Tarulli, 1990).

Professional issues in the outpatient setting include: (a) communication and regard for patient/family input, (b) fostering excellent public relations,

(c) ongoing self- and peer-evaluation, and (d) quality improvement activities. Key to these issues are the ongoing relationships the nurse maintains, particularly with the clients and families she encounters. In the inpatient setting, control often lies with the institution and its personnel; however, power and control of health care issues in the outpatient setting shifts to the client and family. Professional boundaries are less clear and the vulnerability of the provider to litigious situations increases. This in turn promotes a greater need for peer support and critique which can improve the care and decision-making process of each individual nurse.

The overall goals in pediatric outpatient settings include: (a) advocating for the client and family; (b) ensuring client and family awareness of services and programs available to support and promote health; (c) ongoing education concerning care, equipment, and treatments; and (d) encouragement to support or change existing health care practices. Medico-legal risk management in the outpatient setting is emerging. The development of risk-management programs in the outpatient pediatric setting can prevent situations leading to litigation and encourage the identification and ongoing evaluation of care provided in this setting.

This chapter presents three cases of nursing liability in outpatient pediatric care settings. The first case discusses an adolescent who was provided insufficient and ineffective care while participating as a subject in a research protocol. The second case demonstrates how crucial appropriate management and education is to a febrile infant. The last case discusses boundaries and legal responsibilities to advocate for the child in a home care setting.

Case 1

Facts

Nathan was a 15-year-old male who was being followed in an outpatient, research-based facility within a hospital for treatment of his asthma. Nathan had a family history of asthma, known parental smoking in the home, and exposure to a cat and dog. Nathan had a long-term history of asthma which was treated with Theophylline, Albuterol, Cromolyn, Bronkosol, and Vanceril. His parents were separated, but Nathan spent time with both. In his first visit to this facility, at age 11, Nathan was seen for ongoing laryngitis. On exam, it was noted that he had slight swelling of hypopharynx and viral laryngitis with possible upper tracheitis. This diagnosis was validated with laryngoscopy. Nathan was referred back to his private physician for follow-up care.

Four years later, Nathan was seen again at this facility, in the research center, for potential participation in a study. Preliminary skin testing was performed. Positive results for a peanut allergy provided the stage for entrance into a double-blind research study aimed at determining the effects of rush therapy (ongoing exposure to an allergen) in building an immunity towards this allergen over time. This study had three phases: In the first phase, each patient was to receive injections of peanut extract (the allergen). Once the subjects were determined to have sensitivity to the peanut extract, they entered the second phase of the study, where they would be divided into an experimental and control group. The experimental group received peanut extract. The control group would receive a placebo injection which contained a histamine. In the third phase of the study, subjects would receive post-rush therapy through maintenance injections of the peanut extract to build immunity. It was in the third phase of the study that the following incident occurred.

During the first phase of the research, Nathan was determined to have sensitivity to peanuts and also noted to have mild respiratory distress with several injections, requiring rescue treatment with medications (epinephrine and Benadryl). He had no difficulties in the second phase, since he was receiving the placebo. This was unknown to the researchers because of double-blinding.

On a Sunday morning in July, Nathan, accompanied by his mother, came to the research center to receive a third maintenance injection as part of the third phase of this research protocol. The research center was a series of offices in a remote area of the outpatient center, down the hall from the urgent care unit. Two prior maintenance doses had been given a week apart without adverse response. Nathan was to receive the third injection along with two other research subjects. Dr. Odie, a pulmonologist, and his research assistant (a young woman with no medical background) were the only personnel present in this setting with these three subjects. The following sequencing of events occurred:

0900–0915: Nathan and two other study subjects arrived for their injection.
0915: One subject, a female, was given her injection after baseline patient assessment was performed.
0930: Dr. Odie performed baseline vital signs and a peak flow study, then gave Nathan his injection. Nathan had an immediate response to the injection, complaining of shortness of breath. Dr. Odie's response was to perform another peak flow study. After discovering that this peak flow was 130 (1/4 of the beginning measurement, which was 520), indicating extreme respiratory distress, Dr. Odie asked Nathan to self-administer his inhaler. Dr. Odie then applied a tourniquet to the injection site (per protocol) and gave an injection of epinephrine 0.3 mL (at the site of injection).
0932: When Nathan did not respond, Dr. Odie instructed the research assistant to administer another dose of epinephrine 0.3 mL into the other arm.
0935: Dr. Odie then asked the research assistant to call for help. He first asked her to call the adult intensive care unit (rather than the urgent care unit which was a short distance away). Nathan's condition continued to deteriorate, with increased throat tightness, and then he collapsed. Dr. Odie yelled to the research assistant to call a COR-0. The research assistant, unsure of the procedure of calling a COR-0, called the operator by dialing 0 instead of 5555 (which was the COR-0 number at this center). After this, the research assistant dropped the phone and ran to the urgent care unit to summon help. Dr. Odie initiated mouth-to-mouth resuscitation.
0945: Two RNs from the urgent care unit responded, bringing the crash cart.

Upon arrival, one nurse began cardiac compressions and Dr. Odie began to administer bag and mask ventilation. The other nurse applied EKG leads. Minimal electrical activity was captured on the monitor (an indeterminable heart rate). Dr. Odie then told the second RN to call the adult critical care area for back-up assistance.
0950: An adult intensive care nurse responded to the phone call and started an IV line. Meanwhile, because Sam Smith, a technician in the pulmonary department, and Dr. Miller were standing at the phone operator's desk, they overheard the phone call and rushed to the scene. Sam Smith attempted an intubation. Dr. Odie had not attempted intubation, saying he wanted the most skilled individual to try.
0950–1010: Sam Smith continued with several attempts to intubate Nathan. This process was complicated by the extreme edematous state of the patient (to the extent of obliteration of features) and his repeated vomiting.
1010: Dr. Dill, an adult lung specialist, was the next physician to arrive on the scene. When he assessed the difficulty of the intubation process, he decided to perform a tracheostomy and upon request was handed a new tracheostomy setup, one he was not familiar with. He made several attempts, feeling the trachea collapse each time he tried to push through. The estimated length of these attempts was 20–25 minutes.
1025: Dr. Little entered the pediatric critical care unit (several floors away from the research center), heard about the incident, and immediately proceeded to the research center. On the way, he encountered Dr. Mae, a second pediatric critical care intensivist, and asked him to proceed to the center with him.
1030: Upon their arrival, Dr. Mae successfully intubated Nathan on his first attempt with a small endotracheal (ET) tube (*one hour* into the COR-0!). After intubation, breath sounds were unequal and a pleural tap was performed by Dr. Wood, another pulmonary physician, to attempt air evacuation. No pneumothorax was present. Because of the small tube, a large air leak was noted.
1035: One ampule of sodium bicarbonate ($NaHCO_3$) was given via ET tube, without a blood gas reading. A dose of epinephrine was also given by ET tube and attempts for central line placement were made. At this time, ventricular fibrillation was detected on the cardiac monitor. Nathan was then defibrillated four times.
1038: After the fourth shock, a pulse was detected. An arterial blood gas was obtained which revealed a mixed severe respiratory and metabolic acidosis with a pH of 6.7, a low P_{O_2}, and a high P_{CO_2}. Two additional ampules of $NaHCO_3$ were given by ET tube. Ms. Hiliary, the nursing supervisor, arrived on the scene and contacted a local children's hospital to transport Nathan for further care in a tertiary center.
1110: The children's transport team arrived at the research center and further stabilized Nathan for transport.
1130: Nathan was rushed in critical condition to the local children's hospital.
1130–0151: Over the course of the next 14 hours, Nathan received intensive care services at the children's hospital.

Outcome

Nathan died of complications at 0151 (approximately 14 1/2 hours later).

Legal

This case was settled out of court for an undisclosed amount.

Case Commentary

Undesirable Patient Outcome

This outpatient case is an example of a "high risk" situation patients might encounter when they participate in research. This adolescent was willing to participate in the research, yet may not have been thoroughly knowledgeable about the risk factors involved. In this situation, with only a physician present, it is possible that informed consent was not obtained. If the study had been explained thoroughly, perhaps Nathan or his mother may not have consented to an injection of a potentially lethal test dose on a Sunday morning, when fewer medical personnel were present. Dr. Odie, who was carrying out this research protocol, was the only "qualified" medical practitioner present, and yet he was ill-equipped to manage airway difficulties. This alone should have alerted him of the need to perform the injections in a controlled environment where emergency equipment and skilled backup were available. The fact that he was the *lone* medical personnel performing this research is litigious at best. His research assistant didn't even know how to access the COR-0 team through the operator (she called the operator as if she were needing phone assistance).

Assessment The nurses' role in this case was peripheral until the time that they responded and intervened. Seeing the graveness of the situation, the two responding nurses needed to *immediately summon* skilled, *pediatric* medical personnel familiar with pediatric airway management to perform an intubation. They instead followed the request of the physician and called the adult critical care unit. All of the actors in this situation arrived coincidentally as they heard of the issues at hand (i.e., Dr. Miller and Sam Smith became aware of the situation serendipitously as they stood at the desk speaking with the hospital operator; Dr. Dill was on the adult floor and heard about the incident and responded; Dr. Little was told after entering the pediatric critical care unit and, while responding, ran into Dr. Mae and asked him to accompany him). After review of the case, it was revealed that the call to initiate the COR-0 was never appropriately made, therefore no "real" COR-0 was called. Physicians arrived on the scene through word of mouth and phone calls to units.

Diagnosis No nursing diagnosis existed, because there was only emergency contact with this patient. However, prior contact with this patient indicated adverse responses to the allergen and should have resulted in documentation of this history and development of medical diagnoses and nursing diagnoses to alert those performing future injections of this adolescent's potential responses.

Planning Nurses entering the scene did not appropriately respond or summon qualified medical personnel in a timely manner. Nurses did not summon appropriate personnel via the emergency access system which resulted in a *45-minute* delay in obtaining appropriate personnel.

Implementation No planned nursing interventions occurred. Nurses did begin CPR and supported medical intervention, but the documentation of this process was scant, leaving one to wonder what really happened sequentially.

Evaluation Although nurses were not involved initially, upon responding and evaluating the graveness of the situation, they did not access appropriate resources in a timely manner. The nurses did not advocate for safe care of this adolescent.

Desirable Patient Outcome

Assessment An area of liability in medical research is informed consent. While it is the physician who orders treatment, nurses often enter into the responsibility for ensuring that informed consent has been obtained (Chamorro & Tarulli, 1990). No system appeared to be in place that ensured informed consent in this situation. (No nurse was involved in this research project.)

A nurse did not *immediately* assess the skill level of each participant. When the first two nurses arrived, one should have assessed how the COR-0 call had been executed and if skilled help was indeed responding. (One would have to question the medical judgment of a physician who was managing an adolescent who had had prior respiratory responses to injections in a remote area with no other medical backup or emergency equipment.) Although the nurses responded with the COR-0 cart, they should have minimally put in another COR-0 call, and asked someone to call the *pediatric* critical care area to summon help. Nathan should have been moved immediately to the urgent care unit where equipment and personnel were available, and access to him and to equipment could have been optimized. Clearly this adolescent needed a pediatric specialist skilled at intubation!

Standards of Maternal-Child Health Nursing Practice require nurses to promote "an environment free from hazards to reproduction, growth and development, wellness, and recovery from illness" (ANA, 1983, p. 8). The nurse "identifies actual or potential hazards to maintenance of health" (ANA, 1983, p. 8). Conducting research in a remote site for protocols which are potentially life threatening puts the patient at extreme risk. Litigious events happen when nurses fail to assess patients, take adequate histories, observe and monitor patients, and summon appropriate medical personnel (Chamorro & Tarulli, 1990). In litigation, there is an emerging trend toward placing liability upon the individual nurse for this dereliction in duty (Chamorro & Tarulli, 1990).

Diagnosis Upon arrival, the preliminary diagnoses should have been:

Ineffective Airway Clearance related to airway edema
Impaired Gas Exchange related to ineffective ventilatory efforts

Knowledge Deficit of medical personnel related to access and emergency protocol
Risk for Injury

Lack of timely development of nursing diagnoses delayed emergency care.

Planning No plan of care existed, which resulted in life-threatening events due to the nurses' inability to access emergency equipment and personnel.

Implementation This was not a simple protocol testing a "safe" intervention, but one which carried with it a potential for life-threatening reactions. Sound protocols and guidelines are imperative for conducting research. The key to avoiding risk-management issues lies in adherence to tangible guidelines (Chamorro & Tarulli, 1990). The protocol for this research should have included specific guidelines for provision of emergency equipment and personnel to manage an airway in the event of an allergic response. Although guidelines existed for application of a tourniquet and administration of epinephrine (at the site of the original injection), no procedure was outlined that would guide the personnel in accessing emergency care. The physician in this case did not assess the severity of the situation rapidly enough and delayed intervention by doing peripheral testing (i.e., peak flow study) and having the patient self-administer medication in his compromised condition.

Dr. Odie violated the standard of care for subjects in a research study by failing to establish written policies, procedures, and protocols and make them readily accessible to clarify research personnel's roles in the conducting of this research. A trained, informed research assistant with knowledge of systems to access in the event of an emergency would have been able to access a COR-0 team through the hospital operator. The Joint Commission on Accreditation of Healthcare Organizations (1992) have set standards stating that all hospital personnel working in patient care areas have the knowledge necessary to activate emergency systems (e.g., for fire and life safety) in the institution where they work within three working days of employment. Furthermore, Dr. Odie delegated the task of preparing and administering an epinephrine injection to untrained personnel. This too violates the standard of care.

A key nursing intervention in the care of this adolescent was the establishment and ongoing support of cardiopulmonary function. Nurses arriving on the scene found an adolescent with no spontaneous respirations or detectable heart rate. A skilled nurse would have acted on the assessment of absent breath sounds and pulse and, once Nathan was intubated, would have evaluated the quality of his breath sounds (they were decreased on the left side, indicating a misplaced tube or pneumothorax). According to documentation, the physicians were the only ones assessing the condition of this adolescent. Appropriate resuscitation equipment was not available until the nurses arrived with a COR-0 cart. Successful intubation was further delayed because it took almost 45 minutes to access qualified personnel. When the nurses saw that Sam Smith was unsuccessful in his attempts to intubate the patient, they should have advocated for the patient and immediately summoned qualified personnel. They clearly should not have allowed an adult care physician to attempt a tracheostomy with unfamiliar equipment in an uncontrolled environment. The *Code for Nurses* (ANA, 1985) requires nurses to advocate for the client's safety and care. Nursing advocacy was absent during the critical periods in delivery of care, and resulted in the eventual death of this adolescent.

Nursing, in this situation, ultimately had the legal and ethical accountability for actions taken and judgments made (ANA, 1985) regardless of the action or lack of action taken by the physicians. The nurses in this case should have: (a) immediately summoned qualified, skilled, pediatric medical personnel to the scene; (b) questioned, confronted, and challenged the physician wanting to perform a tracheostomy in an uncontrolled environment; (c) operationalized the chain of command when physician response was not occurring; (d) reassessed why the emergency system failed to summon appropriate personnel; and (e) immediately transferred Nathan to an area such as the urgent care unit down the hall where supplies, equipment, and trained personnel were available. Had the nurses carried out these procedures, Nathan may have been intubated and resuscitated in a successful manner.

One final concern lies with the ongoing care of the other two subjects in the study. Existing documentation does not indicate what was happening to these subjects. Nathan's collapse into a COR-0 situation was observed by both his mother and the other two subjects. His mother left the room when it became extremely congested with personnel (the COR-0 had been going on for a long time). If the nurse had assessed the environment appropriately, she would have had the mother escorted to an area where she could wait. The other subjects should have been escorted to the urgent care unit for ongoing assessment and management.

Evaluation Continued hypoxia and lack of spontaneous respirations validate the ineffectiveness of interventions and require the nurse to redirect, reassess, and revise interventions (e.g., to question the resources and personnel conducting the interventions) (ANA, 1991). Nathan's outcome was further complicated by the lack of nursing response and placement of a COR-0 call to summon skilled personnel. Ineffective airway management resulted in progressive deterioration in Nathan's condition. The ongoing symptoms should have resulted in a reassessment and revision of the plan.

Lack of critical thinking and decision-making on the part of the nurses resulted in inappropriate nursing actions. Inappropriate interventions resulted in prolonged patient hypoxia and ultimate nursing accountability for violations in the standard of care. The outcome might well have been avoided had appropriate action ensued. Appropriate, skilled personnel should have been available to care for these research subjects in the event of an adverse response. Large numbers of research studies are being conducted in pediatric outpatient settings. The outcome for this adolescent leads one to question whether research with potentially life threatening treatments should be conducted in a remote setting lacking emergency equipment. This case provides rationale for clearly defining research protocols and for employing qualified personnel to carry out interventions.

Case 2

Facts

On October 16, 9-month-old Jimmy was brought to the emergency room (ER) by his mother, who gave the following history:

1800–1830: Mom took temperature, which was 101 degrees F. She gave the infant five drops of Liquiprin.
1930: Mom rechecked temperature, which was now 103 degrees F.
1945: Mom gave five additional drops of Liquiprin.
2130: Mom brought child to ER and stated that temperature had been 103 degrees for one hour at home; infant had been vomiting and had diarrhea for one hour, and last Liquiprin dose was given at 1945. Admission vital signs: T 40.7 rectally (R).
Time ?: Tepid sponge bath given.
2215: Vital signs: T 104 F, P 150, R 30.
2220: Physician examined infant (Table 12-2) and drew blood for CBC.
2240: T 39.4; CBC results: WBC 3,900, segs 39, bands 3, lymphs 52, monos 5; Hgb 11.3, Hct 33.3.
2330: Discharged from ER with "Fever Instruction Sheet."

Table 12-2 Physician's Physical Examination Documentations

Original Note in ER (10/16)	Organ/System	Dictated Note (10/21)
Clear	**Tympanic membrane**	Not hyperemic; normal appearing
Congested	**Nasal**	Nasal congestion with significant discharge
Clear, moist	**Throat**	Hyperemic; no exudate present; mucous membranes moist
Supple	**Neck**	Supple; 1+ firm cervicle lymphadenopathy; moved neck easily in full range throughout exam, without signs of distress
Soft, flat	**Anterior fontanel**	Still open; soft and flat
Clear, rate 24, no accessory muscle use	**Lungs**	Clear without rales or wheezes; rate 24 when not crying; no grunting or use of accessory muscles
Rate 120; regular rate; no murmur	**Cardiovascular**	Rate 120 when not crying; no murmur heard
Soft, no masses, no tenderness	**Abdomen**	Soft, normal bowel sounds present; no masses palpable; appears no tenderness
(No comments)	**Skin**	Normal turgor and was warm
Physiologic	**Neurologic**	No focal deficits with strong motor response and cry. During exam, alert and reacting in normal pattern to exam. Acting normal throughout day 10/16, with normal activity and feeding pattern. Persisted until he went to bed, then 1 1/2 hours after going to sleep, awoke and vomited x 1. Not toxic appearing and had responded in a normal manner to his physical exam. Withdrew with good strength during parts of the physical exam (ear and throat) and was inquisitive to other aspects of the exam (auscultation of lungs). Motor function strong and strong cry.

On October 18 at 0145, after an apparent seizure, Jimmy again was brought to the ER where he was found to be mottled, tachypneic, febrile, and quite flaccid. An IV was started, diazepam (Valium) given to control his seizures, and a lumbar puncture performed. He was transferred in an ambulance for further management to a second hospital.

On admission, his temperature was 37 degrees C (R), weight 9.75 kg. He had gasping respirations. He looked moribund, peripherally cyanotic, and totally mottled with undetectable blood pressures. His ears were infected, his pupils fixed and dilated, and he was unresponsive to painful stimuli. Jimmy's heart rate (HR) was 160, he was gasping with poor air entry, and he had abdominal distention. A nasogastric (NG) tube was inserted and coffee ground secretions obtained. Because he was continuously seizing, he was given 50 mg of phenobarbital IV × 2, intubated, and bagged with 100% oxygen. Laboratory data included:

- cerebral spinal fluid (CSF): (+) gram-negative bacillus; +1 pus cells; glucose 2; chloride 108; white cell count >600
- blood glucose: 6
- blood urea nitrogen (BUN): 12.8
- electrolytes: Na 125, K 3.8, Cl 85
- CBC: WBC 5,600; Hgb 10
- after infusion of bicarbonate and hyperventilation, ABG: pH 7.13; $Pa\text{O}_2$ 197; $Pa\text{CO}_2$ 15, HCO_3 5, BE –22; O_2 saturation 99%.

A tentative diagnosis of meningitis, most likely due to *Hemophilus influenzae* type a, was made.

Outcome

Despite vigorous resuscitation, Jimmy died on October 18, of *Hemophilus influenzae* meningitis, three hours after admission to the second hospital.

Legal

This case was settled out of court for multiple hundreds of thousands of dollars.

Case Commentary

Undesirable Patient Outcome

Assessment On admission to the first hospital's ER, the nurses took only a temperature instead of a complete set of vital signs (e.g., HR, R, and BP). No BP was *ever* taken. According to the mother's report, the nurse recorded a history of the fever and illness, but the timing of events (e.g., medication administration, recheck of fever) was not documented. The nurse failed to perform or document any physical assessment.

Diagnosis No nursing diagnoses were formulated or documented.

Planning No nursing care plan was formulated or documented.

Implementation No antipyretic was administered in the ER. A tepid sponge bath was given, but was not documented in the chart (the tepid sponge bath was documented by the physician on October 21, in a dictated note, but not in the initial ER note).

Evaluation On Jimmy's admission, the nurse did not evaluate the effectiveness or ineffectiveness of the mother's home interventions for the infant (i.e., whether the doses of Liquiprin were effective in lowering temperature). The nurse never evaluated whether the infant retained the medication, since he had been vomiting prior to his arrival at the ER. Since the tepid sponge bath was not documented by the nurse, other relevant nursing evaluations (e.g., temperature of the water, infant's response to the procedure, time and length of bath, and body temperature before and after treatment) also were not performed or documented.

Desirable Patient Outcome

Assessment Although no nursing assessments were documented, the nurse, in her deposition, described the infant as "lethargic, pale and warm, not very active for a 9-month-old (i.e., very quiet and listless)." In her deposition, the mother described her child as "listless; lying still; whiny; refusing food; and whole body including feet and legs were white." In her deposition, the mother's friend, who accompanied her to the ER, described the infant as "very, very sick; listless and quiet; not active at all; refused supper; slept all the way to the hospital; not himself for a couple of days; listless and whiny on the ride home; very, very pale when unwrapped from blanket at home." These assessments sharply contrast the physician's two notes (Table 12-2).

Incomplete, inadequate, and undocumented nursing assessment violates the Standard of Care to collect client data utilizing appropriate assessment and screening techniques, and to document in a retrievable form (ANA 1983, 1991). Poor assessment results in: (a) poor nursing diagnoses, (b) inadequate/no plan of care, and (c) inadequate/incomplete intervention and evaluation. The professional nurse must assume responsibility and accountability for her incompetent practice (ANA 1985, 1991).

Diagnosis On Jimmy's admission to the ER, the nurse failed to formulate any nursing diagnoses because she had not assessed this infant appropriately or gathered the sufficient data necessary to formulate diagnoses. Potential nursing diagnoses should have included:

Activity Intolerance and/or Fatigue related to poor nutritional status and fever as evidenced by poor tolerance to tepid bath and poor oral intake
Altered Tissue Perfusion: Cardiac related to decreasing respiratory status
Altered Nutrition: Less than Body Requirements related to poor oral intake and vomiting as evidenced by mottled skin, dry mucous membranes
Impaired Gas Exchange related to ineffective ventilatory effort

Appropriate nursing diagnoses based on assessment data should have included:

Altered Tissue Perfusion: Peripheral; Cerebral
Diarrhea
Ineffective Infant Feeding Pattern related to ineffective suck and swallow as evidenced by poor feeding and vomiting
Fluid Volume Deficit (active loss) related to vomiting and increased insensible water loss
Hyperthermia related to presence of infection
Pain related to infected ear
Risk for Infection related to febrile state, altered ear exam
Risk for Injury related to seizure activity secondary to hyperthermia
Knowledge Deficit related to lack of information about hyperthermia management, symptoms of dehydration, and nutrition

Analysis of data, formulation of nursing diagnoses, and documentation of diagnoses and outcome measures constitute competent nursing practice that meets the standards of care as outlined by professional organizations (ANA, 1983, 1985, 1991) and the state nurse practice acts.

Planning Lack of nursing diagnoses prevented Jimmy's nurse from formulating and documenting an appropriate plan of care addressing dependent, independent, and interdependent nursing functions (ANA, 1983, 1991). The nurse was therefore unable to prescribe interventions to attain outcomes (ANA, 1991).

Implementation In this case, dependent nursing actions (i.e., carrying out the physician's orders) included a tepid sponge bath. The nurse performed the procedure but neither documented it nor assessed the infant's behavioral or physiologic response (ANA, 1983, 1991). Treatment of this infant's hyperthermia required interdependent action of both the nurse and physician. If the ER had a policy/protocol about treating hyperthermia with antipyretics, neither nurse nor physician followed it. Neither did the nurse or physician follow the standard of care for treating a fever written in the ER's "Fever Instruction Sheet," given to the mother at discharge. Even though the "Fever Instruction Sheet" instructed parents to treat fever with antipyretics at >101.5 degrees F, no antipyretics were ever given in the ER for Jimmy's hyperthermia.

Education of parents is an extremely important intervention in the management of fevers in infancy. Nurses working in pediatric inpatient and outpatient settings must have and provide sound knowledge and education related to fever management—its definition and meaning, the benefits and disadvantages, when to be concerned about the fever as an indicator of serious illness, home management (including proper dosaging of antipyretics), and when to contact a health care provider. Such education has improved home management and enhanced parental confidence when caring for the child with a fever (Robinson, 1989).

Administration of an adequate dose of antipyretics on admission to the ER would have facilitated adequate assessment of the child, especially neurologic status. Alterations in neurologic status (e.g., irritability, listlessness, poor feeding) may be due to fever or to meningitis. If sensorium clears after a decrease in temperature, then alteration of neurologic status was secondary to hyperthermia and not meningitis. If sensorium does not improve, the infant/child is a candidate for further laboratory evaluation, including a lumbar puncture (Barkin & Rosen, 1990).

This infant was discharged with a temperature of 39.9 without receiving fluids or a septic workup. Infections account for the majority of fevers in all age groups (van der Jagt, 1992). The younger the child, the more difficult it is to diagnose bacterial infection; this is particularly true for infants less than a year of age (van der Jagt, 1992). Standards of practice for the febrile infant recommend that all febrile infants under a year of age minimally have a septic workup and, if the infant is less than six months, include a lumbar puncture (van der Jagt, 1992). The nurses should have advocated for a septic workup for this child to determine the source of the temperature, particularly considering the age of the child.

A nursing diagnosis of *Fluid Volume Deficit* (as evidenced by vomiting and diarrhea as well as increased insensible water losses because of hyperthermia) required independent nursing action. In order to assess current fluid status and evaluate fluid volume deficit, the nurse should have: (a) put a urine bag on the infant or collected urine from the diaper; (b) evaluated the specific gravity with a refractrometer; and (c) dipsticked the urine for pH and for the presence of blood, glucose, and ketones. Was this child currently hydrated or dehydrated? Jimmy's clinical symptoms indicated that he was dehydrated. This should have prompted the nurse to make further assessments and develop interventions to hydrate the child (e.g., to assess whether Jimmy was able to retain ingested fluids, and to provide rehydration fluids to him). In the ER, the mother should have been given clear liquids to offer to her infant. Would he drink orally? Given Jimmy's history of vomiting, was he able to retain oral fluids? Since increased fluid losses are associated with hyperthermia (necessitating an increase of 10% fluid intake for every degree of fever), was this infant able to consume ample fluids above maintenance level? If Jimmy was unable to hydrate himself adequately, he should have been a candidate for hospital admission.

Evaluation In this hospital, nursing services did not create an environment in which the nursing process was the framework for delivery of nursing care (ANA, 1988). Inadequate evaluation was the end-product of an inadequate nursing process. Jimmy's nurse did not evaluate the response or lack of response, or the effectiveness or ineffectiveness of:

1. Mother's antipyretic administration:
   - underdosed medication—a 9-month-old child should have received Liquiprin (60 mg/1.25 mL) 1.6 mL per dose (Schmitt, 1980, p. 78); mother gave five drops × 2 (total 10 drops, 2 mL)
   - temperature 40.9 on admission: 2.2 degrees higher than at 1930, 1–1 1/2 hrs (i.e., peak action of drug) after second underdose of Liquiprin
   - temperature 40.7 on admission: 4.2 degrees higher than at onset of problem (3–3 1/2 hrs earlier)

- did child retain 1800/1830 and 1945 doses, or vomit one or both?

2. Fever treatment in ER: Is fever intractable, or is treatment inadequate?
   - infant unresponsive to Liquiprin dosages by mother
   - no significant decrease in temperature after tepid sponge bath: decreased 1.2 degrees after bath (to 40); decreased only 0.2 degree more than 25 minutes later (to 39.9)
   - infant discharged with temperature of 39.9 degrees
   - temperature decreased only 1.4 degrees from admission temperature of 40.7 degrees
   - still >1.5 degrees higher than 38.5 degrees (i.e., worrisome level for development of seizures)
   - no evaluation 1–2 hours after tepid bath to assess temperature rise or fall
   - no vital signs evaluated before discharge (last temperature 50 minutes before discharge)
3. Baseline hydration status (i.e., specific gravity) or ability/inability to hydrate and retain oral intake.
4. Mother's understanding of written/verbal instructions regarding "Fever Instruction Sheet." Mother stated in her deposition that the physician handed her the instruction sheet but did not explain the instructions to her. The nurse never clarified or asked if the mother had any questions.

The nurse never evaluated the results of the CBC even though this infant: (a) was the classic age (six months to one year) for development of fever; (b) had an upper respiratory infection; and (c) presented with symptoms at the peak time of the year (autumn and early winter) for *Hemophilus* flu meningitis (Whaley & Wong, 1995). Presence of leukopenia (i.e., WBC <5,000) may represent life threatening disease and requires further workup, including a lumbar puncture, to rule out meningitis (Barkin & Rosen, 1990; Berman, 1991). As a patient advocate, the nurse had the responsibility to: (a) evaluate the CBC; (b) realize significant leukopenia was present; (c) advocate for further laboratory workup to diagnose the cause of the fever; and (d) utilize the chain of command if necessary to obtain appropriate medical diagnosis and treatment for this infant (ANA, 1985, 1991).

Often in many outpatient settings (e.g., emergency rooms, outpatient clinics, physician's offices) RNs function as "traffic cops" (i.e., moving patients to and from rooms) or "servants" (i.e., assembling equipment for and cleaning up after the doctor) instead of professional care providers (i.e., utilizing the nursing process and making nursing diagnoses). In many outpatient settings, RNs are being replaced by unlicensed assistive personnel (UAPs), licensed practical/vocational nurses (LPNs, LVNs), or paramedics. "Traffic cop" and "servant" functions can be delegated, but the practice of professional nursing in outpatient settings cannot be delegated or substituted for by UAPs, LPNs/LVNs, or paramedics.

When the RN and the physician act as a complementary and collaborative professional team in outpatient practice, the nurse's professional practice and advocacy benefit the patient. A retrospective review of 25 pediatric cases seen in the ER found quality-of-care issues in 41% of the cases and legal claims made based on failure to diagnose (64%) and inappropriate treatment (24%) (Reynolds, Jaffe, & Glynn, 1991). Over a 10-year period, legal fees in 16 of these cases amounted to $191,677, while total payments to families amounted to $43,850 (Reynolds, Jaffe, & Glynn, 1991). In another study, 32% of febrile infants seen in an ER who were later found to have positive urine cultures had been assigned other diagnoses (Hoberman, et al., 1993). In another case, a four-month-old infant with a temperature of 40.6 degrees waited in the outpatient department for longer than four hours (because she didn't have an appointment) to be examined by a doctor. This delay in diagnosis, coupled with mistakes in the treatment of meningitis, resulted in severe developmental delays and mental retardation. In a US District Court, the federal government was ordered to pay greater than $14,000,000 as compensation for negligence of the hospital staff (McKibben, 1994). Where were the nurses in these outpatient settings? Had the RNs been replaced by paramedics, UAPs, or LPNs? If present, were the RNs functioning as "traffic cops" or "servants"? Were there collaborative-practice protocols to direct nursing and medical practice? Would the presence of an RN, functioning professionally, using the nursing process and nursing diagnoses, have made a difference in the care of these children?

Unfortunately, in Jimmy's case, the nurse's sole attention to dependent nursing functions precluded her attention to not only the nursing process but also independent and interdependent nursing functions. Nursing responsibility and accountability does not end at performance of dependent nursing functions (i.e., carrying out the physician's orders). Nursing responsibility and accountability includes "judgments made and actions taken in the course of nursing practice, and neither physician's orders nor the employing agency's policies relieve the nurse of accountability for actions taken and judgments made" (ANA, 1985, p. 9). A very different outcome for this infant and his family may have occurred if the nurse had: (a) practiced competently and professionally according to the standards of care, and (b) advocated for him to receive the standard of medical care.

Case 3

Facts

Seth, born at 34 weeks gestation with bronchotracheal malacia, had been ventilated since one week of age. Other problems in the NICU included: (a) intraventricular hemorrhage (IVH) (grade III) with shunt placement, (b) necrotizing enterocolitis (NEC) and feeding intolerance, and (c) placement of a gastric button at two months of age. Because they lived about 400 miles from the hospital, had financial problems, and had two other children to care for, Seth's parents (Marie and Jack) visited him only four times during his seven-month hospitalization. Initially they called daily and then monthly while he was hospitalized.

Before Seth was discharged from the hospital, his primary nurse attempted to have his parents "room in" with Seth for at least a weekend to learn his care. Citing distance and the care of their two other children, Seth's parents declined "rooming in." Instead, they chose to come to the hospital early on the day of discharge to learn his care. During their instruction, both parents were extremely nervous. They participated in his care, but did not speak to or initiate holding Seth.

For the first ten days at home, the insurance company paid for 24-hour nursing care on the contingency that Seth's parents work intensively on learning his care. By day 11, Seth's nursing hours were decreased by 2 hours every fifth day. Seth was now 8 months of age and had been home from the hospital for 1 month. Nursing care at this time was 18 hours/day (0730–1700 and 2200–0600) per parental request.

Marie usually returned from work at 1630 and took report from the primary nurse, Nurse Jones. Marie often acted disinterested during report. Although she spoke to Seth, Marie didn't pick him up and her interactions with him lacked warmth. Marie preferred to discuss the clinical aspects of Seth's care with the nurses. Except for Nurse Jones, all other nurses experienced Marie as distant, challenging, and often critical of their care. Marie's 2-year-old daughter, Sydney, who was often cranky and clingy, followed Marie everywhere. Seth's 4-year-old brother, Sam, was often criticized and yelled at by his mother. Seth's father, Jack, a mechanic, was laid off three months ago when the family-owned gas station went out of business. He continued to pay for the health insurance, but as Seth's bills increased and were unpaid, Jack became unsure of how long he could continue paying Seth's premiums. Jack was gone most of the day and participated infrequently in the children's care, particularly in Seth's. Jack was often heard criticizing the care Marie gave the children.

The night nurse, Nurse Young, found Seth in his crib wearing a soaked diaper, crying, and high-pressure alarming his ventilator. Seth was inconsolable, even after suctioning. Nurse Young vented his gastrostomy button and a large amount of air escaped. Since his temperature was elevated, she changed, fed him, gave him Tylenol, and rocked him to comfort him. Marie told Nurse Young to "put him back in bed and let him cry it out. He's just too spoiled by his nurses." Even when Nurse Young verbalized concerns that he had signs of illness, Marie was unsympathetic; she appeared stressed and angry and was attempting to get her two other children to bed.

Marie stated that she didn't do Seth's nebulizer or chest physiotherapy treatments. Nurse Young, having worked the night before, noticed that two bottles were left rather than the usual one. A review of the nurses notes revealed that Seth received all his daytime feedings, and Nurse Young wondered if he missed an evening feeding. When Nurse Young checked the ventilator alarm, she found that the rate alarm had been turned to zero. When confronted, Marie stated, "He kept disconnecting himself and the alarm was driving me crazy. He is fine. He can breathe on his own." Nurse Young explained the danger of overriding an alarm, charted these incidents, reported them to Nurse Jones, the primary nurse (who defended the mother), and discussed them with the pediatric home nursing supervisor, Jill Canby.

One month later, the nursing hours dropped to 14 hours (0630–2030) of care during the day and evening. Marie requested that the family provide care during the night. Nurse Jones, the primary nurse, had become very attached to Marie (e.g., during her shifts, she went outside on the porch and smoked with Marie). Nurse Jones made constant complaints to the supervisor about the "other nurses," and talked to Marie several times a day by telephone.

One of the nurses received, in report, that Seth had been febrile (38.8C) for five hours during the night. When the nurse asked if she gave Seth Tylenol, Marie stated, "I was too tired." After hearing a very different report from Nurse Jones, Jill Canby, the nursing supervisor, made a home visit. During the visit, Jill found: (a) Seth had gained only 2 ounces in the last month, (b) he had two episodes of otitis media and a severe monilial diaper rash, (c) he had developed dark circles under his eyes, was listless and pale, and (d) his siblings also appeared tired with dark circles under their eyes, were pale and thin for their ages, had disheveled clothes, and were often inappropriately dressed for the weather. Jill learned from the evening nurse that the siblings went to daycare and often hadn't had dinner by the time of the evening nurse's departure at 2030.

Outcome

The family and its care of Seth are of ongoing concern to the home care agency.

Legal

As health care reform continues, the venue of care delivery changes from the hospital to home. Litigation involving home health nurses will become more prevalent. The increased autonomy of home care increases legal risks for the agency as well as the individual professional nurse (Sullivan, 1994).

Case Commentary

Undesirable Patient Outcome

Assessment This family evidenced multiple family stressors and inappropriate interactional patterns that increased the risk of parental neglect.

Diagnosis Nursing diagnoses related only to physical needs were formulated and documented:

Ineffective Airway Clearance
Risk for Infection
Risk for Impaired Skin Integrity

Planning Although this family experienced numerous stressors and had aberrant interactional patterns and responses, the primary nurse formulated no social or teaching/learning diagnoses or plan of care.

Implementation No diagnoses were formulated and thus no nursing interventions were developed to intervene with the neglect.

Assessment Data for Case 3

Family Stressors

- Preterm infant with prolonged hospitalization and parent separation
- Minimal contact with family during seven-month hospitalization
- Minimal caretaking instructional experience prior to discharge
- Financial problems
- Home care of chronically ill infant

Interactional Patterns

- Parental lack of warmth and initiation of interaction with child
- Peripheral involvement of father
- Lack of judgment concerning infant's physical/emotional/developmental needs
- Decreased family interactions and increase in negative interactions
- Disorganized family functioning: no routines, no consistency

Family Strengths

- Support system (large extended family; large network of close friends; home health professionals/agency)
- Parents both received nurturing care from their families (no history of neglect or separation of parents as children)
- Parents have been married ten years and are both in their 30's
- Parents in good health
- Live in adequately spacious house which accommodates all members and baby with multiple medical needs and supplies
- All children planned and wanted
- History of supportive parental relationship prior to premature/chronically ill child
- Community with many resources; private health insurance pays for counseling

Evaluation Although some of the nurses recognized and intervened when the mother neglected to care for the infant and/or jeopardized the infant, the primary nurse developed an alliance with the mother, complaining about the "other nurses." Nurse Jones failed to report noncompliance to the nursing supervisor.

Desirable Patient Outcome

Assessment Nurse Jones, the primary nurse, failed to "identify the immediate, interim, and long-term health needs" (ANA, 1983, p. 9) of this infant and family. Failure to collect data about the family's role relationships, interactional patterns, and adequacy or inadequacy of support systems violated the standard of care (ANA, 1983, 1986). An assessment of this family's stressors, interactional patterns, and strengths is shown in the accompanying box. Despite the input of her nursing colleagues, Nurse Jones failed to detect subtle as well as significant changes in this infant's health and developmental status (ANA, 1983, 1986). Being in a unique position to practice crisis intervention, Nurse Jones violated the standard of care. She did not collect family/individual data about experience with stressors (e.g., "high tech" home care and caring for a chronically ill child) (ANA, 1983).

Rather than establishing a professional, empathetic, and therapeutic relationship, Nurse Jones became sympathetic to Marie, the infant's mother. Empathy, an understanding and acceptance of another's life and an accurate perception of feelings, is one of the dimensions of a therapeutic relationship (Potter & Perry, 1994). Sympathy, thinking or feeling like another, is a subjective view of another person's world. Sympathetic relationships may impede the nurse from objectively perceiving another's life, issues, and challenges (Potter & Perry, 1994).

Enmeshment, the lack of clear boundaries (Minuchin, 1974), with this mother prohibited Nurse Jones from objectively assessing pertinent data (as shown in the box). Emotional overinvestment and overidentification with the client or family prevents the professional from: (a) objectively observing critical information, (b) utilizing information to formulate appropriate diagnoses, (c) developing an appropriate plan of care, (d) implementing appropriate interventions, or (e) objectively evaluating, reviewing, and revising the plan. Boundary diffusion (Minuchin, 1974) prevents the nurse from assessing a competent professional role/relationship with the child and family (ANA, 1985). Instead, overidentification with parents results in biased (rather than unbiased), personal (rather than impersonal), prejudiced (rather than impartial), and subjective (rather than objective) assessments and evaluations.

Diagnosis No diagnosis of alterations/disturbances in family relationships and interactional patterns occurred (ANA, 1983). At-risk families have an increased chance of experiencing family difficulties as evidenced by: (a) parental inability to provide basic needs (i.e., food, shelter, clothing; emotional, supportive, and intellectual stimulation) and (b) manifestation in children of signs of tension and stress (e.g., growth failure, emotional/behavioral difficulties such as distraught, withdrawn, aggressive, depressed) (Mott, 1990). Nursing diagnoses related to family stress, coping, attachment, parenting, and role-functioning should have included:

Ego Integrity

Impaired Adjustment
Anxiety
Defensive Coping
Ineffective Individual/Family Coping
Fear
Dysfunctional Grieving
Powerlessness
Personal Identity Disturbance
Situational Low Self-Esteem
Impaired Verbal Communication
Compromised Family Coping
Disabling Family Coping

Altered Family Processes
Parental Role Conflict
Altered Parenting
Altered Role Performance
Impaired Social Interaction
Social Isolation

Teaching/Learning

Altered Growth and Development
Knowledge Deficit related to lack of information about physical, psychosocial, and developmental care of: (a) healthy siblings, and (b) chronically ill infant
Noncompliance related to physical, psychosocial, and developmental care of child and siblings
Ineffective Management of Therapeutic Regimen

Planning In collaboration, the primary nurse, other nursing staff, and nursing supervisor should have formulated and documented a plan of care to include: (a) obtaining consultation, (b) education and/or counseling, (c) behavioral contract, and (d) alteration in nursing hours. Inadequate assessment of stressors and indicators of parenting difficulties, coupled with failure to formulate nursing diagnoses, resulted in lack of a plan. Failure to collaborate, establish goals, and develop a care plan violates the standard of care (ANA, 1983, 1985, 1986, 1991).

Implementation Enmeshment, the blurring of boundaries (Minuchin, 1974) between professional and parent, prevented the primary nurse from advocating for the infant. Although "parenting the parent" (i.e., temporary dependence of the parent on the care provider) is a helpful intervention, it is not similar to enmeshment. "Parenting the parent" proceeds from dependence to interdependence to independence to the ultimate goal of parental empowerment and autonomy. Enmeshment of nurse and parents decreases parental autonomy and empowerment, thus inappropriately binding the nurse to the family. Here, the nurse's needs (i.e., codependence) (Snow & Willard, 1989) take precedence over the family's autonomy, independence, and empowerment. Since child neglect is not easy to define, its identification requires a value judgment, and it includes any form of substandard child care (Mott, 1990). The enmeshed nurse can neither make an objective evaluation nor take an appropriate action on behalf of the child. Appropriate interventions for this family should have begun with obtaining consultation (ANA, 1983, 1985) from: (a) nurse colleagues providing this family's health care, (b) nursing supervisor, (c) social services, and (d) child protective services.

Since child neglect is often caused by ignorance, education and counseling are appropriate nursing interventions (Whaley & Wong, 1995). This family had limited opportunity to prepare for discharge and management of ongoing care for a chronically ill child at home. Educational interventions about the ventilator, signs of illness, adequate nutrition, need for consistency, etc., were warranted for this family (ANA, 1983). Utilizing data on family strengths, nurses should have assisted the parents in identifying resources and supports (e.g., community, friends, family). Provision of care to the older children by these supports could have provided needed respite to the family. Changing the nursing hours so the mother could sleep through the night and involving the unemployed father in child care may have been helpful.

Help with parenting a chronically ill infant, a toddler, and a preschooler may require education beyond the mother's development, strategies to promote growth and development, and alternatives to existing parenting behaviors (ANA, 1983). Positive reinforcement of appropriate parenting and caretaking efforts is essential (ANA, 1983). Parent-to-parent support groups, parenting classes, or counseling support groups may also assist in a change of parenting style and coping (ANA, 1983). Feelings associated with parenting a chronically ill child (e.g., anger, grief, resentment, fatigue, disappointment) need to be discussed in a supportive environment like a support group. When nurses intervene therapeutically, they help parents identify stressors, current and alternative coping strategies, and effective or ineffective coping methods.

Evaluation Failure to assess, plan, diagnose, and intervene appropriately resulted in the nurse failing to help this family: (a) "attain and maintain optimum health" (ANA, 1983, p. 9); (b) "achieve and maintain a balance between the personal growth needs of individual family members and optimum family functioning" (ANA, 1983, p. 11); (c) "prevent potential developmental and health problems" (ANA, 1983, p. 12); (d) "promote an environment free of hazards to . . . growth and development, wellness, and recovery from illness" (ANA, 1983, p. 14); (e) "detect changes in health status and deviations from optimal development" (ANA, 1983, p. 13); (f) "carry out appropriate interventions and treatment to facilitate survival and recovery from illness" (ANA, 1983, p. 16); (g) "understand and cope with developmental and traumatic situations during illness, childbearing, and childhood" (ANA, 1983, p. 18); and (h) "enhance access to and utilization of adequate health care services" (ANA, 1983, p. 20).

A more timely evaluation by the supervisor could have prevented the continued deterioration of the infant's physical and psychological health and development, as well as family dynamics and functioning. Disparate reports of the primary and staff nurses, an enmeshing relationship between the primary nurse and mother, inability of the family to provide safe care, and strained family relationships and functioning should have prompted earlier consultation, referral, and evaluation. The standards of professional performance require the nurse to "systematically evaluate the quality and effectiveness of nursing practice" (ANA, 1991, p. 13). Nurses assess responsibility and accountability for "exercising informed judgment, using individual competency and qualifications as criteria in delegating nursing activities" (ANA, 1994, p. 10). Instead of "continually evaluating" (ANA, 1986) and providing prospective "quality assurance" (ANA, 1988, 1991), this nursing supervisor and health care agency became involved retrospectively, after the infant's condition had deteriorated.

References

Allen, A. (1991). Risk management: A proactive process. *Journal of Post Anesthesia Nursing, 6*(3), 195–196.

American Nurses Association. (1983). *Standards for maternal-child health nursing practice.* Washington, D.C.: Author.

American Nurses Association. (1985). *Code of ethics.* Washington, D.C.: Author.

American Nurses Association. (1986). *Standards of home health care nursing practice.* Kansas City, MO: Author.

American Nurses Association. (1988). *Standards for organized nursing services.* Washington, D.C.: Author.

American Nurses Association. (1991). *Standards of clinical nursing practice.* Washington, D.C.: Author.

American Nurses Association. (1994). *Registered professional nurses and UAPs.* Washington, D.C.: Author.

Barkin, R. & Rosen, P. (1990). *Emergency pediatrics* (pp. 192–198). St. Louis: Mosby-Yearbook.

Berman, S. (1991). *Pediatric decision-making* (pp. 2–9; 276–279). Philadelphia: B.C. Decker.

Chamorro, T. & Tarulli, D. (1990). Strategies for risk management in cancer nursing. *Cancer Nursing Perspectives, 17*(6), 915–920.

Hoberman, A., Chan, H., Keller, D., Hickey, R., Davis, H., & Ellis, D. (1993). Prevalence of urinary tract infections in febrile infants. *Journal of Pediatrics, 123,* 17–23.

Hogue, E. (1992, August). Legalease. *Hospital Home Heath,* pp. 110–112.

Japsen, B. (1994, October). Tracking risk in integration. *Modern Healthcare,* pp. 53–54.

Joint Commission on Accreditation of Healthcare Organizations. (1992). *Standards of nursing practice.* Oakbrook Terrace, IL: Author.

_____. (1990). Nursing practice update. *Texas Nursing, 64*(1), 8–9.

McKibbon, G. (1994, June 16). Brain-damaged girl to get top care. *The Denver Post,* p. 10A.

Minuchin, S. (1974). *Families and family treatment.* Cambridge, MA: Harvard University Press.

Mott, S. (1990). Nursing care of the family at risk. In S. Mott, S. James, & A. Sperhac (Eds.), *Nursing care of children and families,* 2nd ed. Menlo Park, CA: Addison-Wesley Nursing.

Potter, R. & Perry, A. (1994). *Basic nursing theory and practice,* 3rd ed. St. Louis: Mosby-Yearbook.

Reynolds, S., Jaffe, D., & Glynn, W. (1991). Professional liability in a pediatric emergency department. *Pediatrics, 87*(2), 134–37.

Robinson, J. (1989). The impact of fever health education on clinic utilization. *American Journal of Disease in Children, 143,* 698–71.

Schmitt, B. (1980). *Pediatric telephone advice* (p. 78). Boston: Little Brown.

Snow, C. & Willard, D. (1989). *I'm dying to take care of you: Nurses and codependence.* Redwood, WA: Professional Counselor Books.

Sullivan, G. (1994). Home care: More autonomy, more legal risks. *RN*, pp. 63–69.

Sussman, M. & Siegel, P. (1991). Assessing an agency's risks. *Caring Magazine.* pp. 42–45, 67–68.

van der Jagt, E. (1992). Fever. In R. Hoekelman (Ed.), *Primary pediatric care,* 2nd ed. (pp. 923–927). St. Louis: Mosby-Yearbook.

Whaley, L. & Wong, D. (1995). *Nursing care of infants and children,* 5th ed. St. Louis: Mosby-Yearbook.

13

Inpatient Pediatric Care

Mary I. Enzman Hagedorn, RN, PhD, CNS, CPNP
Sandra L. Gardner, RN, MS, CNS, PNP
Elizabeth A. Ely, RN, PhD

Pediatric inpatient health care organizations/settings provide comprehensive, family-centered health care for both children and adolescents with acute and/or chronic illnesses (Whaley & Wong, 1995). Between 10–20% of all children in the US have a chronic illness. These children use 60% of all pediatric inpatient services, thus further complicating provision of care in the pediatric population (Hagedorn, 1993). "The goal of pediatric nursing is to promote the healthy maturation of the child/adolescent as a physical, intellectual, and emotional/social being within the context of family and community" (Betz, Hunsberger, & Wright, 1994, p. 4). Incorporated within this goal are themes of prevention, assessment, and intervention for children and adolescents experiencing alterations in their health patterns. Nurses are in a key position to assess and intervene to preserve the child's physical, cognitive, and emotional/social/cultural well-being. The uniqueness of care for children and adolescents centers around the issues of developmental responses to altered health conditions and need for advocacy by the family and nurse.

Several environmental factors, including place, time, and equipment can contribute to injuries in the child (Whaley & Wong, 1995). Theoretically, all injuries to the child are preventable, and one of the key responsibilities of the nurse is to anticipate and recognize when and where safety measures need to be applied. Injury prevention requires protection, education, and advocacy.

For pediatric nurses who work in acute-care settings, skill acquisition varies depending on whether the facility is a children's hospital or a general hospital. Although pediatric nurses are responsible to themselves, their profession, and the agency where they are employed, primary responsibility lies with the receivers of their nursing care, the child and family (Whaley & Wong, 1995). Furthermore, since nurses spend the most time caring for the child, they are in a unique position to provide insight about the child's condition and response to therapy. The nurse must work with the child and family to identify goals and needs and plan interventions that meet specific, defined problems. Nurses caring for children must have advanced training in the care of children ranging in age from birth to twenty-one years of age.

Care must be aimed at providing for child/family safety, advocacy, and autonomy. As a child/family advocate, the nurse ensures family awareness of available services, provides educational information about treatments and procedures, and encourages the child/family to support or change existing health care practices (Whaley & Wong, 1995). Overall goals in pediatric inpatient nursing include recognition of: (a) developmental characteristics of the child in relation to disease processes, (b) altered health patterns in the child in relation to physical, intellectual, emotional, cultural, social, and political processes, (c) nursing strategies that recognize the unique responses of children to health and illness, (d) educational strategies that effectively address the needs of both the child and family, and (e) child/family advocacy within the health care system (Betz, Hunsberger, & Wright, 1994).

Medical-legal risk management in the pediatric setting is complex. The environment, personnel mix, and family needs differ and the pediatric nurse must provide safe, comprehensive care that addresses principles, skills, and policies specific to children. Legal issues unique to pediatric nursing include state laws governing informed consent for treatment of minors, laws regarding child abuse and maltreatment, and professional issues related to pediatric nursing (Betz, Hunsberger, & Wright, 1994). In most cases, parents decide what procedures will be performed on the child, who may not understand what is being performed or why. Pediatric nurses are in a key role to assist the parents and child in determining the most beneficial or least harmful treatments and care within a framework of societal mores, value systems, professional practice standards, the law, and institution policies and guidelines (Whaley & Wong, 1995). The pediatric nurse must advocate for both the child and family with the goal of safe, comprehensive, pediatric-based care.

This chapter presents cases of nursing liability related to patient safety, recognition of signs and symptoms of impending dangers in patient conditions, safe care related to intravenous therapy in pediatrics, and nursing knowledge related to safe use of equipment. The first case discusses the issues surrounding provision of safety and confidentiality for a hospitalized adolescent. The second case demonstrates how crucial ongoing nursing assessment and intervention are to positive outcomes for a hospitalized child. The third case explores the safety and judgment issues surrounding intravenous therapy.

Case 1

Facts

On April 9 at 0045 a teenager, Catherine Adams, presented to the emergency room (ER) of a community hospital with a 1–2 month history of flu symptoms and dizziness with labyrinthitis (diagnosed two days prior to this visit in a previous hospital admission). This evening Catherine had a large dinner, vomited, and "blacked out"—she did not remember the ride to the hospital. An intravenous (IV) of D5LR at 150 mL/hr was started in the ER. When admitted to the pediatric area by Jean Knott, RN, Catherine was in no acute distress, alert, oriented, and said she felt "light headed." Nurse Knott explained the procedure for intake/output and the need to call for assistance when out of bed. For the first two days of hospitalization, Catherine was out of bed only with assistance because of her dizziness, and she felt intermittently nauseated and "woozy."

On the 11 to 7 A.M. shift of April 11, Catherine still had an IV at 100 mL/hour, and she was visiting with her family as Nurse Knott came onto the floor, entered the room, and spoke to her. At 2400, Nurse Knott noted that the patient was asleep and the television on; her IV site was without redness or swelling. At 0100 the television was noted to be off. While checking on the patient every hour (on the half hour), at 0130, Nurse Knott noticed the light off over the sink and a pile of items (gown, towel, and washcloth) on the chair at the foot of the patient's bed. At 0200 and 0400, she entered notations of "sleeping." At 0600, Nurse Knott awakened Catherine for the *only set of vital signs* on the shift. The patient stated that she was "still a little dizzy, and unsteady on her feet." Asked if she got up to the bathroom by herself during the night, she said she had. The only urine output noted for the shift was 200 mL at 0600; total IV intake (charted on the hour) was 800 mL. At 0700, Nurse Knott stepped out of the nurses' station and happened to see a male orderly go into Catherine's room. As Nurse Knott started walking toward the room to advise him to leave (because she knew he was not supposed to be there), he came out almost immediately. He approached the nurse and asked if she wanted water and juice passed. She said she did not and he went to the next nurses' station.

At 0845 on April 12, Catherine asked Trixie Potts, RN, if she had had a male nurse during the night. Nurse Potts told Catherine that Nurse Knott was her nurse. Catherine stated that a man dressed in light green scrubs came into her room every hour during the night, identified himself as her nurse, took her temperature, and stated that the doctor had told him to rub lotion on her body. Catherine stated that he kept touching her face and hair and rubbed her thighs with lotion. She said, "I thought he was my nurse." In the morning when he entered her room, he told her that she needed to remove her gown and put on a hospital gown. She refused to comply and he did not force her to remove it. Catherine described the intruder as a short, small, Hispanic male with coarse, dark, curly, shoulder-length hair. He had no name tag on, and was wearing light green scrubs and shoes that made a squeaking noise when he walked.

Nurse Potts paged the clinical manager and related the incident to her. She reassured Catherine that she would be moved closer to the nurses' station. At 0920, the patient related the same account to Sally Radisson, RN, the clinical manager, and added, "He rubbed lotion on my back and down under my panties. I tried to wiggle to keep him away from my front. I told him he was making me uncomfortable and he stopped and told me to just relax and fall asleep." The clinical manager notified the assistant director of nursing and the patient's doctor of the incident.

At 1030, a magnetic resonance imaging (MRI) information booklet was given to Catherine's mother, and at 1115 Catherine was taken by ambulance to receive the MRI at another hospital.

That evening, after consulting with family members, Catherine's father contacted the police and reported a sexual assault on a minor. Catherine's account to police detectives included:

April 10:
2330–2340: A Hispanic male dressed in light green scrubs entered her room and said, "I need to take your temperature and pulse." He turned her bracelet and read her name, then patted her on the head and said, "I'm gonna turn off the light and close the door so you can get some sleep." Patient told him to leave the light on. He said "No," turned the light off, and shut the door as he walked out.

April 10–11:
2400–0010: He returned and Catherine noted a squeaky noise from his shoes as he entered the room. (This noise differed from the clicking noise of the nurse's shoes on the wooden floor.) He told her that he had to put cream on her for the tests in the morning. He rubbed cream on her back, legs, across her buttocks and close to her vaginal area. Catherine tensed when the touching got close to her vaginal area and tried to roll onto her back, but he said, "Relax. Just go to sleep. This is going to help you." While she was still on her stomach, he reached around and began rubbing and massaging her breasts. He turned her over and started massaging, squeezing, and fondling her breasts. She asked, "Is this necessary?" He said, "Yes it is."

April 11:
Third Encounter: Since she had been asleep, Catherine was unsure what time he returned, but she was awakened by the squeaking sound of his shoes. He stood at the end of the bed watching her for almost ten minutes. She faked sleep, hoping that he would just leave her alone.

After watching her for ten minutes, he walked over and started rubbing her back and front again. She tensed and tried to roll away, but he rolled her back and started rubbing her front, her stomach, and down towards her crotch area, where he went underneath her panties and started touching her vaginal area. She tensed her legs together to try to keep his hands away from her vagina and asked, "Why are you doing that?" He responded, "I'm helping you. Don't worry. Just relax." He left the room, leaving the lights off and closing the door.

She stated that she was definitely afraid of him now and thought he was the nurse that was taking care of her all night. She was afraid to push the call button because he would return and do more fondling. She was also afraid to call on the phone. She thought he would overhear or catch her and would do something to her physically. She was afraid to go to the bathroom during the night.

About 0300: He returned with a hospital gown and told her to take off her gown and put on the hospital gown for the morning test. She refused and said

she'd put it on in the morning and that she wanted to be left alone. He then started grabbing the gown she had on, trying to pull it off, but she refused and resisted. He finally relented, put the gown beside the bed and told her, "I'll leave it here and you can put it on later," and he then left the room.
About 0430: He entered, stood at the end of the bed, and watched her for a long time. She thought he'd left but evidently he had walked into the bathroom. She heard another pair of foot steps come in (possibly the nurse due to the clicking of the shoes). The other party entered, checked some charts, and then left. She then heard the squeaking shoes walking around in the room, then going to the door, and then she heard the door close slowly.
Sixth Encounter: He woke her and said he had to look in her eyes. After probing open her eyes, he then grabbed her with both hands, pulled her head towards him and started kissing her. She tried to push him away but didn't have enough strength. He tried pushing his tongue into her mouth. She tried to pull away but wasn't strong enough and he held her head with both hands.
Seventh, Eighth, and Ninth Encounters: He came back to the room two to three more times, fondled her for short periods of time, and then left. She was very afraid of this person, afraid to do anything. She was relieved when the new nurse came, but was still afraid to say anything.
0700: He entered, awakened her, and said, "I just want you to know, you're a beautiful girl and it was a pleasure to meet you."
After 0700: She called her boyfriend and told him what had happened, and he advised her to tell a nurse. She called the morning nurse, told her what had happened, and stated that she knew Nurse Knott but had seen her only once during the night.

Outcome

Catherine received short-term counseling.

Legal

Civil: A nursing malpractice suit was settled out of court to the plantiff's satisfaction.
Criminal: The perpetrator was sentenced to four years in prison for sexual assault on a minor.

Case Commentary

Undesirable Patient Outcome

Assessment Nurse Knott made continuous nursing notes about light headedness, dizziness, "woozy," nausea, and "a little sleepy."

Diagnosis Preliminary nursing diagnoses were completed on admission. These included:

Risk for Sensory/Perceptual Alteration
Risk for Fluid Volume Deficit
Risk for Injury

Planning The nursing care plan noted "up with assistance," but this patient had been up without assistance since admission.

Implementation Despite planned activity of "up with assistance," Nurse Knott found the lights out and door closed at 0130. She did not awaken the patient to inquire and reinstruct her to get out of bed only with help. Intravenous intake was charted every hour on the hour, but Nurse Knott stated in her deposition that she checked Catherine every hour on the half hour. Vital signs were assessed and documented *only once* that shift, at 0600, and the only output (200 mL) was charted at the end of the shift. Nurse Knott did not assist the patient to the bathroom or reinstruct her concerning the need for assistance.

Evaluation Although Nurse Knott was the only care provider assigned to pediatrics, she noticed a pile of linens in the patient's room at 0130. She did not investigate who was going into this young girl's room.

Desirable Patient Outcome

Assessment Because the pediatric area was being renovated, pediatrics had been moved to the last four rooms at the end of the geriatric floor. The pediatric nurses' station consisted of a desk and chart rack placed inside the treatment room directly across the hall from the first pediatric room. The nurse's ability to view up and down the hall was totally blocked except for the area directly in front of the door.

The *Code for Nurses* requires the nurse "to safeguard the client's right to privacy by judiciously protecting information of a confidential nature" (ANA, 1985, p. 4). The *Standards of Clinical Nursing Practice* requires the nurse to "maintain client confidentiality" (ANA, 1991, p. 15). The *Standards of Organizational Nursing* (ANA, 1988) also requires nursing administration to provide records that are accessible to nurses but are maintained in a confidential manner. Pediatric charts were accessible to the staff in a mobile, open (i.e., unlocked) chart rack. Staffing with only one nurse left the medical records of all patients unsecured, therefore accessible to anyone, while the nurse was in the patients' rooms administering care. The patient's medical record is a confidential document and only those directly concerned with the client's care should have access to it. The orderly assigned to the geriatric floor knew about the scheduled test for the following morning because he had unauthorized access to Catherine's kardex and/or medical record. There were no security safeguards for, nor surveillance of, confidential patient records. This violated the facility's (JCAHO, 1995) and organized nursing service's duty to provide "a structure . . . to maintain care within ethical and legal guidelines" (ANA, 1988, p. 7). Although these were paper-based records, restricting access to online data and maintaining confidentiality of computerized records is also essential (Frawley, 1994).

Diagnosis *Standards of Maternal-Child Health Nursing Practice* require the nurse to promote "an environment free of hazards to reproduction, growth and development, wellness, and recovery from illness" (ANA, 1983, p. 14).

The nurse "identifies actual or potential hazards to maintenance of health" (ANA, 1983, p. 14). Positioning pediatrics at the end of the geriatric floor placed four pediatric rooms next to the floor's unsecured rear exit. Since a nurse in the nurses' station had no visual access to the hall in front of the rooms, she had no way of monitoring entrance and/or exit from the children's rooms. Staffing with one nurse left all other patients vulnerable (i.e., to abduction, molestation, etc.) when the nurse was in another patient's room administering care.

The "old" pediatric area was a closed unit—a cluster of rooms around a central nursing station all secured behind two closed doors. Compared to the "old" area, the temporary pediatric unit was not conducive to the children's physical safety or nursing vigilance. Since the security of the pediatric area was compromised by the temporary arrangements, all pediatric patients placed in any of these rooms should have had the nursing diagnosis: *Altered Protection.* This diagnosis would have heightened the awareness of the nursing staff and increased their level of suspicion because of the unsafe conditions of the physical environment. Other relevant nursing diagnoses should have included:

Knowledge Deficit related to lack of information about safety/assistance when getting out of bed

Knowledge Deficit related to lack of information about MRI testing

Planning The *Standards of Clinical Nursing Practice* requires nurses to "develop a plan of care that prescribes interventions to attain expected outcomes" (ANA, 1991, p. 10). A plan to increase vigilance and surveillance, which may have included moving the nursing desk into the hall and locking the medical records in a file cabinet, would have partially addressed the nursing diagnosis of *Altered Protection.* A plan to monitor who went in and out of this patient's room was also warranted, since only one nurse was the designated nighttime care provider for all three pediatric patients. A plan to address this patient's knowledge deficits should have resulted in awakening her to reiterate the need for assistance when out of bed, and instructions regarding MRI.

The excellent security of the "old" pediatric area was not considered in planning temporary pediatric bedspaces. The institution did not provide an appropriate physical environment, nor did it provide a mechanism to review and revise staffing patterns to implement plans of care for *Altered Protection* adequately (ANA, 1988). To prevent a hazardous environment for pediatric patients, nursing administration should have demanded that the hospital either secure the temporary pediatric area with prefabricated walls and doors, or provide adequate nursing staff to scrutinize access to patient rooms and records.

Implementation To promote an environment free of hazards, the nurse monitors hazardous environments, teaches personnel practices that minimize or eliminate environmental hazards, and intervenes to minimize or eliminate environmental hazards (ANA, 1983). Since the institution's temporary physical layout did not accommodate pediatric safety, organized nursing services should have encouraged independent nursing interventions to minimize hazards to all pediatric patients (ANA, 1988). In carrying out appropriate interventions and treatments to facilitate survival and recovery, the nurse provides a physical and psychological environment conducive to recovery and achievement of health (ANA, 1983). The total lack of challenge to the orderly as he freely roamed the hallway in the pediatric area, to which he was not assigned, demonstrates the nurse's lack of surveillance of patient rooms and independent nursing interventions to minimize hazards. The lack of an established nurse-patient relationship enabled this teenager to develop a relationship with the perpetrator (who posed as her night nurse). Opportunities to establish and continue a relationship between Nurse Knott and Catherine were lost in the nurse's failure to intervene by: (a) assessing vital signs at the beginning of the shift; (b) teaching Catherine about her impending MRI test and any patient preparation needed; and (c) awakening Catherine to reiterate the need for assistance in getting out of bed. These missed opportunities enabled this patient to establish a closer relationship with her abuser than with her caretaker.

All 50 states require health care providers, including nurses, to report any suspected child abuse. Failure to report is a criminal offense (in all but Mississippi, North Carolina, Wyoming, and Maryland) or may result in forfeiture of professional license (in Maryland) (Tammelleo, 1988). Both direct (i.e., the child's eyewitness description) and circumstantial (i.e., physical or psychological) evidence constitute grounds for reporting. The *Child Abuse and Prevention Act* (P.L. 100–294) defines sexual abuse as the use, persuasion, or coercion of any child to engage in sexually explicit conduct (or any simulation of such conduct) for producing any visual depiction of such conduct, or rape, molestation, prostitution, or incest with children (Whaley & Wong, 1995). When a person responsible for the child's care (e.g., parent, babysitter) commits such acts, it is considered child abuse; when a stranger commits such acts, it is considered sexual assault and is handled by police and criminal courts (National Center on Child Abuse and Neglect, 1989). Only after consultation with family members did the father call the police to report sexual assault on a minor. No professionals (staff or administration) reported this incident to the police. Since a report is a request for an investigation and not an accusation, all persons reporting in good faith are immune from criminal prosecution and civil liability. If the family had not reported the attack, would the hospital or its professional employees have done so? Were the "best interests" of the minor child or the "best interests" of the hospital being protected? Would this perpetrator ever have been brought to justice? How many defenseless geriatric patients had this perpetrator molested?

Evaluation Children should be safe (i.e., secure, protected, unendangered, unharmed) at school, at church, and in a hospital. Outcome criteria to measure a hazard-free environment include fewer complications due to hazards in the hospital environment (ANA, 1983). This child suffered both physical and psychological complications as a result of nursing's lack of surveillance and vigilance regarding patient safety. During the six to seven months of this inappropriate physical layout for pediatrics, it is amazing that an abduction did not occur!

Case 2

Facts

Six-week-old Tanya was brought by her mother to the ER of a children's hospital for an axillary temperature of 38.9 of 1 1/2 hours duration and a decreased appetite for three to four days. ER records also noted: a birth weight of 6 lbs 5 oz (2860 grams), an admission weight of 9 lbs 13 oz (4460 grams), oral thrush, and a history of frequent vomiting since birth, at times projectile. A sepsis workup included: urinalysis; blood and urine culture and sensitivity; CBC; blood glucose, and lumbar puncture. A peripheral IV was started, the first dose of Ampicillin given, and the infant admitted to a semiprivate room.

At admission, Sally Jones, RN, recorded the following on the nursing data base:

- Vital signs: T 37.8 C (R), P 180, R 36; BP 84/P
- History of current health problems: has been irritable and has had decreased appetite for several days. Spiked temperature to 38.9 today. Her mother called private pediatrician who told her to bring baby to ER. Has past history of vomiting.
- Nutrition: Similac with Iron, takes 4–5 oz. every 3–4 hours; eats well.

Nurse Jones also wrote the nursing assessment summary:

Six-week-old female admitted with history of vomiting, decreased appetite, fever, and irritability. Admitted for urinary tract infection (UTI). Is alert but fussy; is well hydrated.

Nurse Jones also wrote the nursing care plan in Table 13-1.

Table 13-1 Identified Problems and Nursing Care Plan

Date	Patient/Family Problems	Nursing Plan of Care	Goals
June	UTI	• Assess and document urinary status q shift for odor, amount. • Push fluids. • Cleanse perineum front to back. • IV maintenance and antibiotics as ordered. • Call HO for increase temperature. Sponge prn and give acetaminophen as ordered.	Void fully. No increase in temperature. Parental knowledge.
June	Discharge teaching	• Follow-up care. • Administration of medications at home. • Proper pericare and cleansing.	Parental knowledge of care of child.

The medical admitting note read: baby was 37 weeks at birth; at four days was readmitted for cyanosis. An echocardiogram revealed a persistent foramen ovale. Rice cereal begun two weeks ago.

After results of laboratory data were obtained, this infant's medical diagnoses were: UTI and sepsis (positive for *E. coli* in blood culture). Tanya was hospitalized for seven days, during which time she received IV antibiotics and fed orally. During these seven days, she remained in a semiprivate room with another infant. Tanya's chart contained 16 RN documentations of vomiting and four MD citations of vomiting—all by a third-year medical student. On the seventh day of hospitalization, two RNs were in the room at 1520 giving/receiving shift-to-shift report. At 1530, the 3–11 RN found Tanya lying in a 35–40 mL pool of vomited formula, with no heart beat or respirations. There was no suction equipment (i.e., bulb or wall suction) in the room; CPR wasn't begun until the RN removed the baby and equipment to the treatment room. The first set of arterial blood gases showed severe respiratory acidosis (pH 6.89).

Outcome

An upper gastrointestinal (GI) series revealed gastroesophageal reflux (GER). The child is now profoundly retarded with severe developmental delays and cerebral palsy.

Legal

This case was settled out of court for $900,000.

Case Commentary

Undesirable Patient Outcome

Assessment Both the ER nurse and the ward's staff nurse collected and recorded data about this infant's history of vomiting.

Diagnosis On admission to the hospital, this infant's differential medical diagnoses included: septicemia, UTI, and meningitis. Only after lab data was obtained were the diagnoses of UTI and sepsis certain. All pertinent and potential nursing diagnoses were not considered or documented. "UTI" is a medical diagnosis, *not* a nursing diagnosis. Assignment of a medical diagnosis narrowed the nursing approach to care and focused the nurse on actions outside nursing's domain.

Planning In planning the physical environment (e.g., room assignment, use of monitors, risk of apnea/seizures), the admitting nurse did not consider all potential problems. Inappropriate diagnosis (i.e., use of medical instead of nursing diagnoses) creates inaccuracy in the planning and implementation of care. Independent nursing responsibilities (i.e., providing a safe physical environment that is developmentally appropriate) were not addressed in the plan or implementation of care. The resultant plan of care was not specific: parameters for practice—how often, how much, when, by whom—were not delineated.

Implementation The implemented plan did not meet patient needs because *all* preceding steps did not accurately define patient needs/problems.

Evaluation Evaluation was not carried out because no measurable outcomes were defined throughout this infant's hospitalization. Also, this infant's history of vomiting and continuation to vomit in the hospital did not prompt Nurse Jones to evaluate her nursing plan or her implementation of care. In this setting, nursing care was nondirectional.

Desirable Patient Outcome

Assessment Pertinent data about a history of vomiting was available but did not enter into nursing diagnosis, planning, implementation, or evaluation (ANA, 1983, 1991).

Diagnosis Nurse Jones failed to identify any nursing diagnoses (ANA, 1983). None of Tanya's nurses reviewed diagnoses in a resource text, prioritized possible diagnoses, or consulted with nurse colleagues or clinical nurse specialists initially or throughout this infant's hospitalization (ANA, 1991). Given the assessment data, potential nursing diagnoses for this infant should have included those in Table 13-2.

Planning The nursing plan of care in Table 13-1 does not meet the standard of care because it does not identify expected outcomes derived from the diagnoses nor prescribe interventions to attain expected management of a vulnerable client (ANA 1983, 1991). The nursing care plan in Table 13-2 utilizes the assessment data; prioritizes nursing diagnoses; and enables care to be planned, implemented, and evaluated based on nursing diagnoses.

Implementation Nurses were unable to implement appropriate and therapeutic interventions because the plan of care (Table 13-1) was *not* based on the assessment data and nursing diagnoses (ANA, 1991). A review of the admission care plan in Table 13-2 illustrates this infant's potential for apnea and/or seizures related to sepsis, UTI, and meningitis. The plan also illustrates the risk of suffocation (secondary to aspiration) because of her history of vomiting, addition of rice cereal to formula feedings (used in gastroesophageal reflux) and vomiting that may accompany sepsis, UTI, and meningitis. The standard of care requires that interventions be implemented in a safe and appropriate manner (ANA, 1991). Considering these risk factors for potentially fatal complications, Tanya's nurses should have provided for a safe physical environment by implementing the following measures:

- A review of environmental safeguards in the hospital's policies and procedures for care of infants would reveal that infants are *never* left alone in rooms without frequent assessment and monitoring. At-risk infants are always monitored (with alarms on) since choking, seizures, and apnea are silent phenomena that may occur when staff are present but otherwise occupied. Since these life threatening events are accompanied by heart rate and respiratory changes, the monitor will sound and summon care.
- A review of environmental safeguards on pediatric floors will reveal that pediatric patients (according to developmental abilities) are given a "call

Table 13-2 Nursing Care Plan

Patient Needs/ Nursing Diagnosis	Patient Goals/Outcomes	Nursing Interventions/ Collaborative Actions	Evaluation
Hyperthermia related to infection (rule out: sepsis, UTI, meningitis)	Maintain temperature between 36.5 and 37.5 degrees C.	• Take axillary temperature q 2 hours. • Dress appropriately. • Call HO for > temperature - sponge. • Administer acetaminophen and document response prn.	Axillary temperature between 36.5 and 37.5 degrees C.
Altered Tissue Perfusion: Cerebral as evidenced by > irritability and < appetite for 3–4 days *High Risk for Suffocation* (secondary to apnea-seizures) related to sepsis /meningitis	Maintain/preserve neurologic integrity.	• Keep stimulation to a minimum; provide quiet environment. • If irritability continues or increases, obtain order for analgesic (acetaminophen) or sedative (chloral hydrate). • Set cardiorespiratory monitors with following settings: apnea 20 sec, low alarm 90, high alarm 200. • Resuscitation equipment (bag, mask, oxygen) setup at bedside.	No apnea. No pain behaviors: crying irritability restlessness >HR, R, BP. No seizure behaviors: nystagmus tongue thrust hyper/hypotonicity apnea tonic/clonic movements.
Ineffective Infant Feeding Pattern related to history of vomiting since birth, addition of rice cereal at 4 weeks of age *High Risk for Aspiration* related to history of vomiting	Maintain/continue adequate nutrition. Parents utilize appropriate feeding techniques.	• Observe parent-infant feeding behavior. • Feed infant and note timing of vomiting (type, amount, color, consistency). • Chalasia regime: HOB up 30–45 degrees at least 1 hour after feedings; prone after feedings. • Cardiorespiratory monitors (with settings as above). • Suction equipment at bedside (bulb; wall suction and #8 and #10 fr. catheters and gloves).	Intake 110–120 kcal/kg/day. Weight gain: 20–30 gm/day. Output 1–3 mL/kg/hr. Specific gravity 1.002 to 1.012. Parents able to position and burp infant while feeding and position infant correctly after feeding. Decrease in number of vomiting episodes. No aspiration or apnea secondary to vomiting.
Altered Family Processes related to infant's hospitalization	Parents remain involved in infant's care. Minimal/no increase in family stress.	• Encourage parent visits and participation in care. • Instruct and assist in feeding techniques.	Parents visit and participate in care. Parents ask appropriate questions.
Altered Urinary Elimination related to infection	Maintain/preserve urinary tract integrity.	• Strict I & O. • Urinary dipstick and specific gravity q void. • Weigh daily. • Monitor temperature q 4 hrs. • Administer medications and monitor for effect, adverse reactions.	Output 1–3 mL/kg/hr. Specific gravity 1.002 to 1.012. Weight gain: 20–30 gm/day. Temperature: 36.5–37.4 C Ax. Cultures: negative. Urinalysis: WNL.

light" to summon the nurse. Children who are sick enough to be hospitalized are at risk for potentially fatal events. An at-risk infant who cannot call for help with a "call light" must be provided some way (i.e., cardiorespiratory monitor) to summon help. For infants on a pediatric floor, the standard of care for safety cannot be any lower than the standard practiced for infants of the same age and acuity in the level II-III nurseries. Provision of a safe physical environment is an independent nursing function, a professional duty to the patient that does not require a physician's order. The *Standards of Maternal-Child Health Nursing Practice* (ANA, 1983) cites a safe environment as a standard of care for pediatric nurses. Hospital policies and protocols should reflect room/bed assignments for pediatric patients that are safe and developmentally appropriate. However, "neither a physician's order nor the employing agency's policies relieve a nurse of accountability for actions taken and judgments made" (ANA, 1985, p. 9). In this situation, the nurses were not relieved of their duty and accountability because they failed to make judgments and take appropriate action.

Evaluation Over a seven-day hospital stay, 16 nursing documentations of vomiting did not result in any evaluation or alteration of the plan of care (ANA, 1983, 1991). Every nurse who cared for Tanya in the week she was hospitalized should have evaluated the implementation of her nursing care plan. For example: Since she continued to vomit, was there suction equipment at the bedside? Was the room assignment safe? Should cardiorespiratory monitors be initiated? A proactive model of active, ongoing, dynamic evaluation at every step of the nursing process would have prevented the tragic outcome of this case and enabled the discharge of a healthy infant to her parents.

Case 3

Facts

Three-week-old Sarah was admitted from a clinic to a community hospital pediatric unit on November 2 at 1300 with the medical diagnoses of bacterial meningitis and rule out Group B beta-hemolytic strep. According to her mother, Sarah awoke during the night "screaming as if she was in pain, and real hot." Sarah's mother brought her to the clinic.

An assessment of Sarah in the clinic revealed a rectal temperature of 38.9 and a very irritable child. A lumbar puncture was performed with the following results: cloudy cerebral spinal fluid (CSF) with 1,400 WBCs, 95% neutrophils, glucose 14, and protein 318 (CSF and blood cultures were positive for *E. coli* 24 hours later). The decision was made by the clinic staff to admit Sarah to the hospital.

Upon admission, Susan Broad, RN, noted the following:

- Vital signs: T 38.4C (R), P 200 and regular, R charted as infant crying, BP 120/80.

- Weight 9 lb. 10 oz. (4500 grams) (birth weight 8 lbs. 5 oz. [3770 grams]).
- Nutrition: breastfeeds every 3–4 hours with supplemental feedings of Enfamil with iron formula via an Evenflo nipple.
- Infant alert and very fussy on admission. Eyes puffy and glazed, but PERL with some apparent sensitivity to light.
- No previous illness or hospitalization.

Physician orders on admission were as follows:

- IV D5.2NS at 15 mL/hr.
- Ampicillin 500 mg IV now and q 8 hrs.
- Gentamicin 10 mg IV now and q 8 hrs.
- Dexamethasone 0.6 mg IV q 6 hrs × 4 days.

November 2:
At 1400, Nurse Broad inserted a 24-gauge angiocath into Sarah's left hand to begin administration of medications ordered by Sarah's physician. An IV infusion pump was used to deliver the fluid at 15 mL/hr and medications were added to the IV tubing at regular intervals. (Throughout her hospitalization, from 1300 on November 2 to 1000 on November 6, when she was prepared for transport to a tertiary hospital, nurses repeatedly documented problems with intravenous access and maintenance of IV sites in both the nurses' notes and the IV flow sheet.)

November 3:
At 1330, the IV pump alarmed and Nurse Broad found an infiltrated IV site in Sarah's left hand. Nurse Broad discontinued the angiocath and applied a "warm pack" to the swollen hand. Thirty minutes later, when the pack (now cold) was removed, Nurse Broad documented that the swelling had "decreased." Nurse Broad then inserted a 24-gauge angiocath into Sarah's right antecubital space and secured it on an armboard with tape and gauze.

November 4:
At 1400, Nurse Broad again found Sarah's IV infiltrated with localized swelling in her right antecubital area. She again applied a "warm pack." She restarted the IV in Sarah's left foot at 1500.

November 5:
At 0130, Nurse Smith, the night-shift nurse, found Sarah's angiocath half out of her foot when she went into Sarah's room to respond to the IV pump alarm. Nurse Smith was unable to restart Sarah's IV and held Sarah's IV medications until 0600, when she called the physician about the IV. At 0600, the physician ordered the medications to be given intramuscularly (IM) until another IV could be inserted. At 0645, Nurse Broad arrived on the floor, was told about this order, and successfully restarted an angiocath in Sarah's right hand at 0800.

November 6:
This angiocath remained in place until 1000, when Sarah's physician, assessing her for transfer to a tertiary center, unwrapped the gauze covering the IV site and found a "significant infiltration" into the soft tissue of Sarah's right

hand and forearm. Sarah's left index finger and dorsal side of hand were noted to be "severely swollen with broken blisters on the anterior surface and whitened skin on the dorsal surface of her hand, extending almost to her elbow." A "warm pack" was again applied. A Telfa dressing was applied after consultation with a dermatologist, and Sarah was transferred to a tertiary care hospital for placement of a central line to continue the IV antibiotic therapy.

Over the next few days, the IV infiltrate was treated as a "chemical burn" at the tertiary center, and Sarah was discharged from the hospital after completion of the antibiotic therapy. For almost three weeks, Sarah was followed as an outpatient for ongoing care of the infiltration site.

Outcome

One year later, Sarah has a large scar on the inner aspect of her right arm resulting from the IV infiltration.

Legal

Sarah's parents have filed a lawsuit against the community hospital and the nurses who cared for Sarah. Sarah's parents contend that Sarah received inadequate care for IV maintenance and drug therapy and, as a result, is scarred. The case is under litigation at this time.

Case Commentary

Undesirable Patient Outcome

Assessment As documented in the IV-site maintenance record, nursing assessment of Sarah's IV site was sporadic throughout her hospitalization. Within the 24-hour period following the start of the first IV site (left hand), medications were administered into the IV line ten times and nurses documented checking the site only seven times: at 1800, 2400 (November 4), 0200, 0400, 0600, and 1400 (November 5), when an infiltration was discovered. During the 24-hour period following the start of the second IV site (right antecubital), medications were administered into the line ten times, while the nurses documented checking the IV site a total of four times: at 2400, 0200, 0600, and 1400, when the IV infiltrated.

Documentation of the third IV site in Sarah's left foot was made a total of six times: at 1600, 1800, 2000, 2200, 2400, and 0130, when the IV was dislodged. Medications were added to this line ten times. Sarah's fourth IV site in her right hand was inserted at 0800 on November 5 and an assessment of the site occurred only once, at 0200 on November 6, even though seven doses of medications were administered through that line.

Diagnosis Nurse Broad initiated a standardized care plan for this infant at the time of admission which included two diagnoses: infection (meningitis) and discharge planning. She used a plan of care that was formulated for adult patients, and modified it for Sarah by inserting "parents" for "patient" at key spots in the care plan (Table 13-3).

Table 13-3 Standard Care Plan

Diagnosis	Goals	Related Interventions
Infection	1. To prevent complications and eliminate infection. 2. Patient (Parent)* learns measures to prevent contamination of others. 3. To return to optimal health.	1. Assess signs and symptoms of infection on admission and every shift. 2. Obtain lab work as ordered; explain all procedures to patient (parents).* 3. Give antibiotics as ordered to maintain therapeutic blood level; monitor for side effects. 4. Monitor TPR every 4 hours and record; report elevations; monitor as ordered. 5. Monitor I & O. 6. Isolate if communicable. 7. Use appropriate isolation techniques. 8. Explain necessary precautions to patient (parents).* 9. Monitor lab results. 10. Medicate as ordered for pain (fussiness).*
Discharge Planning	1. Patient (Parents)* to perform necessary procedures satisfactorily prior to discharge. 2. Patient (Parents)* to receive written information for use at home.	1. Teach medications ordered: name, purpose, dose, frequency, precautions, side effects. 2. Teach steps of all procedures to be done at home; observe patient (parents)* practice. 3. Teach patient (parents)* symptoms that require medical attention. 4. Tell patient (parents)* where and when to return for follow-up care. 5. Answer any questions and respond to any concerns. 6. Provide written information to take home: identify other available resources.

*Indicates where adult standardized care plan was altered to fit "parent" and "fussiness" as pediatric parameters.

Planning The nursing care plan, designed for use with adult patients, addressed only the diagnoses of infection and discharge planning. A medical diagnosis of infection (meningitis) created inaccuracies in the planning and implementation of nursing care. Independent responsibilities (e.g., monitoring for hyperthermia, supporting families, providing ongoing education, providing adequate fluids, and monitoring skin integrity, particularly at the IV site for signs of infiltration) were not addressed in the care plan. The resultant plan of care addressed only two of the multiple needs of this infant, no nursing diagnoses were formulated, and interventions were not specific for parameters for practice: how often, how much, when, and by whom were not delineated.

Implementation The implemented plan did not comprehensively address Sarah's needs. *All* steps of the nursing process were not accurately carried out to define this child's needs or used to develop nursing interventions.

Evaluation Evaluation of the interventions was incomplete since all of the interventions were related to medical diagnoses and resultant treatments. Sarah's nurses did not evaluate or intervene for her ongoing hyperthermia and problematic intravenous therapy. They did not evaluate their plan of care to change or alter their nursing interventions.

Desirable Patient Outcome

Untold nursing hours are spent obtaining and maintaining vascular access in the neonate, infant, and child. The intravenous route offers a direct and rapid means of fluid, blood, and drug administration. Despite the multiple benefits of IV therapy, serious consequences can result when infiltrations occur. A number of factors have been identified that increase the risk of IV infiltration: (a) age, (b) type of cannula, (c) site of IV, (d) method of stabilizing the IV, (e) ability to visualize the IV site, (f) type of IV solution, (g) administration of IV medications, (h) use of IV infusion pumps, and (i) experience of personnel starting and caring for the IV site (Batton, Maisels, & Applebaum, 1982; Bostrom-Ezrati, Dibble, & Rizzuto, 1990; Brown, Hoelzer, & Piercy, 1979; Fay, 1983; Hagedorn & Yucha, 1994; Petit & Hughes, 1993; Phelps & Cochran, 1989; Phelps & Helms, 1987).

Up to 11% of IV lines have been reported to infiltrate in the pediatric population. These can result in significant sequelae including tissue necrosis, pain and discomfort, scarring, loss of function of an extremity through nerve damage or contractures, and amputation (Brown, Hoelzer, & Piercy, 1979; Dunn, 1984; Upton, Mulliken, & Murray, 1979). Treatment for the sequelae of an IV infiltration in the pediatric patient often results in a longer hospital stay, surgical debridement, skin grafting, and in some cases, amputation of the limb (Brown, Hoelzer, & Piercy, 1979; Dunn, 1984; Upton, Mulliken, & Murray, 1979). In addition to the increased length of hospitalization for the infant or child, cases involving infusion-related injuries are frequently litigated (Johnson & Sipos, 1987). Patients most at risk to develop extravasation and resultant necrosis are very young children who are unable to communicate the pain produced by the extravasated fluid (Phelps & Helms, 1987). A reported increase in the incidence of infiltration in neonates and infants, ranging from 58–78% (Batton, Maisels, & Applebaum, 1982; Johnson & Donn, 1988; Phelps & Cochran, 1989; Phelps & Helms, 1987), reflects the lack of a standard clinical definition and the variation in reporting IV failure. In addition, more extravasation/infiltration injuries occur at night than during the day, due in part to the decreased ability to visualize the site in the night hours (Johnson & Donn, 1988). Furthermore, inexperienced personnel may take several attempts to establish venous access and may predispose the vein to early infiltration; or they may attempt to "preserve" a line fearing they will not successfully restart an IV.

Infants and children receiving medications via an IV infusion pump have two additional factors that increase the risk of infiltration and resultant tissue damage. Most medications introduced into an IV line are irritants and decrease the longevity of the IV (Petit & Hughes, 1993). Furthermore, occlusion alarms on IV infusion pumps are often not helpful in the detection of infiltrations, because infiltration has already occurred (a degree of back pressure must occur to activate the alarm).

Lastly, the positioning of the extremity on an IV board and massive taping rituals can also lead to infiltration (Petit & Hughes, 1993). Inadequate visualization, due to the taping, impedes the identification of an infiltration until it has progressed to a level that often leads to tissue sloughing. Taping a bony prominence to an unpadded, rigid board can lead to tissue breakdown and resultant blistering and eschar development (Petit & Hughes, 1993).

Once an infiltration is detected in a child, the nurse must know the institutional policies and standards of care surrounding management of the infiltration. For years, pediatric nurses have wrapped the infiltration site in "warm/hot" packs, believing that this intervention increases circulation to the area, thereby relieving the infiltration. In fact, literature has documented untoward effects of heat on an infiltrated IV site in the pediatric patient. Moist heat has reportedly led to maceration and subsequent necrosis (Brown, Hoelzer, & Piercy, 1979; Door, Alberts, & Stone, 1989; Few, 1987). Rudolph and Larson (1987) suggested that the application of warmth increases the metabolic demand of the surrounding tissues, thereby increasing tissue necrosis that often occurs with vesicants. Clinical case studies also indicate that massive damage can occur when heat is applied to tissues already filled with fluid. Heat actually raises the metabolic demands of the tissue and the temperature of the fluid, ultimately leading to a blistering burn that often sloughs leaving eschar (Brown, Hoelzer, & Piercy, 1979; Hagedorn & Yucha, 1994).

Larson (1982) advocated the application of cold in addition to elevation to treat infiltrations. Robson & Tompkins (1989) treated IV infiltrations in pediatric ICU patients (n=15) with gauze soaked in ice-water/slush solution. The immediate identification and treatment with ice/slush resulted in 100% resolution of tissue injury in these patients.

Repeated infiltrations of IV sites in the child may indicate the need for placement of a percutaneous catheter or central line to provide necessary fluid and drug therapy. Nurses are the health care professionals who care for and monitor these intravenous lines, and therefore must have appropriate knowledge and skill to recognize and manage infiltrations and advocate for the child when a percutaneous or central line is indicated. This case is a primary example of the lack of independent decision-making by the nurse and an inability to follow prudent standards of care.

Assessment Pertinent data about the history of hyperthermia, "screaming as if in pain," and sudden change in health status did not enter into the plan of care for this infant. Given the assessment data revealed in the clinic, ongoing assessment of hyperthermia, fluid status (including IV management), and nutritional status would be particularly important.

Sarah had several factors that increased her risk of IV infiltration: age, type of cannula, site of IV, method of stabilizing the IV cannula, ability to visualize the IV site, type of IV solution, administration of IV medications, use of IV infusion pump, and inexperienced personnel caring for the IV site (Bostrom-Ezrati, Dibble, & Rizzuto 1990; Brown, Hoelzer, & Piercy, 1979; Fay, 1983). An ongoing, hourly assessment of the IV was indicated to avoid extensive infiltration of the site.

Standards of pediatric care, hospital policies, and the plan of care for an infant with an IV via an infusion pump endorse an hourly assessment and documentation of the IV site and condition to detect swelling, redness, or infiltration (Brown, Hoelzer, & Piercy, 1979; Hagedorn & Yucha, 1994; Fay, 1983; Petit & Hughes, 1993; Zenk, 1980). In addition, administering medication through an IV line further necessitates the ongoing hourly assessment of an IV site in an infant or child (Petit & Hughes, 1993; Hagedorn & Yucha, 1994).

Sarah was receiving both IV fluids and two antibiotics (known to irritate veins when administered). The IV site was not assessed on an hourly basis. In addition, massive taping and gauze placed at the IV site occluded the nurse's visualization of the site.

Diagnosis The *Standards of Maternal-Child Health Nursing Practice* (ANA, 1983) requires the nurse to promote "an environment free of hazard to reproduction, growth and development, wellness, and recovery from illness" (p. 8). Failure to diagnose adequately this child's alterations in health led to inadequate development and implementation of nursing interventions. Appropriate nursing diagnosis rather than medical diagnosis would have alerted the nurse to pertinent problems requiring ongoing assessment and evaluation. Appropriate nursing diagnoses for this child should have included:

Hyperthermia related to increased metabolic rate, illness, and fluid losses as evidenced by elevated temperature

Risk for Infection related to presence of pyrogens in blood as evidenced by increased temperature, irritability, positive blood culture

Altered Tissue Perfusion: Cerebral related to inflammatory process as evidenced by irritability

Risk for Injury related to developmental level, restlessness, unfamiliar environment

Fluid Volume Deficit related to decreased fluid intake, increased insensible water loss, SG 1.020, dry mucous membranes, no tears

Altered Nutrition: Less than Body Requirements related to anorexia, fatigue, and vomiting as evidenced by poor oral intake

Risk for Impaired Skin Integrity related to immobility, diaphoresis, presence of an IV catheter

Pain related to meningeal irritation, phlebitis or infiltration, as evidenced by inconsolable cry, irritability

Anxiety, parental, related to unexpected hospitalization of child as evidenced by parental questions, body language

Knowledge Deficit, parental, regarding lack of information about illness, treatments, IV management, home care

Impaired Physical Mobility related to armboard placement for IV, restraints

Planning The *Standards of Clinical Nursing Practice* requires nurses to "develop a plan of care that prescribes interventions to attain expected outcomes" (ANA, 1991, p. 10). A plan to increase assessment of the IV site, nutritional and fluid status, and parental knowledge and anxiety was indicated. For nurses to simply alter an adult care plan to the pediatric setting by putting "parent" in place of "patient" (Table 13-3) violates the standard of clinical nursing practice (ANA, 1983, 1991). Standardized care plans are often helpful to the clinical nurse in divising a plan of care, but the standardized plan of care must be formulated for that specific population and modified for the individual patient. In planning and carrying out appropriate interventions and treatment to facilitate the child's recovery, the nurse must have the knowledge and skill to recognize threats to the child's safety and design appropriate plans of care related to these factors (ANA, 1983, 1991).

Implementation Nurses were unable to implement appropriate and therapeutic interventions because the plan of care was *not* based on assessment data or nursing diagnosis (ANA, 1991). In addition, nurses providing Sarah's care clearly lacked adequate knowledge and skill to monitor intravenous therapy, or they simply failed to institute appropriate institutional policies regarding maintaining IV infusions in pediatrics (i.e., failing to assess and document condition of IV site hourly). Sarah's IV access was difficult to establish and maintain. This should have alerted the nurses to more prudent surveillance of these lines. Massive tape and gauze not only impeded the assessment of the site, but may have contributed to IV infiltration. Furthermore, each time a medication was added to the IV line, the IV site should have been reassessed to ensure appropriate administration of the drug and integrity of the line. Lack of reassessment of the site on two occasions, prior to medication administration, resulted in significant infiltrations later being discovered.

Once Sarah's IV infiltrations were detected, little was done to manage the resultant effects. What was instituted, the warm pack, may have actually led to tissue damage and maceration (Brown, Hoelzer, & Piercy, 1979; Few, 1987; Hagedorn & Yucha, 1994; Rudolph & Larson, 1987).

Evaluation Over several days, Sarah's nurses administered multiple medications into her IV line that may have contributed to IV infiltration, yet the nurses failed to assess, evaluate, or document the integrity of the line hourly. Perhaps much of Sarah's irritability was related to these infiltrations. Every nurse caring for Sarah should have evaluated the implementation of her care plan (e.g., hyperthermia, infection, fluid volume status, nutritional status, pain [including ongoing assessment of the IV], parental knowledge, and anxiety). The impending transport of this infant should not have been the avenue for detecting this massive IV infiltration. A proactive model of ongoing, skilled evaluation, at every step of the nursing process, would have alerted these nurses to the issues surrounding safe IV administration of fluids and medications. Inadequate independent nursing judgment led to the sequelae presently plaguing this child.

Sequelae related to IV infiltration constitute the most common reason for litigation in pediatric nursing (Johnson & Sipos, 1987; Mahoney & Goldstein, personal communications, 1995). Although this case occurred in a community hospital, similar incidents have occurred in tertiary centers (e.g., university-based pediatric units or children's hospitals). Typically, in these incidents, the nurse fails to institute the standards of care and institutional policies for children receiving intravenous therapy. This results in tissue damage, grafting, patient suffering, and/or amputation of the limb. In addition, once the infiltration is discovered, the nurse often manages it inappropriately (i.e., uses "warm/hot" packs and fails to give an antidote such as Wydase or Regitine).

References

American Nurses Association. (1983). *Standards of maternal-child nursing practice.* Washington, D.C.: Author.

American Nurses Association. (1985). *Code for nurses.* Washington, D.C.: Author.

American Nurses Association. (1988). *Standards of organizational nursing.* Washington, D.C.: Author.

American Nurses Association. (1991). *Standards of clinical nursing practice.* Washington, D.C.: Author.

Batton, D., Maisels, M., & Applebaum, P. (1982). Use of peripheral intravenous cannulas in premature infants: A controlled study. *Pediatrics, 70,* 487–490.

Betz, C., Hunsberger, M., & Wright, S. (1994). *Family-centered nursing care of children* (2nd ed.). Philadelphia: Saunders.

Bostrom-Ezrati, J., Dibble, S., & Rizzuto, C. (1990). Intravenous therapy management: Who will develop insertion site symptoms? *Applied Nursing Research, 3,* 146–152.

Brown, A., Hoelzer, D., & Piercy, S. (1979). Skin necrosis from extravasation of intravenous fluid in children. *Plastic Reconstructive Surgery, 64,* 145–150.

Door, R., Alberts, D., & Stone, A. (1989). Cold protection and heat enhancement of doxorubicin skin toxicity in the mouse. *Cancer Treatment Reports, 69,* 431–437.

Dunn, D. (1984). Median and ulnar nerve palsies after infiltration of intravenous fluid. *Southern Medical Journal, 77*(10), 1, 345.

Fay, M. (1983). The special challenges of pediatric IVs. *Dimensions in Critical Care Nursing, 2,* 23–29.

Few, B. (1987). Hyaluronidase for treating intravenous extravasations. *Maternal-Child Nursing, 2,* 23–29.

Frawley, K. (1994, July). Confidentiality in the computer age. *RN,* 59–60.

Hagedorn, M. (1993). *A way of life: A new beginning each day. The family's lived experience of childhood chronic illness* (Doctoral dissertation, University of Colorado). University Microfilms International No. 9324737.

Hagedorn, M. & Yucha, C. (1994). *IV extravasations in pediatrics: A self-instruction module.* Denver, CO: Author.

Johnson, R. & Donn, S. (1988). Life span of intravenous cannulas in a neonatal intensive care unit. *American Journal of Diseases in Children, 142,* 968–971.

Johnson, J. & Sipos, L. (1987). The art of self-defense: Litigation and the neonatal nurse. *Journal of Perinatal Neonatal Nursing, 1,* 61–67.

Joint Commission on Accreditation of Healthcare Organizations. (1995). *Manual on Hospital Accreditation:* Standards. Oakbrook Terrace, IL: Author.

Larson, D. (1982). Treatment of tissue extravasation by antitumor agents. *Cancer, 49,* 1796–1799.

National Center on Child Abuse and Neglect. (1989). *Child abuse and neglect: A shared community concern* (DHHS Publication No. OHDS 89-30531). Washington D.C.: US Government Printing Office.

Petit, J. & Hughes, K. (1993). Intravenous extravasation: Mechanisms, management, and prevention. *Journal of Perinatal Neonatal Nursing, 6*(4), 69–79.

Phelps, S. & Cochran, E. (1989). Effect of the continuous administration of fat emulsion on the infiltration of peripheral intravenous lines in infants receiving parenteral nutrition solutions. *Journal of Parenteral Enteral Nutrition, 13,* 628–632.

Phelps, S. & Helms, R. (1987). Risk factors affecting infiltration of peripheral venous lines in infants. *Journal of Pediatrics, 111,* 384–390.

Robson, L. & Tompkins, J. (1989, October). *Management of caustic intravenous infiltrations in pediatric patients: A pilot study.* Paper presented at the meeting of Omicron, Iota/Delta Chapters of Sigma Theta Tau International, Syracuse, NY.

Rudolph, R. & Larson, D. (1987). Etiology and treatment of chemotherapeutic agent extravasation injuries: A review. *Journal of Clinical Oncology, 5,* 1116–1126.

Tammello, A. (1988, July). If you suspect child abuse. *RN,* 57–59.

Joint Commission on Accreditation of Heathcare Organizations. (1995). *Manual on Hospital Accreditation* Standards. Oakbrook Terrace, IL: Author.

Upton, J., Mulliken, J., & Murray, J. (1979). Major intravenous extravasation injuries. *American Journal of Surgery, 137,* 497–506.

Whaley, L. & Wong, D. (1995). *Nursing care of infants and children* (5th ed.). St. Louis: Mosby-Yearbook.

Zenk, K. (1980). Management of intravenous extravasations. *Infusion, 5*(4), 77–79.

14

Intensive Pediatric Care

Mary I. Enzman Hagedorn, RN, PhD, CNS, CPNP
Sandra L. Gardner, RN, MS, CNS, PNP

Pediatric patients are a particularly vulnerable population within critical care nursing (Kinney, 1992). Children are emotionally and cognitively immature, and this affects their comprehension and response to critical illness. Often the child's communication skills are unrefined or absent because of an early developmental level or intubation. The nurse must be able to anticipate the child's needs and concerns and be especially sensitive to the child's nonverbal communication. Astute surveillance, rapid response to changes, and creative, effective, patient-centered interventions are key to the care of the child in a critical care setting.

Families constitute an essential part of the child's support system and nurses must assess family dynamics and establish positive communication with family members. Parents particularly must be at the center of the decision-making process. Emotional support must be provided for concerns about their child's survival, often uncertain, cause ongoing anxiety, stress, fear, and worry for parents. Communication with parents must be clear, frequent, and consistent (Hazinski, 1992). If communication does not follow this pattern, the relationship between nurse and parent may become divisive and directly affect the care of the child.

"The critical care setting, while replete with wonderful gadgets and skilled professionals, presents many risks to the child" (Kinney, 1992, p. xi). Hazards of instrumentation can be disastrous; adverse sequelae from nutritional support occur frequently; susceptibility to nosocomial infections is of particular concern; intubation and mechanical ventilation pose particular threats; and little is known about the psychological hazards of this technological environment (Kinney, 1992). Technological innovations have brought improved surveillance techniques which in turn have improved the nurse's response time to changes in the child's condition; however, these machines, monitors, and instruments can malfunction and lead to injury. Therapeutic options have become increasingly sophisticated, and many children that a few years ago would have died are now surviving; however, some children emerge impaired, requiring long-term community support for ongoing survival. Pediatric critical care nursing has thus become a rich practice area for litigation.

Education provided for nurses to obtain the skill to care for a child in the critical care setting is often piecemeal and learned at the bedside from a variety of books and journals (Hazinski, 1992). Risk managers, administrators, and nurses may fail to update protocols used in the critical care setting, and individual nurses may fail to maintain their expertise with ongoing classes, inservices, and other training. This may lead to poor outcomes for patients.

As the medical and nursing care of children in the intensive care setting becomes more complex, "the role of the sensitive and compassionate nurse becomes more essential" (Hazinski, 1992, p. xiii). Although technology can increase the efficiency of care or the precision of the delivery of care, it cannot take the place of astute observations, skilled interventions, and personal warmth provided by a competent, compassionate, pediatric, critical care nurse (Hazinski, 1992).

This chapter presents four cases describing care given in pediatric critical care settings that led to the demise or impaired outcome of the child and ultimate litigation. In each instance, the nurse caring for the child failed to make the valuable assessments and interventions needed to provide safe, competent care. Any nurse caring for a seriously ill or injured child must be prepared to modify assessment skills and intervention techniques, so that the child's individual needs are met. This requires expertise, experience, knowledge, compassion, and astute observational skills on the part of the nurse.

Case 1

Facts

On March 5, Michael, an eight-year-old male, arrived at a city hospital via ambulance after being hit by a car while walking home from school. The driver of the car was drunk and driving at an unknown speed. The car ran up on the curb and hit Michael.

Upon arrival on the scene, the paramedics provided stabilization treatment and intubated Michael after bag and mask ventilation with an adult-size ambu bag. Upon arrival at the emergency room (ER), bilateral tension pneumothoraces were diagnosed and chest tubes placed. Two rib fractures were noted on the left side. A cervical collar remained in place until X rays were obtained later that day to rule out cervicle spine fractures.

After stabilization in the ER, Michael was admitted to the Pediatric Intensive Care Unit (PICU) for ongoing trauma care. Because of the multiple trauma from this incident, he had bilateral chest tubes, was intubated, both arms and his left leg were fractured, and he was responding only to painful stimuli, having sustained a closed head injury.

Michael was volume-ventilated throughout the night and most of the next day. Late in the afternoon, a chest X ray was obtained to assess the status of the tension pneumothoraces. The reading of the chest X ray indicated a resolution bilaterally, and his physician wrote an order to place Michael's chest tubes to water seal in preparation for removal later that evening or the next day. Nurse Rich transcribed the order and proceeded to place the chest tubes to water seal. Unfamiliar with the Pleura-vac system, she removed the outlet tube from wall suction and crimped the tube over on itself, covered it with a 4 × 4, and secured it with a rubber band. Approximately one hour and thirty minutes later, Michael's cardio/respiratory alarm sounded. This summoned Nurse Rich to his bedside. The high pressure alarm on the ventilator was alarming. Michael's heart rate was 30. Nurse Rich immediately summoned help and began CPR. The pediatric intensivist arrived in approximately three minutes, assessed the patient, followed the chest tube to the Pleura-vac setup and discovered the crimped outlet tube which was supposed to be open to air. He immediately removed the rubber band and 4 × 4 and hooked the tubing back to wall suction. Meanwhile, the response team had arrived; bagging and cardiac massage continued. A STAT chest film was taken and revealed extensive bilateral pneumothoraces as well as cardiac tamponade. After twenty minutes of intensive effort and multiple drugs, Michael was pronounced dead.

Outcome

This case resulted in pediatric death.

Legal

The case was settled out of court for an undisclosed amount.

Case Commentary

Undesirable Patient Outcome

Assessment Nurse Rich failed to assess Michael after the changes to his chest tube setup prior to his arrest. She documented the changes made to the Pleura-vac system as "chest tube placed to water seal" along with a set of vital signs and the present ventilator settings. At the time that Nurse Rich placed Michael's chest tubes to water seal, she documented his status as "stable."

Diagnosis Several nursing diagnoses were formulated for this child at the time of admission. These included:

Impaired Gas Exchange related to decreased aeration of lungs secondary to bilateral pneumothoraces and rib fractures
Altered Nutrition: Less than Body Requirements related to NPO status
Pain related to multiple abrasions, fractures, and contusions
Altered Family Processes related to unexpected hospitalization secondary to trauma
Anxiety related to unfamiliar surroundings and personnel

Planning The plan of care was developed after initial assessment and was not updated after that time. No new diagnosis was made once Michael's chest tubes were changed to "water seal."

Implementation No interventions were performed after the chest tubes were placed on "water seal." Nurse Rich did not change the existing interventions to identify problems from placing a child's chest tubes on "water seal" while the child continued to be volume ventilated.

Evaluation No evaluation was made of the child's condition after Michael's chest tubes were changed to "water seal."

Desirable Patient Outcome

Assessment The most important nursing responsibility in the care of the child receiving mechanical ventilation is the assessment of the adequacy of the ventilatory support. Whenever a change in ventilatory variables (i.e., changes in chest tube from suction to water seal) is made, frequent reassessment of the patient is necessary to determine his or her responses to the change (Hazinski, 1992). The nurse should ask the following questions (Hazinski, 1992):

- Is the child fighting the ventilator?
- Are there any changes in the vital signs now that a change has been made?
- Is the child's color and perfusion acceptable?
- Is the chest rising symmetrically with each cycle?
- Are the breath sounds equal and adequate bilaterally?
- Is the child's level of consciousness appropriate for his condition?

Once Nurse Rich changed the setup, she failed to document any assessment of Michael's condition until the time of his arrest. According to standards and institution protocols, changing the chest tubes to water seal would warrant a need for closer observation and assessment over the next few hours, to determine if any reaccumulation of air occurred (ANA 1983, 1991).

The more critical issue was the nurse's lack of knowledge concerning chest tube setup and management. Nurse Rich did not identify her own lack of knowledge related to the Pleura-vac and how to change the patient's tubing from suction to water seal. She also did not do appropriate follow-up assessments of the patient once the switch from suction to water seal occurred. Inappropriate nurse monitoring put Michael in great danger of reaccumulation of tension pneumothoraces and cardiac tamponade.

Diagnosis Appropriate nursing diagnoses did exist for the care of this child; however, no new diagnoses were developed with the change in chest tube setup. Nurse Rich should have developed a new diagnosis of *Risk for Injury.* A child receiving mechanical ventilation is at a greater risk for developing pneumothoraces, particularly when the chest tube is malfunctioning. In this instance, the malfunction occurred because the water seal setup was inappropriately carried out (i.e., Nurse Rich occluded the exit site for water seal).

Planning Nurse Rich did not develop a plan for increased surveillance of this child with the change in chest tube setup nor was she knowledgeable about the chest tube setup and policies and procedures related to the maintenance of chest tubes. Despite her lack of knowledge about chest tubes, she could have consulted other expert staff to assist her in properly setting up the system. Although Nurse Rich did have a policy available to her, she did not consult the policy when changing the system from suction to water seal. Failure to consult expert colleagues and policies is in direct violation of the standards of clinical practice (ANA, 1985, 1991).

Implementation Nurse Rich's failure to increase her surveillance of Michael's condition violated the institution's policies and procedures. Nurse Rich's lack of consultation with colleagues and failure to follow institutional policies led to the unfortunate death of this child (ANA, 1985, 1991).

Evaluation Nurse Rich's failure to perform ongoing evaluation of each step of the nursing process led to this unfortunate outcome and was in direct violation of standards for clinical practice (ANA, 1991). Evaluation must be systematic and ongoing.

In summary, the complications related to Michael's death began when he was resuscitated with inappropriate equipment by the paramedics (i.e., use of an adult ambu bag). This incident led to bilateral tension pneumothoraces. However, this complication was reversed in the next few hours. The tragedy of this situation lies with the incompetent care given by Nurse Rich which contributed to the overall deterioration and death of this child. She had the support of colleagues with a greater knowledge base, as well as hospital policies and procedures, but chose not to seek their consultation.

Case 2

Facts

Terry, a six-month-old male, was admitted to the PICU secondary to nonaccidental trauma inflicted by a babysitter. Terry had been with this babysitter for only one week. The story the babysitter told was that Terry was in his walker and fell down the stairs. On CAT scan, Terry was found to have a subdural hematoma, believed to be secondary to head trauma. No skull fracture was present. Terry was admitted to the PICU for ongoing care of the subdural hematoma that included: placement of a ventriculostomy, intubation and mechanical ventilation, and placement of a femoral central venous line (CVP) to administer and monitor fluids. Terry's mother was devastated and became teary several times during the first day of hospitalization, stating, "If only I had not gone back to work, this would never have happened."

On the third night after admission, Nurse Lucas noted that Terry's left leg (the leg with the central line) was swollen and had decreased capillary refill. She mentioned these findings to the resident when he came in on rounds, and was instructed to place a "hot pack" on the leg to increase perfusion. Nurse Lucas prepared the "hot pack" by saturating a diaper with water and putting it in the microwave for one minute to heat. She then placed the diaper directly on the leg. When checking the leg 45 minutes later, she found a large fluid-filled blister on the leg and one on the dorsal surface of the foot. She called the physician, who instructed her to remove the "hot pack" and said he would look at the leg when he came through on rounds. Two hours later, the physician arrived in the unit, and ordered Bacitracin to be applied to the blister and a dermatology consult to rule out staph bullous.

Dermatology arrived the next day at 1000 for consult. In reviewing the chart, the dermatologist noted Nurse Lucas's documentation of the placement of a "hot pack" and asked if anyone knew how this "hot pack" was applied. The nurse caring for the child told the physician that the nurse had prepared a diaper with hot water and wrapped the leg for approximately 45 minutes. Finding no other fluid-filled lesions, the dermatologist ruled out staph bullous and asked for a surgical consult for burn management. He told the mother he was not sure of the origin of the lesions, but felt that they would be best treated "like a burn" with Silvadene cream applied twice a day with dressing changes.

Surgeons arrived in the unit one hour later and, after assessing the foot and leg, debrided the burns and ordered dressing changes with Silvadene cream. Over the next few days, burn dressings were applied and a dark eschar formed on the dorsal aspect of the foot and leg. In the meantime, Terry's condition had improved dramatically and he was extubated and on nasogastric feedings of Pediasure. A transport to the local children's hospital for ongoing rehabilitation was ordered.

Terry's nurses at the children's hospital quizzed his mother about the "burns" on his leg. She told them that the physicians were unsure what caused them and ordered dressing changes, which nurses were still doing. A surgeon assessed the child and told his mother that the burns needed debridement and skin grafting under general anesthesia. This procedure was performed and the wounds healed with scarring.

Outcome

Terry sustained a full-thickness burn with resultant grafting and scarring.

Legal

This case was settled out of court for an undisclosed amount.

Case Commentary

Undesirable Patient Outcome

Assessment Nurse Lucas assessed the leg, determined the change in size and color, and attributed these findings to altered perfusion rather than the obvious reason, infiltration. Based on this assessment, she summoned physician assessment and orders.

Diagnosis The following diagnoses were developed on admission to the unit:

Altered Tissue Perfusion: Cerebral
Altered Nutrition: Less than Body Requirements related to NPO status

Anxiety, maternal, related to child's injury
Impaired Gas Exchange related to requirement for mechanical ventilation

Planning Inadequate assessment of the rationale for the signs and symptoms of infiltration led to a failure to develop a nursing diagnosis identifying the problem. No plan of care based on assessment data and nursing diagnosis was established to direct nursing interventions.

Intervention The child's lesions were not assessed or treated by a staff physician until the following morning. It was at that time that the physician began to question the nurse on duty about the "hot packs." The dermatologists were under the impression that they were to assess the child for rule out staph bullous. They determined a cause of the lesions after reading the documentation by Nurse Lucas. Although nursing interventions were related to care of a burn, no one communicated the source or causation of the burns to the mother.

Evaluation Lack of ongoing evaluation of burn management occurred and resulted in skin grafts for this child. Nurses performed dressing changes as ordered but failed to do ongoing evaluation of this treatment. This ultimately resulted in a need for skin grafting. Nurse Lucas failed to realize that her intervention resulted in the iatrogenic burns this child experienced.

Desired Patient Outcome

Assessment In gathering information about a patient's condition, the professional nurse is not only responsible for assessment of clinical conditions but also for interpretation of these findings (ANA, 1991). Complete nursing assessment of a child with a femoral central line must include: (a) clinical manifestations, (b) placement and ongoing condition of the site and extremity, and (c) ongoing assessment of skin integrity. Recognizing the significance of the leg swelling and color change, the nurse should have been suspicious of infiltration or leakage in the line and utilized the nursing process to formulate a plan of care (ANA, 1991).

Diagnosis Because the nurse failed to recognize the problem of infiltration, no diagnosis was formulated that directed nursing actions for this problem. Instead, the nurse sought physician advice and was directed to place a hot pack, which further compromised skin integrity of the site and heated the fluid which had accumulated under the skin (Hagedorn & Yucha, 1994). Appropriate diagnoses might have included:

Impaired Skin Integrity related to placement of a central line
Risk for Infection related to placement of a central line

Planning The nursing care plan did not include the need for surveillance of an extremity where a central line was placed. Nurse Lucas failed to develop interventions that addressed the ongoing monitoring of the IV site and inaccurately diagnosed the swelling in the extremity as a perfusion issue. If she had identified the swelling early and treated this with discontinuance of the line and elevation, these iatrogenic outcomes may never have occurred.

Implementation Once the extremity swelling was detected, Nurse Lucas should have consulted the physician regarding potential discontinuance of the line rather than an order to "hot pack" the extremity. Central lines at the femoral site should be temporarily placed and monitored closely for signs of infiltration (e.g., swelling, changes in color or temperature of extremity, and irritability/pain expressed by child). A femoral catheter placement carries with it a higher incidence of infection (secondary to fecal contamination), dislodgment and infiltration (secondary to the dampness of the area), and embolism (secondary to impeded blood flow to the extremity) (Hazinski, 1992). Nursing interventions must be directed at identification and management of these complications. Application of heat to an already compromised extremity increases the metabolic demands of the surrounding tissues, thereby increasing the incidence of tissue necrosis (Rudolph & Larson, 1987). As in this case, heat actually raises the temperature of the fluid trapped under the skin and ultimately leads to blistering burns that often slough leaving eschar (Brown, Hoelzer, & Piercy, 1979; Hagedorn & Yucha, 1994).

Furthermore, Nurse Lucas failed to recognize that her interventions for extremity swelling led to the iatrogenic burns this child experienced. The child, who was intubated, was unable to express his pain verbally. This made it even more critical that Nurse Lucas perform ongoing assessments of this extremity for altered integrity. By failing to assume responsibility and accountability for individual nursing judgments and actions, Nurse Lucas delayed treatment of these burns and violated the standard of care (ANA, 1985). Nurse Lucas had the responsibility to identify the ineffectiveness and potential danger of hot-packing an infiltration. Nurses are accountable for judgments made and actions taken. "Neither physician's orders nor the employing agency's policies relieve the nurse of accountability for actions taken and judgments made" (ANA, 1985, p. 9).

Finally, the complete information surrounding this child's burns was never disclosed to the mother until the child's arrival at another institution. The nurse had an ethical duty to inform the mother of the cause of these burns and the resultant treatment. Nurses must participate in the "profession's effort to protect the public from misinformation and misrepresentation" to maintain high quality nursing care (ANA, 1985, p. 1).

Evaluation A proactive approach to an ongoing, skilled evaluation, at every step of the nursing process, might have altered the issues surrounding the detection and treatment of this line infiltration. Inadequate independent nursing judgment actually led to the sequelae present in this child. Failure to disclose information to the mother is an example of breach of practice standards on the part of nursing (ANA, 1991) and medicine. Many litigations result from the lack of disclosure of information which is later detected when a parent seeks specialized care for the child or reads the contents of the hospital chart while transporting the child to a clinic or office visit (see Chapter 4).

Case 3

Facts

Tony, a 15-month-old, was admitted to the PICU with the diagnosis of near drowning. Earlier in the day, Tony's mother was scrubbing the kitchen floor with Pinesol and was distracted by a phone call. When she returned to the kitchen, she found Tony immersed in the pail of water. She immediately summoned the paramedics who stabilized, intubated, and transported the child to the local city hospital. Tony was mechanically ventilated and treated with prophylactic antibiotics to avoid secondary infection.

On Tony's third day of hospitalization, Nurse Hammond was doing her routine assessment and documentation of ventilator settings. When checking the thermometer at the mouthpiece of the endotracheal (ET) tube, she noted the temperature to be 39.5 degrees C. Perplexed by the fact that the temperature sensor failed to alarm for this temperature, she paged the respiratory therapist to check the ventilator. At the same time, she noted a reddened area on Tony's cheek under the path of the ventilator tubing. She placed a washcloth between the skin and the ventilator tubing.

The respiratory therapist arrived in a few minutes and validated her findings. He told her that this was a new ventilator with complex software and that he too was concerned that the ventilator had not alarmed with this high temperature. After examining the ventilator, he told Nurse Hammond that someone had diverted the temperature sensor alarm and that he wanted to check with his colleagues to determine the rationale for these actions. He returned in 30 minutes with another ventilator and switched the patient. He took the ventilator with him stating, "I'll have to have my boss look at this."

When the physicians came in on rounds, Nurse Hammond asked them to check the child's cheek. Upon exam, they determined that the child had a second degree burn and ordered burn care to the cheek.

Two days later, Dr. Nott, the chief of pulmonary medicine, came to the unit and questioned Nurse Hammond about the incidents surrounding Tony's burn on his cheek. He confided that the ventilator was found to be malfunctioning and the heat sensor was inadvertently bypassed to remedy a faulty heat sensing alarm. He assured her that the ventilator would be returned to the manufacturer for servicing.

Outcome

Tony sustained a full-thickness burn requiring treatment.

Legal

This case was settled out of court for an undisclosed amount. The suit was directed at the respiratory personnel who diverted the heat sensor.

Case Commentary

Undesirable Patient Outcome

Assessment Nurse Hammond detected a potential malfunction of the ventilator during routine assessment of her patient. She was uncertain why this malfunction was occurring, but summoned assistance from a respiratory therapist to determine the cause for the high-temperature reading.

Diagnosis The following diagnoses were developed on Tony's admission to the unit:

Impaired Gas Exchange related to iatrogenic lung damage secondary to immersion into pail of cleaning solution
Altered Nutrition: Less than Body Requirements related to NPO status
Ineffective Family Coping related to incidents surrounding near drowning

Planning A plan was developed addressing the above diagnoses. Interventions were specific and updated daily.

Implementation Immediately after discovering the high temperature within the ventilator tubing, Nurse Hammond summoned the assistance of a respiratory therapist. When she identified the red cheek, she buffered the child's skin from further contact with the overheated tubing.

Evaluation Even after the incident, Nurse Hammond followed up on the incident by speaking with the chief of the pulmonary department.

Desirable Patient Outcome

Assessment When providing care that involves the use of technological equipment (e.g., mechanical ventilation) the nurse has a responsibility to assess the function of this equipment with each assessment she makes of the patient. This assessment is performed to determine any problems or malfunctioning of the equipment. When determining the significance of data assessed, the nurse is responsible for consulting with appropriate personnel to alleviate the problem identified. Nurse Hammond followed the appropriate chain of command in reporting the malfunction of the ventilator.

Diagnosis Another diagnosis pertinent to this child's care included:

Risk for Impaired Skin Integrity related to placement and securing of ET and NG tubes

Planning A plan of care was inclusive of the key problems but failed to include a diagnosis for skin integrity that would have guided other nurses in assessing the ongoing condition of the child's skin, particularly around the ET tube.

Implementation Nurse Hammond appropriately managed the situation and sought appropriate personnel for input.

Evaluation Nurse Hammond's timely identification and implementation of interventions prevented further sequelae for this child. When collaborating with other health care providers (in this instance, respiratory therapy) the nurse must coordinate and continually assess the effect of treatment provided by these personnel for safeguarding the patient (ANA, 1985).

Despite the fact that Nurse Hammond was asked to provide testimony in the form of a deposition for this case, she served as a fact witness rather than a defendant. The respiratory therapist who altered the equipment and the hospital as his employer assumed full liability for this patient's injury/harm. The manufacturer was excluded as a defendant because the equipment had been altered rather than serviced as directed by the manufacturer (FDA, 1987; HIMA, 1984) (see Chapter 4).

Case 4

Facts

On November 13, 2-year-old Nelson Little was admitted to the local children's hospital for repair of his mitral stenosis and ventricular septal defect. As an infant, he had his patent ductus arteriosus and coarctation of the aorta repaired. Nelson had hypoplastic left heart variant and pulmonary hypertension. His oral intake was supplemented by gastrostomy feedings and his daily medications included: Lanoxin (digoxin), Lasix (furosemide) Kaochlor, Gantrisin, benzothiazide sulfisoxazole, and 1–5 L of oxygen.

After tolerating the surgical procedure well, Nelson was admitted in stable condition to the PICU with bilateral chest tubes and a mediastinal tube, and on volume ventilation. On the night shift of November 14/15, Nelson spiked a temperature to 38.5 C rectally, and was placed on a cooling blanket. Tracheal aspirate revealed gram negative diplococcus. Antibiotics were started. On November 15, the ventilator was gradually weaned with special caution to avoid hypercapnia ($>PaCO_2$), and hypoxia ($<PaO_2$) because of the child's pulmonary hypertension. After excellent arterial blood gases, extubation was accomplished in the evening of November 15. No increased respiratory distress occurred, and Nelson continued to have adequate blood gases and continued on 1 L of oxygen per nasal cannula. On November 16, Nipride, nitroprusside, and Dopamine were slowly weaned. On November 17, Nelson's oral diet was advanced though he remained febrile with slight pulmonary edema validated on chest X ray.

On November 18, during routine monitoring of electrolyte status at 0200, Nurse Downs discovered a potassium level of 2.9 meq/L. From 0300 to 0600 she administered three doses of potassium phosphate 3 meq IV, each over one-hour intervals. At 0545, repeat electrolyte values were obtained and the potassium level was 3.5 meq/L and the calcium level was 3.9 meq/L. At approximately 0615, Nurse Downs began administering 1.25 mL of 100 mg/mL calcium chloride solution. At 0635, Nurse Downs documented: "Nurse at the bedside, pushing a small amount (0.3 mL) of calcium chloride, when the child took a deep sigh, and stopped breathing. Heart rate was 80 beats per minute."

The pediatric resuscitation sheet timed the above events at 0630, and cardiac massage began at 0635. The ongoing resuscitation was documented as follows:

0637: Intubated and bagged with 100% oxygen. Meds: atropine, sodium bicarbonate.
0638: Meds: epinephrine.
0640: Heart rate (HR) 94.
0645: HR 69, atropine repeated.
0646: External pacemaker attached and heart was paced at a rate of 129. No measurable blood pressure was obtained.
0647: HR 118 with pacer not capturing. Sodium bicarbonate repeated.
0648: Epinephrine repeated.
0650: BP 50/29, HR 111.
0651: BP 32/24, HR 108.
0652: Chest opened, and open cardiac massage started. BP 25/14, HR 185. Since the heart was at a complete standstill, it was defibrillated × 2 and more medications administered.
0653: BP 77/32, HR 104.
0705: Idioventricular rhythm established and compressions stopped.
0715: After placement of a left femoral central line and an aortic arterial line through the open chest wound, the child was taken to the operating room for chest closure.

Outcome

Nelson suffered hypoxic encephalopathy with persistent vegetative state.

Legal

This case is currently under litigation.

Case Commentary

Undesirable Patient Outcome

Assessment Nurse Downs correctly interpreted the child's laboratory values as hypocalcemia and hypokalemia.

Diagnosis No nursing diagnoses were documented on the patient's record.

Planning Nurse Downs correctly calculated the amount of replacement potassium and calcium for this 12.5 kg child.

Implementation Through the central venous catheter placed in the internal jugular vein, potassium phosphate was administered for three hours via a buretrol system. At 0615, Nurse Downs began to administer calcium chloride in 0.1 mL bolus increments via "slow push" from a 3 mL syringe and needle inserted in the IV port.

Evaluation While Nurse Downs was "pushing" calcium chloride (0.3 mL) or the third of three 0.1 mL boluses, the child had a cardiopulmonary arrest requiring extensive resuscitation for 45 minutes.

Desirable Patient Outcome

Assessment The *Standards of Maternal-Child Health Nursing Practice* (ANA, 1983) and the *Standards of Clinical Nursing Practice* (ANA, 1991) require the professional nurse to collect data using appropriate nursing techniques. Nurse Downs appropriately assessed and interpreted the laboratory values of her patient as hypocalcemia and hypokalemia requiring replacement therapy.

Diagnosis Nursing diagnoses are derived from assessment data (ANA 1983, 1991) and identify "actual and potential hazards to the maintenance of health" (ANA, 1983, p. 14). Appropriate nursing diagnoses for this child should have included:

> ***Risk for Injury*** related to muscle weakness and dysrhythmias secondary to hypocalcemia and hypokalemia

Upon making the decision to administer electrolyte replacement, an additional nursing diagnosis should have been formulated:

> ***Risk for Impaired Tissue Integrity*** related to intravenous infusion of potassium and calcium

Planning "The nurse develops a plan of care that prescribes interventions to attain expected outcomes" (ANA, 1991, p. 10). "Formulating a plan of care for risk management of vulnerable clients" (ANA, 1983, p. 13), Nurse Downs should have planned to administer intravenous electrolytes safely according to the hospital protocol.

Implementation Interventions identified in the plan of care must be "implemented in a safe and appropriate manner" (ANA, 1991, p. 11). In order to "promote an environment free of hazards" (ANA, 1983, p. 14), the registered nurse must: (a) "administer preventative measures according to protocols" (ANA, 1983, p. 14), and (b) "intervene to minimize or eliminate environmental hazards to the client" (ANA, 1983, p. 14).

Nurse Downs violated the hospital's eight-page protocol for safe administration of electrolyte boluses in nonemergent situations. The protocol required RNs to: (a) administer through a central line; (b) filter solution; (c) place patient on cardiac monitor; (d) deliver bolus over one hour (*Do not push*), by calculating volume to be given per hour: total volume/hour = mL of medication and dilutant; (e) place calculated hourly volume in a syringe with extension tubing and filter, prime the system, and label and place on syringe pump "to be delivered in one hour"; and (f) monitor for ECG changes (bradycardia, AV block, asystole, cardiac arrest, and ventricular fibrillation), changes in vital signs or insertion site, altered neurologic status, anuria/oliguria, and proper delivery by pump.

Evaluation The nurse is required to evaluate a patient's response to interventions for effectiveness and progress toward stated goals (ANA 1983, 1991). In her deposition five years after this incident occurred, Nurse Downs stated that "she still administers electrolytes without using the hospital protocol." The institutional purpose in promulgating the protocol is to ensure safe administration of electrolytes. Nurse Downs violated and continues to violate the standard of care by administering replacement electrolyte solutions in direct violation of the hospital's procedure/protocol (i.e., she continues to give undiluted electrolyte solutions by her "slow push" manual method). The competent nurse needs to know that concentrated electrolyte solutions have direct action on muscle contractility (i.e., cardiac contractility), renal function, and central nervous system function, and are quite caustic to tissue if infiltrated (ANA, 1985).

The hospital protocol provided a drug table for calcium, potassium, and magnesium. The drug-interactions column on the calcium table specifically cited calcium's incompatibility with sodium bicarbonate and phosphate. Calcium precipitates as a crystal in the presence of phosphates, carbonates, sulfates, and tartrates (Lehne, 1994). In addition, calcium precipitates in an alkaline medium and is never added to intravenous fluids with an alkaline pH (Corbett, 1987). Since Nurse Downs administered the potassium phosphate for three hours through the IV setup and tubing (instead of through the medication port of the IV tubing with a syringe pump), she effectively contaminated the entire IV setup and line with an alkaline solution (with the phosphate). Upon administration of the calcium chloride (again *undiluted* and without a syringe pump as the protocol required) into the alkalinized line, the calcium chloride and potassium phosphate formed a precipitate in the line and ultimately resulted in this child's cardiac arrest (Lehne, 1994). Since the central line was the child's only IV access, calcium chloride, potassium phosphate, and the precipitate were still in the intravenous line interacting with the drugs used to resuscitate the child.

Deviation from the protocol is incompetent practice and resulted in Nurse Downs assuming (through legal liability) the responsibility and accountability for her nursing judgment and actions (ANA, 1985). Institutional liability insurance covers "the nurse employee for acts that are within the scope of employment" (TAANA, 1989, p. 4). Clinical nursing practice that deviates from institutional policy and constitutes actions not authorized by the institution may not be covered by the institution's insurance. Although this institution is legally defending Nurse Downs, since her actions deviated from the institution's written policy and procedure, she might have found herself in the position of having to access and pay for her own legal defense. Lastly, because Nurse Downs stated in her deposition that she continues this negligent approach to administering supplemental intravenous electrolytes, she is accountable to the state board of nursing for these actions.

References

American Nurses Association. (1983). *Standards of maternal-child nursing practice.* Washington, D.C.: Author.

American Nurses Association. (1985). *Code for nurses with interpretive statements.* Washington, D.C.: Author.

American Nurses Association. (1991). *Standards of clinical practice.* Washington, D.C.: Author.

Brown, A., Hoelzer, D., & Piercy, S. (1979). Skin necrosis from extravasation of intravenous fluid in children. *Plastic Reconstructive Surgery, 64,* 145–150.

Corbett, J. (1987). *Laboratory tests and diagnostic procedures with nursing diagnosis* (2nd ed.). Norwalk, CT: Appleton Lange.

Food and Drug Administration. (1987). *Compliance policy guidelines: Devices.* Washington, D.C.: Author.

Hagedorn, M. & Yucha, C. (1994). *IV extravasations in pediatrics: A self-instruction module.* Denver, CO: Author.

Hazinski, M. (1992). *Nursing care of the critically ill child* (2nd ed.). St. Louis: Mosby-Yearbook.

Health Industry Manufacturer's Association. (1984). *The reuse of single-use medical devices.* Washington, D.C.: Author.

Kinney, M. (1992). Foreword. In M. Hazinski (Ed.), *Nursing care of the critically ill child* (2nd ed.). St. Louis: Mosby-Yearbook.

Lehne, R. (1994). *Pharmacology for nursing care* (2nd ed.). Philadelphia: Saunders.

Rudolph, R. & Larson, D. (1987). *Etiology and treatment of chemotherapeutic agent extravasation injuries: A review. Journal of Clinical Oncology, 5,* 1116–1126.

The American Association for Nurse Attorneys, Inc. (1989). *Demonstrating financial responsibility for nursing practice.* Baltimore, MD: Author.

Appendix A
NANDA Nursing Diagnoses

North American Nursing Diagnosis Association, 1995/1996

Activity Intolerance
Activity Intolerance, Risk for
Adaptive Capacity: Intracranial, Decreased
Adjustment, Impaired
Airway Clearance, Ineffective
Anxiety
Aspiration, Risk for

Body Image Disturbance
Body Temperature, Risk for Altered
Breastfeeding, Effective
Breastfeeding, Ineffective
Breastfeeding, Interrupted
Breathing Pattern, Ineffective

Caregiver Role Strain
Caregiver Role Strain, Risk for
Communication, Impaired Verbal
Community Coping, Potential for Enhanced
Confusion, Acute
Confusion, Chronic
Constipation
Constipation, Colonic
Constipation, Perceived

Decisional Conflict (Specify)
Decreased Cardiac Output
Defensive Coping
Denial, Ineffective
Diarrhea
Disorganized Infant Behavior
Disorganized Infant Behavior, Risk for
Disuse Syndrome, Risk for
Diversional Activity Deficit
Dysfunctional Grieving
Dysfunctional Ventilatory Weaning Response
Dysreflexia

Energy Field Disturbance
Environmental Interpretation Syndrome, Impaired

Family Coping: Compromised, Ineffective
Family Coping: Disabling, Ineffective
Family Coping: Potential for Growth
Family Process: Alcoholism, Altered
Family Processes, Altered
Fatigue
Fear
Fluid Volume Deficit
Fluid Volume Deficit, Risk for
Fluid Volume Excess

Gas Exchange, Impaired
Grieving, Anticipatory
Grieving, Dysfunctional
Growth and Development, Altered

Health Maintenance, Altered
Health-Seeking Behaviors (Specify)
Home Maintenance Management, Impaired
Hopelessness
Hyperthermia
Hypothermia

Incontinence, Bowel
Incontinence, Functional
Incontinence, Reflex
Incontinence, Stress
Incontinence, Total
Incontinence, Urge
Infant Feeding Pattern, Ineffective
Infection, Risk for
Injury, Risk for

Knowledge Deficit (Specify)

Loneliness, Risk for

Management of Therapeutic Regimen: Community, Ineffective
Management of Therapeutic Regimen: Families, Ineffective
Management of Therapeutic Regimen: Individual, Effective
Management of Therapeutic Regimen: (Individuals), Ineffective
Memory, Impaired

Noncompliance (Specify)
Nutrition: Less than Body Requirements, Altered
Nutrition: More than Body Requirements, Altered
Nutrition: Potential for More than Body Requirements, Altered

Oral Mucous Membrane, Altered
Organized Infant Behavior, Potential for Enhanced

Pain
Pain, Chronic
Parent/Infant/Child Attachment, Risk for Altered
Parental Role Conflict
Parenting, Altered
Parenting, Risk for Altered
Perioperative Positioning Injury, Risk for
Peripheral Neurovascular Dysfunction, Risk for
Personal Identity Disturbance
Physical Mobility, Impaired
Poisoning, Risk for
Post-Trauma Response
Powerlessness
Protection, Altered

Rape-Trauma Syndrome
Rape-Trauma Syndrome: Compound Reaction
Rape-Trauma Syndrome: Silent Reaction

Relocation Stress Syndrome
Role Performance, Altered

Self-Care Deficit
- Bathing/Hygiene
- Feeding
- Dresssing/Grooming
- Toileting

Self Esteem, Chronic Low
Self Esteem, Situational Low
Self Esteem Disturbance
Self-Mutilation, Risk for
Sensory/Perceptual Alterations (Specify) (visual, auditory, kinesthetic, gustatory, tactile, olfactory)
Sexual Dysfunction
Sexuality Patterns, Altered
Skin Integrity, Impaired
Skin Integrity, Risk for Impaired
Sleep Pattern Disturbance
Social Interaction, Impaired
Social Isolation
Spiritual Distress
Spiritual Well-Being, Potential for Enhanced
Suffocation, Risk for
Sustain Spontaneous Ventilation, Inability to
Swallowing, Impaired

Thermoregulation, Ineffective
Thought Processes, Altered
Tissue Integrity, Impaired
Tissue Perfusion, Altered (Specify Type) (renal, cerebral, cardiopulmonary, gastrointestinal, peripheral)
Trauma, High Risk for

Unilateral Neglect
Urinary Elimination, Altered
Urinary Retention

Violence, High Risk for: Self-Directed or Directed at Others

Appendix B
Professional Nursing Organizations

American Nurses Association (ANA)
600 Maryland Avenue SW
Suite 100 West
Washington, DC 20024-2571
(202) 651-7000

Association of Women's Health, Obstetrics, and Neonatal Nurses (AWHONN)
700 14th Street NW
Suite 600
Washington, D.C. 20005
(800) 673-8499

National Association of Neonatal Nurses (NANN)
1304 Southpoint Boulevard
Suite 280
Petaluma, CA 94954-6859
(800) 451-3795

National Association of Pediatric Nurse Associates and Practitioners (NAPNAP)
1101 Kings Highway North
Suite 206
Cherry Hill, NJ 08034
(609) 667-1773

American College of Nurse Midwives (ACNM)
818 Connecticut Avenue NW
Suite 900
Washington, DC 20006
(202) 728-9860

Appendix C

Antepartal, Intrapartal, and Postpartal High-Risk Factors

Antepartal High-Risk Factors

Factor	Maternal Implication	Fetal/Neonatal Implication
Social-Personal		
Low income level and/or low education level	Poor antenatal care Poor nutrition ↑ risk of preeclampsia	Low birth weight Intrauterine growth retardation (IUGR)
Poor diet	Inadequate nutrition ↑ risk anemia ↑ risk preeclampsia	Fetal malnutrition Prematurity
Living at high altitude	↑ hemoglobin	Prematurity IUGR
Multiparity >3	↑ risk antepartum/postpartum hemorrhage	Anemia Fetal death
Weight < 45.5 kg (100 lb)	Poor nutrition Cephalopelvic disproportion Prolonged labor	IUGR Hypoxia associated with difficult labor and birth
Weight >91 kg (200 lb)	↑ risk hypertension ↑ risk cephalopelvic disproportion	↓ fetal nutrition
Age <16	Poor nutrition Poor antenatal care ↑ risk preeclampsia ↑ risk cephalopelvic disproportion	Low birth weight ↑ fetal demise
Age >35	↑ risk preeclampsia ↑ risk cesarean birth	↑ risk congenital anomalies ↑ chromosomal aberrations
Smoking one pack/day or more	↑ risk hypertension ↑ risk cancer	↓ placental perfusion → ↓ O_2 and nutrients available Low birth weight IUGR Preterm birth
Use of addicting drugs	↑ risk poor nutrition ↑ risk of infection with IV drugs	↑ risk congenital anomalies ↑ risk low birth weight Neonatal withdrawal Lower serum bilirubin
Excessive alcohol consumption	↑ risk poor nutrition Possible hepatic effects with long-term consumption	↑ risk fetal alcohol syndrome

Factor	Maternal Implication	Fetal/Neonatal Implication
Preexising Medical Disorders		
Diabetes mellitus	↑ risk preeclampsia, hypertension Episodes of hypoglycemia and hyperglycemia ↑ risk cesarean birth	Low birth weight Macrosomia Neonatal hypoglycemia ↑ risk congenital anomalies ↑ risk respiratory distress syndrome
Cardiac disease	Cardiac decompensation Further strain on mother's body ↑ maternal death rate	↑ risk fetal demise ↑ perinatal mortality
Anemia: hemoglobin <9 g/dL (White) <29% hematocrit (White) <8.2 g/dL hemoglobin (Black) <26% hematocrit (Black)	Iron deficiency anemia Low energy level Decreased oxygen-carrying	Fetal death Prematurity Low birth weight
Hypertension	↑ vasospasm ↑ risk CNS irritability → convulsions ↑ risk CVA ↑ risk renal damage	↓ placental perfusion → low birth wieght Preterm birth
Thyroid disorder Hypothyroidsm	↑ infertility ↓ BMR, goiter, myxedema	↑ spontaneous abortion ↑ risk congenital goiter Mental retardation, cretinism ↑ incidence congenital anomalies
Hyperthyroidism	↑ risk postpartum hemorrhage ↑ risk preeclampsia Danger of thyroid storm	↑ incidence preterm birth ↑ tendency to thyrotoxicosis
Renal disease (moderate to severe)	↑ risk renal failure	↑ risk IUGR ↑ risk preterm birth
DES exposure	↑ infertility, spontaneous abortion ↑ cervical incompetence	↑ spontaneous abortion ↑ risk preterm birth
Obstetric Considerations		
Previous Pregnancy Stillborn	↑ emotional/psychologic distress	↑ risk IUGR ↑ risk preterm birth
Habitual abortion	↑ emotional/psychologic distress ↑ possibility diagnostic workup	↑ risk abortion
Cesarean birth	↑ possibility repeat cesarean birth	↑ risk preterm birth ↑ risk respiratory distress
Rh or blood group sensitization	↑ financial expenditure for testing	Hydrops fetalis Icterus gravis Neonatal anemia Kernicterus Hypoglycemia
Large baby	↑ risk cesarean birth ↑ risk gestational diabetes	Birth injury Hypoglycemia

Antepartal High-Risk Factors *(Continued)*

Factor	Maternal Implication	Fetal/Neonatal Implication
Current Pregnancy		
Rubella (first trimester)		Congenital heart disease Cataracts Nerve deafness Bone lesions Prolonged virus shedding
Rubella (second trimester)		Hepatitis Thrombocytopenia
Cytomegalovirus		IUGR Encephalopathy
Herpesvirus type 2	Severe discomfort Concern about possibility of fetal infection	Neonatal herpesvirus type 2 2° hepatitis with jaundice Neurologic abnormalities
Syphilis	↑ incidence abortion	↑ fetal demise Congenital syphilis
Abruptio placenta and placenta previa	↑ risk hemorrhage Bed rest Extended hospitalization	Fetal/neonatal anemia Intrauterine hemorrhage ↑ fetal demise
Preeclampsia/eclampsia (PIH)	See hypertension	↑ placental perfusion → low birth weight
Multiple gestation	↑ risk postpartum hemorrhage	↑ risk preterm birth ↑ risk fetal demise
Elevated hematocrit >41% (White) >38% (Black)	Increased viscosity of blood	Fetal death rate 5 times normal rate
Spontaneous premature rupture of membranes	↑ uterine infection	↑ risk preterm birth ↑ fetal demise

Intrapartal High-Risk Factors

Factor	Maternal Implication	Fetal/Neonatal Implication
Abnormal presentation	↑ Incidence of cesarean birth ↑ Incidence of prolonged labor ↑ Hypertension risk ↑ Nausea and vomiting	↑ Incidence of placenta previa Prematurity ↑ Risk of congenital abnormality Neonatal physical trauma ↑ Risk of intrauterine growth retardation
Multiple gestation	↑ Uterine distension ↑ risk of postpartum hemorrhage ↑ Risk of cesarean birth ↑ Risk of preterm labor	Low birth weight Prematurity ↑ Risk of congenital anomalies Feto-fetal transfusion
Hydramnios	↑ Discomfort ↑ Dyspnea ↑ Risk of preterm labor Edema of lower extremities	↑ Risk of esophageal or other high alimentary tract atresias ↑ Risk of CNS anomalies (myelocele)

Factor	Maternal Implication	Fetal/Neonatal Implication
Oligohydramnios	Maternal fear of "dry birth"	↑ Incidence of congenital anomalies ↑ Incidence of renal lesions ↑ Risk of IUGR ↑ Risk of fetal acidosis ↑ Risk of cord compression Postmaturity
Meconium staining of amniotic fluid	↑ Psychologic stress due to fear for baby	↑ Risk of fetal asphyxia ↑ Risk of meconium aspiration ↑ Risk of pneumonia due to aspiration of meconium
Premature rupture of membranes	↑ Risk of infection (chorioamnionitis) ↑ Risk of preterm labor ↑ Anxiety Fear for the baby Prolonged hospitalization ↑ Incidence of tocolytic therapy	↑ Perinatal morbidity Prematurity ↓ Birth weight ↑ Risk of respiratory distress syndrome Prolonged hospitalization
Induction of labor	↑ Risk of hypercontractility of uterus ↑ Risk of uterine rupture ↑ Length of labor if cervix not ready ↑ Anxiety	Prematurity if gestational age not assessed correctly Hypoxia if hyperstimulation occurs
Abruptio placentae, placenta previa	Hemorrhage Uterine atony	Fetal hypoxia/acidosis Fetal exsanguination ↑ Perinatal mortality
Failure to progress in labor	Maternal exhaustion ↑ Incidence of augmentation of labor ↑ Incidence of cesarean birth	Fetal hypoxia/acidosis Intracranial birth injury
Precipitous labor (<3 hours)	Perineal, vaginal, cervical lacerations ↑ Risk of PP hemorrhage	Tentorial tears
Prolapse of umbilical cord	↑ Fear for baby Cesarean birth	Acute fetal hypoxia/acidosis
Fetal heart aberrations	↑ Fear for baby ↑ Risk of cesarean birth, forceps, vacuum Continuous electronic monitoring and intervention in labor	Tachycardia, chronic asphyxic insult Bradycardia, acute asphyxic insult Chronic hypoxia Congenital heart block
Uterine rupture	Hemorrhage Cesarean birth for hysterectomy ↑ Risk of death	Fetal anoxia Fetal hemorrhage Neonatal morbidity
Postdates (>42 weeks)	↑ Anxiety ↑ Incidence of induction of labor ↑ Incidence of cesarean birth ↑ Use of technology to monitor fetus ↑ Risk of shoulder dystocia	Postmaturity syndrome ↑ Risk of fetal-neonatal mortality and morbidity ↑ Risk of antepartum fetal death ↑ Incidence/risk of large baby

Intrapartal High-Risk Factors *(Continued)*

Factor	Maternal Implication	Fetal/Neonatal Implication
Diabetes	↑ Risk of hydramnios ↑ Risk of hypoglycemia or hyperglycemia ↑ Risk of pregnancy-induced hypertension	↑ Risk of malpresentation ↑ Risk of macrosomia ↑ Risk of intrauterine growth retardation ↑ Risk of respiratory distress syndrome ↑ Risk of congenital anomalies
Pregnancy-induced hypertension	↑ Risk of seizures ↑ Risk of stroke ↑ Risk of HELLP	↑ Risk of small for gestational age baby ↑ Risk of preterm birth ↑ Risk of mortality
AIDS/STD	↑ Risk of additional infections	↑ Risk of transplacental transmission

Postpartal High-Risk Factors

Factor	Maternal Implication
PIH	↑ Blood pressure ↑ CNS irritability ↑ Need for bed rest ↑ risk thrombophlebitis
Diabetes	Need for insulin regulation Episodes of hypoglycemia or hyperglycemia ↓ Healing
Cardiac disease	↑ Maternal exhaustion
Cesarean birth	↑ Healing needs ↑ Pain from incision ↑ Risk of infection ↑ Length of hospitalization
Overdistention of uterus (multiple gestation, hydramnios)	↑ Risk of hemorrhage ↑ Risk of anemia ↑ Stretching of abdominal muscles ↑ Incidence and severity of afterpains
Abruptio placentae, placenta previa	Hemorrhage ↑ anemia ↓ Uterine contractility after birth ↑ infection risk
Precipitous labor (<3 hours)	↑ Risk of lacerations to birth canal ↑ Risk of hemorrhage
Prolonged labor (>24 hours)	Exhaustion ↑ Risk of hemorrhage Nutritional and fluid depletion ↑ Bladder atony and/or trauma
Difficult birth	Exhaustion ↑ Risk of perineal lacerations ↑ Risk of hematomas ↑ Risk of hemorrhage anemia
Extended period of time in stirrups at birth	↑ Risk of thrombophlebitis
Retained placenta	↑ Risk of hemorrhage ↑ Risk of infection

From: Olds, S., London, M., & Ladewig, P. (1996). *Maternal-newborn nursing.* 5th ed. Menlo Park, CA: Addison-Wesley Nursing. Reprinted with permission.

Index